Compendium of Histology

Anders Rehfeld • Malin Nylander
Kirstine Karnov

Compendium of Histology

A Theoretical and Practical Guide

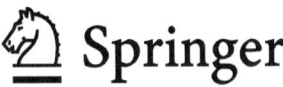 Springer

Anders Rehfeld, MD, PhD
Faculty of Health and Medical Sciences
University of Copenhagen
Copenhagen
Denmark

Kirstine Karnov, MD
Faculty of Health and Medical Sciences
University of Copenhagen
Copenhagen
Denmark

Malin Nylander, MD, PhD
Faculty of Health and Medical Sciences
University of Copenhagen
Copenhagen
Denmark

ISBN 978-3-319-41871-1   ISBN 978-3-319-41873-5   (eBook)
DOI 10.1007/978-3-319-41873-5

Library of Congress Control Number: 2017933277

Printed on acid-free paper

This Springer imprint is published by Springer Nature
The registered company is Springer International Publishing AG
The registered company address is: Gewerbestrasse 11, 6330 Cham, Switzerland

Preface

The scope of this book is to help students of medicine and biology to succeed with their histology classes and earn good grades while using less time on studying the histology curriculum.

Almost all text of this book is written in bullets and put into lists, structured tables, and diagrams, which make it quick and easy to read and understand, and gives a good overview of the curriculum. Additionally, this organization of the text makes it easy to locate specific information, such as the dimensions of cellular structures or functions of cells and tissues.

Most chapters include illustrations covering parts of the curriculum, which are otherwise difficult to interpret. Additionally, the book includes guides to practical histology, including simplified illustrations of histological specimens side by side with photomicrographs of the specimen. The guides follow the respective chapters and help the reader to distinguish between the different histological specimens and describe which characteristics distinguish one specimen from other similar specimens, which can be presented during a practical histology exam. The simplified illustration of the specimen additionally helps the student recognize the important characteristics in the microscope. Finally, the book is filled with "memo-boxes" in which parts of the curriculum are put into rhymes and acronyms.

This book is based on our top-selling Danish edition, which we wrote while teaching histology at the University of Copenhagen.

Due to our fascination of anatomy and especially histology, the three of us started to teach histology, when halfway through medical school. As we were then teachers and medical students at the same time, we had a great understanding of which parts of the curriculum were difficult and which were not. And even though none of us started out as histology experts, the experience gained through years of teaching gave us an insight of how this complex curriculum could be presented in an easy and intuitive way. It was this understanding that made us write our first Danish edition of the book.

With this new, English book, we wish to share these principles as well as our enthusiasm for histology, with students all over the world. This book covers the same curriculum as the classical textbooks, from basic tissue histology to the histology of specific organs, but in a more simple and intuitive way. It can be used as a supplement to classical full-curriculum textbooks, to lectures, or on its own—a quick, easy, and comprehensible way to learn histology, e.g., before class or when brushing up for an exam.

Nowadays, where biological curricula are growing, due to the increasing amount of knowledge gained through research, we believe that it is necessary and often helpful for the understanding to focus on the basics, as students are often overwhelmed by the enormous amounts of information presented to them in textbooks.

Since the fields of histology, cell biology, and physiology are still being explored, the literature is constantly evolving and is in some areas inconsistent. We have tried to present the most recent and the most accepted facts in this book, all in a well-organized and structured way.

The book is divided into two main parts, "histology of tissues" and "histology of organs," as we believe that the structure of the organs is easier to comprehend when first knowing the structures of the basic tissues. Different cells and tissues are described as they appear in hematoxylin and eosin staining, unless otherwise stated. We hope you will enjoy reading this book and that it will help you with your studies.

Copenhagen, Denmark   Anders Rehfeld
                                                                 Malin Nylander
                                                                 Kirstine Karnov

Acknowledgments

All authors: We would like to thank our editors at Springer, Richard Hruska and Susan Westendorf, for the guidance during the writing of this book; the team of illustrators at SPI Publisher Services, Divya Ashokan and Selvaraju Periyasamy, for the professional help with the illustrations; the production staff at SPI Publisher Services, Mr. Pradeepkumar, Project Manager and Mr. Dhanapal Palanisamy, Springer Production Co-ordinator, for their patience with typesetting the book; Katie Taylor for her valuable suggestions to improve the book; Professor Jørgen Tranum-Jensen and Associate Professor Steen Seier Poulsen of the Department of Cellular and Molecular Medicine, University of Copenhagen, for giving us permission to use photomicrographs of their unique collection of histological specimens; and lastly our editors at Munksgaard, Britta Østergaard and Lis Maaløe, for allowing us to base this book on our original Danish book.

AR: I would like to thank my family for their support during the writing of this book, especially my wife Tine and my sons August and Victor. Without your help, this would not have been possible. I would also like to thank Direktør Ib Henriksens Fond for granting me a stay in their villa in Castellaras, where a large part of the work in this book has been done. Lastly, I would like to thank my coauthors Malin and Kirstine, for embarking on this time-consuming project with me, for the second time. The sparring with you has always been encouraging.

KK: First, I would like to thankfully acknowledge my family who continuously helped me with support during the process of making this book, especially Niclas for his endless patience and understanding. Furthermore, I would like to thank the many people who have encouraged me, including my cowriters for an extraordinary teamwork.

MN: I would like to thank my dear parents for their all-time support. I would also like to thank Anders and Kirstine for an inspiring cooperation during the writing of this book.

Abbreviations

⌀	Diameter
3D	Three dimensional
ACTH	Adrenocorticotropic hormone
ADH	Antidiuretic hormone
ADP	Adenosine diphosphate
ANP	Atrial natriuretic peptide
APCs	Antigen-presenting cells
ATP	Adenosine triphosphate
AV	Atrioventricular
BALT	Bronchus-associated lymphatic tissue
BCR	B-cell receptor
BNP	Brain natriuretic peptide
CD	Cluster of differentiation
CDK	Cyclin-dependent kinase
CNS	Central nervous system
DNA	Deoxyribonucleic acid
ECM	Extracellular matrix
ER	Endoplasmic reticulum
FSH	Follicle-stimulating hormone
G_0	Resting phase
G_1	Gap phase 1
G_2	Gap phase 2
GFAP	Glial fibrillary acidic protein
GH	Growth hormone
GnRH	Gonadotropin-releasing hormone
G_{TD}	Terminally differentiated
H2A	Histone H2A
H2B	Histone H2B
H3	Histone H3
H4	Histone H4
hCG	Human chorionic gonadotropin

HE	Hematoxylin and eosin
HEV	High endothelial venules
ICAM-1	Intercellular adhesion molecule 1
Ig	Immunoglobulin
IgE	Immunoglobulin E
LH	Luteinizing hormone
M	Mitosis
MHC	Major histocompatibility complex
mRNA	Messenger RNA
mtDNA	Mitochondrial DNA
MTOC	Microtubule-organizing center
NK	Natural killer
NO	Nitric oxide
OX	Oxytocin
PAS	Periodic acid–Schiff
pCO_2	Partial pressure of carbon dioxide
PNS	Peripheral nervous system
pO_2	Partial pressure of oxygen
PRL	Prolactin
PTH	Parathyroid hormone
rER	Rough endoplasmic reticulum
RNA	Ribonucleic acid
rRNA	Ribosomal RNA
S	Synthesis
SA	Sinoatrial
sER	Smooth endoplasmic reticulum
T_3	Triiodothyronine
T_4	Thyroxine
TCR	T-cell receptor
TDLU	Terminal duct lobular unit
TSH	Thyroid-stimulating hormone
UV	Ultraviolet

Contents

Part III   Histology of Tissues

Author Biography

Kirstine Karnov In 2013 Kirstine Karnov obtained her MD from the University of Copenhagen. She is in residency to become an otorhinolaryngologist and is currently doing a PhD on oral cancer. She began teaching histology during the 3rd year of her medical studies and has taught multiple classes of anatomy, dissection, and histology at the University of Copenhagen during a period of 5 years. Teaching has been one of her most enjoyable and learning experiences in her professional career, and the fun in teaching culminated in 2012 when the first compendium on histology *Histologi kompendium* (in Danish) was published by the authors.

Malin Nylander Malin Nylander graduated as a MD from the University of Copenhagen in 2012 and earned her PhD in gynecological endocrinology from the University of Copenhagen in 2017. With a great interest in human biology, she started teaching anatomy and histology halfway through medical school and has taught several classes of anatomy, histology, and human biology at the University of Copenhagen. Using a systematic approach combined with simple, schematic drawings on the black board, she tried to make the, at times, complicated curriculum comprehensible to all—something she implemented in the first compendium on histology *Histologi kompendium* (in Danish) published by the authors in 2012.

Anders Rehfeld Anders Rehfeld finished his MD from the University of Copenhagen in 2014 and earned his PhD in male reproductive biology from the University of Copenhagen in 2017. He began teaching histology during the 3rd year of his medical studies and has since taught 19 classes of histology of tissues and basic cell biology at the University of Copenhagen. From the beginning of his teaching period, he has been eager to help his students comprehend the large curriculum in a smarter and faster way, and in 2012 his efforts culminated with the publishing of the first compendium on histology *Histologi kompendium* (in Danish) by the authors.

Part I
Introduction

Chapter 1
From Cells to Tissues

Contents

Human Anatomy

General

Anatomy is the study of the structure of the organism.

Divided into
- Macroscopic anatomy
  - The study of structures visible to the naked eye
- Microscopic anatomy
  - The study of structures only visible with the use of microscopes
  - Divided into:
    - Cytology: the study of cells
    - Histology: the study of tissues and organs

© Springer International Publishing Switzerland 2017
A. Rehfeld et al., *Compendium of Histology*, DOI 10.1007/978-3-319-41873-5_1

Consists of
The organism consists of:
- Cells
  ↓
- Tissues
  ↓
- Organs
  ↓
- Organ systems
  ↓
- Organism

CELLS

General
- The smallest living basic structural and functional unit of the human body.
- There are more than 250 different types of human cells.

Consist of
- Nucleus
  - Nucleoplasm containing the nuclear DNA (main part of the genome)
  - Surrounded by a nuclear envelope, separating the nucleoplasm from the cytoplasm
- Cytoplasm
  - Cytosol containing organelles
  - Surrounded by a plasma membrane, separating the cytoplasm from the extracellular space

Divided into
- Germ cells:
  - The only human cell type, which undergoes meiosis
  - Give rise to oocytes or sperm cells (gametes)
- Somatic cells:
  - All non-germ cells

Physiological Properties of Cells

Divided into
- Absorption: uptake of extracellular substances
- Secretion: release of products formed within the cell
- Excretion: release of waste products
- Respiration: energy production through oxidation
- Irritability: ability to react to stimuli
- Conductivity: ability to transmit an impulse
- Contractibility: ability to shorten in a specific direction
- Reproduction: renewal of cells by growth and cell division
- Automaticity: ability to initiate an impulse in the absence of external stimuli

TISSUES

Structure
Organized groups of cells that together perform specific functions

Divided into
Four basic types based on the morphology and function:
1. Epithelial tissue: closely interspaced cells facing free surfaces
2. Connective tissue: separated cells in an extracellular matrix
3. Muscle tissue: contractile cells
4. Nerve tissue: neurons and glial cells

ORGANS

Structure
Functional units composed of several different tissues, which together perform specific functions

Consist of
- Parenchyma
  - Functional (specific) tissue of the organ
  - Commonly epithelial tissue
- Stroma
  - Supporting tissue of the organ
  - Commonly connective tissue

MEMO-BOX
- Parenchyma **P**erforms the specific actions of an organ.
- Stroma is the **S**upporting tissue of an organ.

ORGAN SYSTEMS

Structure
- Functional units composed of multiple organs that together perform specific functions
- For example, the urinary system

Formation of Tissues (Histogenesis)

General
The developmental process, from undifferentiated stem cells in a germ layer to specialized cells of a tissue

Formation
- In the early embryo cells are organized into three germ layers:
  - Ectoderm
  - Mesoderm
  - Endoderm
- The cells of the germ layers develop into specialized cells of tissues by:
  - Undergoing cell divisions (cell proliferation)
  - Specializing structurally and functionally (cell differentiation)
  - Undergoing apoptosis (regulated type of cell death):
    - Apoptosis controls the removal of certain cells/tissues, e.g., the tissue between the fingers in the developing hand.

Origin of the Four Basic Tissues

Divided into
- Epithelial tissue:
  - Derived from cells of all three germ layers
    - Ectoderm → e.g., epidermis of the skin
    - Mesoderm → e.g., mesothelium of peritoneum
    - Endoderm → e.g., epithelium of the intestines
- Connective tissue:
  - Mainly derived from cells of the mesoderm
- Muscle tissue:
  - Mainly derived from cells of the mesoderm
- Nerve tissue:
  - Mainly derived from cells of the ectoderm

Cell Differentiation

General
The development of less specialized cells into more specialized cells

Formation
Changes in gene expression give rise to cell differentiation:
- Genes are expressed in specific patterns in different cell types.
- Gene expression is regulated at any step from the transcription of the DNA to the modification of the final protein product:
  - Mainly regulated at the transcriptional level
  - Affected by multiple factors, e.g., epigenetic marks (Chap. 4)

Cell Potency

General
The ability of a cell to differentiate into other cell types

Divided into
- Totipotent cells
  - Can differentiate into all cell types, including those of extraembryonic tissues, e.g., the placenta
  - For example, the zygote

- Pluripotent cells
  - Can differentiate into all cell types, except those of extraembryonic tissues
  - For example, embryonic stem cells
- Multipotent cells
  - Can differentiate into multiple, but not all, cell types
  - For example, mesenchymal stem cells
- Unipotent cells
  - Can only differentiate into a single cell type
  - For example, erythrocyte progenitor cells

MEMO-BOX
- **TOT**ipotent cells can differentiate into the **TOT**al amount of human cell types.
- "Uni" means one: unipotent cells can differentiate into only one cell type.

Genes

General
- A segment of DNA encoding a functional protein or RNA product, e.g.:
  - A mRNA molecule, which can be translated into a protein
  - A rRNA molecule, which make up a part of the ribosome.
- The molecular unit of heredity

Divided into
- Tissue-specific genes
  - Code for proteins with specialized functions
  - Only expressed at certain times and in certain cells
  - $\approx 80\%$ of all genes
- Housekeeping genes
  - Code for proteins necessary for maintaining basic cell function
  - Expressed in almost all cell types
  - $\approx 20\%$ of all genes

Induction

General
- Interaction between differentiating cells
- A developing cell/tissue affects adjacent cells/tissues to differentiate in a certain direction

Divided into

Induction by:
- Cell–cell contact
- Cell–extracellular matrix (ECM) contact
- Diffusion of signaling molecules, which creates a concentration gradient:
  - Different levels of the signaling molecule induce different effects in cells.

Morphogenesis

General

The arrangement of differentiated cells into tissues and organs

Consist of
- Cells recognize and adhere to cells of the same type.
- Cells are affected by signaling molecules, called morphogens:
  - Form concentration gradients → affect the differentiation of cells according to their spatial position
  - For example, proteins encoded by homeotic genes:
    - Induces differentiation and morphogenesis
    - Are only expressed in certain areas of the embryo

References

5, 33, 34.

Chapter 2
Histological Methods

Contents

Microscopy

General

Several types of microscopy exist, each with their advantages and specific uses, e.g.:
- Light microscopy:
  - Brightfield: fixed, stained cells and tissues
  - Phase contrast: living, unstained cells and tissues
  - Fluorescence: living or fixed fluorescence-stained cells and tissues
- Electron microscopy: fixed and contrasted cells and tissues

© Springer International Publishing Switzerland 2017
A. Rehfeld et al., *Compendium of Histology*, DOI 10.1007/978-3-319-41873-5_2

Resolution

General

Smallest distance between two points, at which they can still be distinguished from each other:

- Resolution of the eye: ≈0.2 mm
- Resolution of light microscopy: ≈0.2 μm
- Resolution of electron microscopy: ≈0.2 nm

LIGHT MICROSCOPY

Magnification

General

- The magnification of structures by use of the microscope
- Calculated by eyepiece magnification multiplied with objective magnification (Table 2.1)

Field of View

General

- Area of the specimen viewed through the eyepieces.
- Field of view ⊘ is calculated by field of view number (written on eyepiece) divided by objective magnification (Table 2.2).

Table 2.1 Magnification in light microscope

Eyepiece magnification	Objective magnification	Total magnification
10×	4×	40×
10×	10×	100×
10×	40×	400×

Table 2.2 Field of view in light microscope

Field of view number	Objective magnification	Field of view ⊘
18 mm	4×	4.5 mm
18 mm	10×	1.8 mm
18 mm	40×	450 μm

PREPARATION OF TISSUE FOR LIGHT MICROSCOPY

General
- Most tissues are colorless and soft and have to be prepared to be examined using a microscope, e.g., by staining the tissue to enhance the visual contrast.
- To avoid autolysis (self-digestion), the tissue specimen should immediately after removal be either fixed or frozen.

Divided into (Table 2.4)
- Standard (routine) preparation
- Frozen section
- Smear

Standard preparation

Consists of (Table 2.3, Fig. 2.1)
1. Fixation
2. Embedding
3. Cutting
4. Staining

Frozen section

Consists of
1. Freezing of specimen
    - Tissue is embedded in cryoprotective medium and frozen quickly:
        - Inactivates enzymes → terminates metabolism and inhibits autolysis
        - Hardens the tissue
        - Preserves lipids
2. Cutting of frozen specimen (cryosectioning)
    - The hard frozen tissue can be cut directly in ≈ 5 μm thin slices.
3. Fixation (optional) and staining
    - I. Slices are mounted on glass slides.
    - II. Specimen is fixed shortly, e.g., with ethanol.
    - III. Specimen is stained, covered with a mounting solution and a coverslip.

Table 2.3 Standard preparation

	Process	Function	Commonly using
1. Fixation	Tissue specimen is bathed in fixative	• Inactivates enzymes → terminates metabolism and inhibits autolysis • Kills microorganisms • Denatures or cross-binds proteins → stabilizes and maintains structure of the tissue	Formalin
2. Embedding	1. Specimen is dehydrated using organic solutions, as paraffin is not water-soluble • Organic solutions also leach out lipid contents (causing an artifact) 2. Specimen is embedded in, e.g., paraffin	Provides hardness to the tissue allowing it to be cut in thin slices	Paraffin
3. Cutting	Embedded specimen is cut in ≈5 μm thin slices	Makes tissue thin enough to allow light to shine through	A microtome
4. Staining	1. Slices are mounted on glass slides 2. Paraffin is dissolved out 3. Specimen is then rehydrated, stained, and dehydrated 4. Stained specimen is covered with a mounting solution and a coverslip	Enhance the visual contrast	Hematoxylin and eosin (HE)

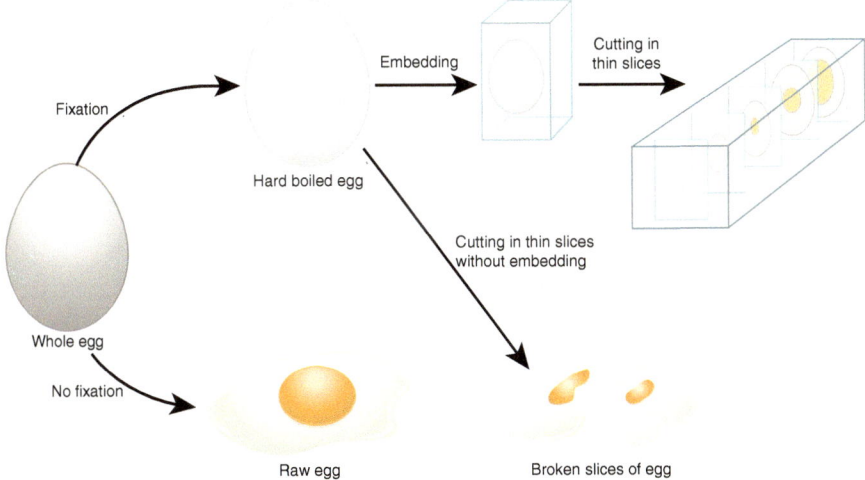

Fig. 2.1 Standard preparation. *Left*: fixation of tissue acts in a similar way as boiling an egg, as it denatures the proteins and thus stabilizes the structure. *Center*: embedding of the tissue makes it hard enough to be cut in μm thin slices. Similarly a boiled egg would have to be embedded to be cut in μm thin slices. *Right*: the μm thin slices of the egg differ according to the origin of the slice. Similarly the single section used for a specific tissue specimen only represents a small part of a much larger 3D structure

Smear

General
Some specimens, e.g., epithelial scrapes, soft tissues, and body fluids, can be prepared as a smear.

Consists of
1. Smear
   - Small amount of the specimen is smeared out on a glass slide.
2. Fixation (optional) and staining
   I. Specimen is fixed shortly, e.g., with ethanol.
   II. Specimen is stained, covered with a mounting solution and a coverslip.

Table 2.4 Tissue preparation types

	Standard preparation	Frozen section	Smear
Tissue structure	Conserved	Conserved	Not conserved
Morphological detail	High	Medium	Low
Procedure duration	Long	Short	Short
Procedure difficulty	Medium	High	Low
Preservation of antigens	Low	High	High
Conservation of lipids	Low	High	High

Artifacts

General
Errors introduced in the tissue during preparation

Divided into
Artifacts can be divided into, e.g.:
- Structural artifacts, e.g.:
    - Contractions
    - Foldings
    - Autolysis (self-digestion)
- Leaching of cellular components, e.g.:
    - Lipids:
        - Can be preserved by:
            - Making frozen sections of formalin-fixed specimens
            - Using a fixative that fixes lipids, e.g., osmium tetroxide
    - Glycogen:
        - Can be preserved by using nonaqueous fixatives

STAINING

Function
- Enhance the visual contrast
- Illustrate structures of interest (Table 2.5)

Divided into
Multiple types of stains exist, e.g.:
- Acidophilic and basophilic staining
- Histochemical staining
- Immunohistochemical staining
- In situ hybridization

Acidophilic and Basophilic Staining

General

General staining with acidic and basic dyes:

- For example, hematoxylin (acts similar to a basic dye) and eosin (acidic dye) staining, the most common type of histological staining
- Acidic dyes:
  - Negatively charged
  - Binds to material, containing positively charged components:
    - Material is termed acidophilic "acid liking."
      - Often called eosinophilic, due to the common use of eosin.
    - For example, most cytoplasmic proteins.
- Basic dyes:
  - Positively charged
  - Binds to material, containing negatively charged components:
    - Material is termed basophilic "base liking."
    - For example, RNA/DNA (due to PO_4^{3-} groups of backbone).

Metachromasic staining

General

- Some basic dyes can stain in different colors, as they change color when polymerizing, e.g., toluidine blue:
  - Monomeric toluidine blue → blue
  - Polymeric toluidine blue aggregates → red
- Metachromatic staining requires:
  - Closely interspaced binding spots for the dye on the stained molecule, e.g., polyanionic groups in glycosaminoglycans
  - A high enough concentration of the dye to form polymeric dye aggregates
    - Higher dye concentration → higher probability of polymeric aggregate formation

Histochemical Staining

General

Staining of certain components, e.g.:

- Periodic acid–Schiff (PAS) stain, which stains carbohydrate-rich molecules, e.g., in mucus and the basal lamina

Immunohistochemical Staining

General
- Specific staining with the use of antibodies, coupled to, e.g., a fluorescent dye.
- The antibody binds very specifically to a certain antigen and is used to illustrate a structure of interest in the tissue, e.g., tumor markers.

In Situ Hybridization

General
Specific staining of RNA/DNA sequences of interest using complementary RNA/DNA probes, coupled to, e.g., a fluorescent dye.

Table 2.5 Commonly used stains

Name	Stains	Color	Used for staining, e.g.	Photomicrograph example
Hematoxylin	Basophilic material (negatively charged), e.g., RNA and DNA	Blue	Nucleus	
Eosin	Acidophilic material (positively charged), e.g., most cytoplasmic proteins	Red/pink	Cytoplasm	
Periodic acid–Schiff (PAS)	Carbohydrate-rich molecules, e.g., in mucus and the basal lamina	Pink/magenta	Goblet cells	
Sirius red	Cytoplasm	Yellow	Dense connective tissue	
	Collagen	Red		
Van Gieson	Nucleus	Blue	Dense connective tissue	
	Cytoplasm	Yellow		
	Collagen	Red		
Masson's trichrome	Nucleus	Blue/black	Dense connective tissue	
	Cytoplasm	Red		
	Collagen	Blue/green		

(continued)

Table 2.5 (continued)

Name	Stains	Color	Used for staining, e.g.	Photomicrograph example
Mallory's trichrome	Nucleus	Red	Dense connective tissue	
	Cytoplasm	Pale red		
	Collagen	Blue		
Mallory–Azan	Nucleus	Red	Dense connective tissue	
	Cytoplasm	Pink		
	Collagen	Blue		
Toluidine blue	Basophilic material (negatively charged), e.g., RNA and DNA	Blue	Ground substance in cartilage	
	Glycosaminoglycans	Metachromasic (red/blue)		
Alcian blue	Mucin	Blue	Mucous glands	
	Cartilage			
Orcein	Elastin	Red/brown	Elastic fibers	
Weigert's (resorcin-fuchsin)	Elastin	Blue/black	Elastic fibers	
Silver	Reticular fibers and basal lamina	Black/brown	Reticular connective tissue	
Osmium tetroxide	Lipids	Black/brown	Myelin sheets	

Courtesy of photomicrographs, professor Jørgen Tranum-Jensen and associate professor Steen Seier Poulsen, University of Copenhagen

MEMO-BOX
- Hematoxylin stains **B**asophilic material, e.g., RNA/DNA, **B**lue
- **PAS** stains carbohydrate-rich molecules, e.g., glycoproteins, **P**ink
- Or-ce-in stains e-la-stin
- Osmium tetrox**ID**e fixes and stains lip**ID**s

Introduction to the Guides to Practical Histology

General
The purpose of the guides to practical histology is to help with the identification of selected histological specimens:
- Selected characteristic morphological features for each specimen will be described in the guides.
- In addition, a simplified illustration in black and white, emphasizing the characteristic features and a photomicrograph of the specimen, is shown for each specimen.
- For more detailed information about the specimens, please refer to the initial parts of the chapters.
- The guides do not help with the identification of individual cells or cellular contents, which is why there are no guides in Chaps. 3 and 4.

Divided into
The guides to practical histology are:
- Divided into smaller parts based on specimen category and placed at the end of the corresponding chapters.
- Categorized into two parts:
  - Guides to practical histology of the tissues:
    - Aid the identification of the tissues
    - Include an example of where the specific tissue can be found
    - In Chaps. 5, 6, 7, 8, 9, 10, 11, 12, 13, and 14
  - Guides to practical histology of the organs:
    - Aid the identification of organs and organ parts
    - Tissues are often only mentioned by name in this part, not described in detail.
    - In Chaps. 15, 16, 17, 18, 19, 20, 21, 22, 23, 24, 25, 26, 27, 28, and 29

Staining
- The guides to practical histology describe how to identify a given specimen stained with hematoxylin–eosin (HE), as this type of staining is the most commonly used:
  - Hematoxylin:
    - Stains basophilic material blue
    - For example, RNA and DNA
  - Eosin:
    - Stains acidophilic material light red
      - Acidophilic material is also called eosinophilic, as it stains with eosin.
    - For example, most cytoplasmic proteins
- For some specimens, other types of staining are mentioned in addition.

Microscopy of Histological Specimens

General
- Histological specimens are most commonly inspected using a light microscope (Fig. 2.2) or using virtual microscopy.
- If a light microscope is used, proper setup of Köhler illumination on the microscope can aid the identification of the specimen.
- When inspecting the specimen, follow a simple sequence from macroscopic inspection → microscopic inspection:
  - Most specimens can be identified macroscopically or at low magnification microscopically.
  - Always try to identify more than one characteristic feature of the given specimen.
  - Think about other specimens, which can be mistaken for the given one, and how to distinguish between them.

Setting up Köhler illumination on a light microscope:
- Focus the light source on the specimen (Fig. 2.3):
  1. Open aperture diaphragm (on condenser) completely.
  2. Narrow luminous-field diaphragm (on the light source) until the diaphragm is seen within the field of view.
  3. Move the condenser up/down until the edge of the luminous-field diaphragm is seen as a sharp image.
  4. Move the condenser in the horizontal plane, until the luminous-field diaphragm is centered in the field of view.
  5. Open up the luminous-field diaphragm, until the edge is just outside of the field of view.

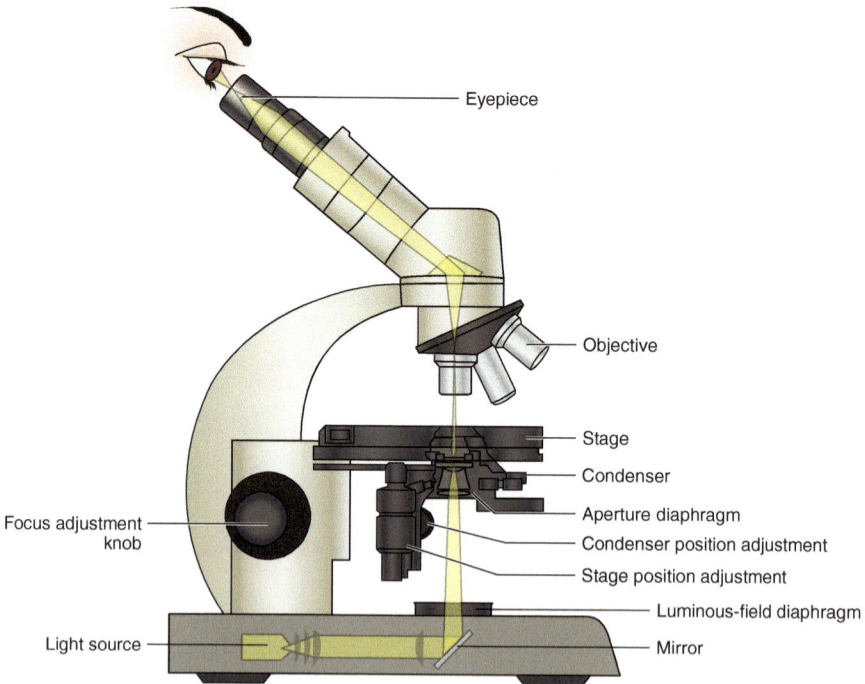

Fig. 2.2 The light microscope

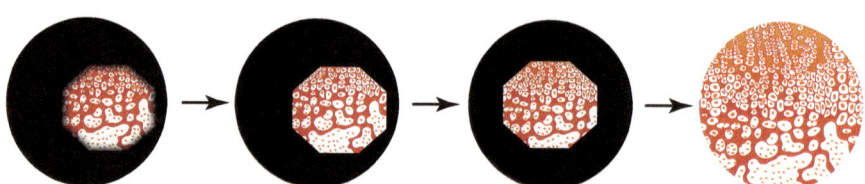

Fig. 2.3 How to focus the light source on the specimen in the light microscope

- Set up the optimal contrast (Fig. 2.4):
  6. Remove one eyepiece and look down the tube directly, with the eye
     10–20 cm away from the opening of the tube.
  7. Narrow the aperture diaphragm until only the central ≈ 80 % of the tube
     ⊘ is illuminated.
  8. Insert the eyepiece again.

- When changing to a new objective:
  - 9. Adjust the luminous-field and aperture diaphragms:
    - Luminous-field diaphragm should be opened/closed, so the edge is just outside of the field of view.
    - Aperture diaphragm should be adjusted so only the central $\approx 80\,\%$ of the tube $\oslash$ is illuminated.

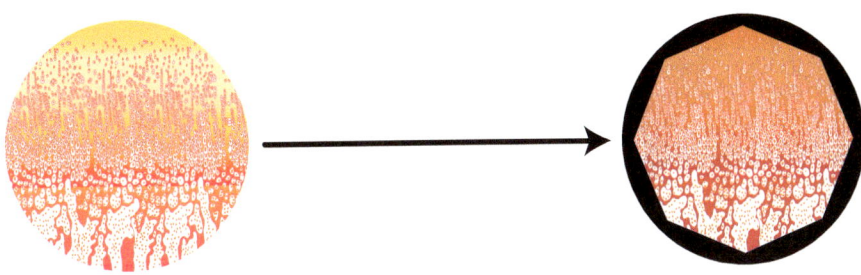

Fig. 2.4 How to set up the optimal contrast in the light microscope

Sequence during identification of specimens

1. Inspect the specimen macroscopically:
   - (a) Place the glass slide on a white background and inspect it with the naked eye or use the lowest possible magnification in the virtual microscope.
   - (b) Note the shape and appearance, e.g.:
     - (i) A part of or a whole ring-shaped structure is seen when tubular structures have been cross sectioned, e.g., large blood vessels.
     - (ii) Other characteristic shape, e.g., the cauliflower-shaped structures seen when sectioning the cerebellum.
   - (c) Note if more than one piece of tissue is seen on the microscopic glass slide:
     - (i) Commonly seen for, e.g.:
       1. The bladder, both in contracted and relaxed state
       2. Skeletal muscle tissue, both in cross and longitudinal sections
   - (d) Note the staining of the specimen:
     - (i) Some specimens are weakly stained → adjust the condenser optimally to obtain good contrast in image.
   - (e) Note the homogeneity of the specimen:
     - (i) Remember to inspect the different areas at higher magnification in non-homogenous specimens.

2. Inspect the specimen microscopically:
  (a) Begin with the lowest magnification
    (i) Browse through specimen to obtain an overview.
      1. Note the microscopic homogeneity of the specimen.
        (a) Remember to inspect the different areas at higher magnification
          in non-homogenous specimens.
      2. Select an appropriate area to inspect at higher magnification:
        (a) For example, an area of longitudinal sectioned muscle cells in
          skeletal or cardiac muscle tissue, to see the cross-striations.
  (b) Inspect specimen at high magnification:
    (i) In most specimens erythrocytes can be found and used as a
      "histological ruler" of $\oslash \approx 7.5$ µm to measure the size of other cells
      and structures in the specimen.

> **MEMO-BOX**
> In histological specimens, one can often find an erythrocyte ($\oslash \approx 7.5$) and
> use it as a ruler to estimate the sizes of other cells and structures.

References

5, 28, 33, 34, 45.

Part II
Cytology

Chapter 3
The Cytoplasm

Contents

General

The cytoplasm is the part of the cell located outside the nucleus:

- Enclosed by the cell membrane
- Contains the organelles of the cell

Consist of

- Organelles, $\approx 50\%$
- Cytosol (cytoplasmic matrix), $\approx 50\%$
- Inclusions, few %

© Springer International Publishing Switzerland 2017
A. Rehfeld et al., *Compendium of Histology*, DOI 10.1007/978-3-319-41873-5_3

Organelles

General

The functional subunits of cells (Fig. 3.1)

Divided into

- Membranous organelles
  - ○ Nucleus, the largest organelle (Chap. 4)
  - ○ Plasma membrane (cell membrane)
  - ○ Endoplasmic reticulum
  - ○ Golgi apparatus
  - ○ Transport vesicles
  - ○ Endosomes
  - ○ Lysosomes
  - ○ Mitochondria
  - ○ Peroxisomes
- Nonmembranous organelles
  - ○ Cytoskeleton
  - ○ Ribosomes
  - ○ Proteasomes
  - ○ Centrioles

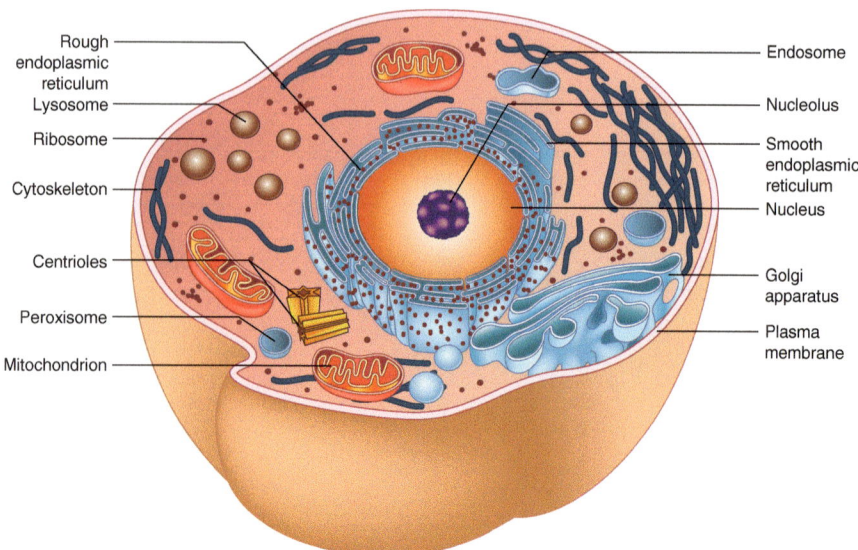

Fig. 3.1 Cell with organelles: cross section through a cell showing the morphology and organization of the organelles

Membranous Organelles

General
- Organelles containing a plasma membrane are called membranous organelles
- Plasma membranes surround:
  - The cell, as the cell membrane
  - The membranous organelles, dividing the cytoplasm into compartments

PLASMA MEMBRANE (CELL MEMBRANE)

Structure (Fig. 3.2)
- Lipid bilayer, with an inner and outer leaflet:
  - ≈8 nm thick
  - Contains membrane proteins
- Trilaminary (three layered) structure:
  - Inner hydrophilic layer
  - Central hydrophobic layer
  - Outer hydrophilic layer
- Glycocalyx (cell coat):
  - Covers the extracellular surface of the cell membrane
  - Formed by the glycosylations (carbohydrates) of membrane glycolipids, glycoproteins, and proteoglycans

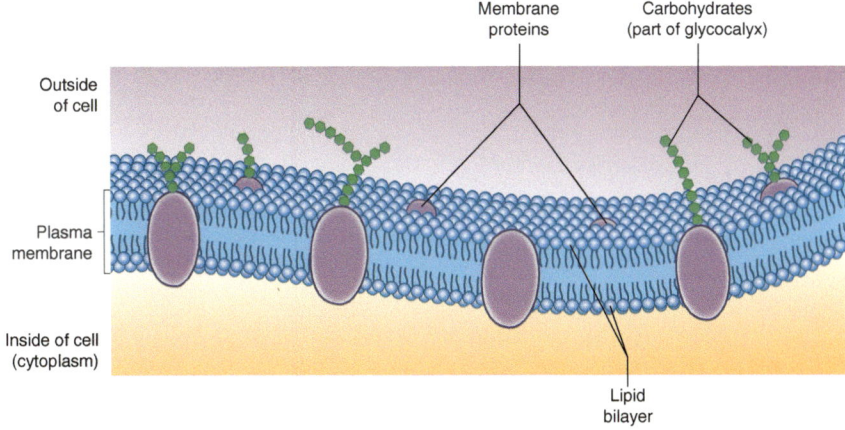

Fig. 3.2 Plasma membrane: cross section through the plasma membrane showing the trilaminary structure of the lipid bilayer and the associated membrane proteins. Note that glycosylations (carbohydrates) are only seen on the extracellular surface

Function
- Lipid bilayer:
  - Forms the cell boundary:
    - A relatively impermeable barrier between the cytoplasm and the extracellular space.
    - Substances must transverse the cell membrane to enter the cell.
  - Forms the boundary of membranous organelles, separating interior organelle environments from the cytosol:
    - Enzymes are kept apart from their substrates → control of metabolic processes.
    - Intracellular concentration gradients are obtained.
- Membrane proteins:
  - Perform various physiological functions, e.g., as ion channels
- Glycocalyx:
  - Covers and protects the cell
  - Takes part in the formation of different cell surface receptors

Consist of
- Membrane lipids, ≈50 %
  - Phospholipids
  - Cholesterol
  - Sphingolipids
- Membrane proteins, ≈50 %
  - Integral membrane proteins
  - Peripheral membrane proteins

MEMO-BOX
PLasma membrane consists of Proteins and Lipids.

Divided into
- Outer leaflet: towards the extracellular space
- Inner leaflet: towards the cytoplasm

Light Microscopy
- The plasma membrane is too thin to be visualized in the light microscope.
- It is however often seen as a thin dark line surrounding cells, as it has, e.g., been cut obliquely during preparation.

Formation

Components are delivered to the plasma membrane as vesicles:

- Membrane lipids:
    1. Produced in the smooth endoplasmic reticulum (sER).
    2. Transported through the Golgi apparatus.
    3. Brought to the plasma membrane as vesicles (membrane lipids make up the vesicle membrane).
    4. Vesicles fuse with the plasma membrane, and the membrane lipids of the vesicle membrane are incorporated into the plasma membrane.
- Membrane proteins:
    1. Produced in the rough endoplasmic reticulum (rER).
    2. Transported through the Golgi apparatus.
    3. Brought to the plasma membrane as part of the vesicle membrane (membrane proteins are situated within the vesicle membrane).
    4. Vesicles fuse with the plasma membrane, and the membrane proteins of the vesicle membrane are incorporated into the plasma membrane.

Membrane Lipids

General

- Float freely within each leaflet of the plasma membrane bilayer by lateral diffusion → liquid two-dimensional lipid sheet (fluid mosaic).
- Spontaneous movement from one leaflet to the other (flip-flop) rarely occurs.
    ○ This maintains an asymmetry between the two leaflets, such that, e.g., glycolipids only are found in the outer leaflet.
- Certain membrane lipids aggregate in microdomains, called lipid rafts:
    ○ Thicker and less fluid membrane regions
    ○ Certain integral membrane proteins can only be located in lipid rafts

Divided into

- Phospholipids, ≈50 %
- Cholesterol, ≈50 %
- Sphingolipids, few %

Phospholipids

Structure

Amphipathic, i.e., with one hydrophobic and one hydrophilic end:

- Hydrophobic ends from each leaflet face each other in the center of the membrane.
- Hydrophilic ends are facing the intra- and extracellular surfaces of the membrane.

→ trilaminary structure

Cholesterol

General
Situated between the hydrophobic ends of the phospholipids

Function
Stabilizes the viscosity of the membrane, i.e., more cholesterol makes the membrane less fluid

Sphingolipids

General
Amphipathic lipids, which take part in lipid raft formation

Membrane Proteins

General
1. Float freely within the membrane by lateral diffusion.
   ◦ Except the membrane proteins, which are anchored to intracellular or extracellular structures, e.g., the cytoskeleton.
- In some cells the cell membrane is divided into domains by tight junctions (Chap. 5) → lateral diffusion is confined to a single domain.
- Certain integral membrane proteins can only be located in lipid rafts → the lipid rafts control the movement and distribution of these proteins.

Divided into
- Integral membrane proteins
- Peripheral membrane proteins

Integral membrane proteins

Divided into
- Transmembrane proteins
  ◦ Amphipathic proteins:
    ▪ Hydrophobic parts (alpha-helixes) cross the plasma membrane (single- or multi-pass).
    ▪ Hydrophilic parts are on the intra- and extracellular side of the plasma membrane.

- Monolayer-associated proteins
  - Amphipathic proteins:
    - Hydrophobic parts (alpha-helixes) are embedded within the plasma membrane.
    - Hydrophilic parts are located on the intra- or extracellular side of the plasma membrane.
- Lipid-linked proteins
  - Covalently bound to membrane lipids

Peripheral membrane proteins

General

Localized externally to the plasma membrane, non-covalently bound to other membrane proteins or lipids

Transport Through the Plasma Membrane

General
- To enter the cell, molecules must transverse the plasma membrane.
- Permeability of the plasma membrane:
  - Permeable to:
    - Fat-soluble molecules
    - Small, uncharged water-soluble molecules

    Transverse the membrane by simple diffusion.
  - Relatively impermeable to:
    - Large water-soluble molecules
    - Charged water-soluble molecules

    Require membrane transport proteins to transverse the membrane.

Divided into
- Passive transport: driven by the electrochemical gradient
  - Simple diffusion
  - Facilitated diffusion
- Active transport: coupled to an energy source, e.g., ATP

Passive transport

Consists of
- Simple diffusion:
  - Fat-soluble molecules
  - Small, uncharged water-soluble molecules
- Facilitated diffusion:
  - Channel proteins
    - Makes hydrophilic pores through the membrane, where large or charged water-soluble molecules can pass
    - Can open/close in response to stimuli, e.g., change in membrane potential, binding of ligand or phosphorylation
    - For example, ion channels
  - Carrier proteins
    - Does not create pores in the plasma membrane but binds a specific molecule as a ligand and changes conformation → transporting the molecule through the membrane
    - Carriers are divided into:
      - Uniporters: transport one molecule
      - Symporters: transport two or more molecules in one direction
      - Antiporters: transport two or more molecules in opposite directions
    - For example, glucose carriers

Active transport

Consists of
Carrier proteins (pumps):
- Usually transport molecules through the plasma membrane against the electrochemical gradient
- Can build up electrochemical gradients, which drive the passive transport of secondary molecules via sym- and antiporters (secondary active transport)
- For example, the Na^+/K^+ pump

ENDOPLASMIC RETICULUM

Structure
- Anastomosing network of flattened membranous tubes, sheets, and sacs
- Membrane is continuous with the outer membrane of the nuclear envelope.
- Lumen of the endoplasmic reticulum (ER) is continuous with the perinuclear cistern of the nuclear envelope.

Divided into
Two regions, which are continuous with each other:
• Rough endoplasmic reticulum (rER)
• Smooth endoplasmic reticulum (sER)

Rough Endoplasmic Reticulum

General
Associated with multiple ribosomes on its surface:
• Stains basophilic because of the ribosomal RNA

Function
• Production of proteins:
  ○ The membrane-bound ribosomes synthesize proteins directly into the lumen of the rER:
    ▪ Secretory proteins
    ▪ Integral membrane proteins
    ▪ Luminal proteins for membranous organelles
  ○ Cells with a large production of these proteins have a large rER.
  ○ All proteins produced in rER are sent to the Golgi apparatus with vesicles.
• Modification of proteins:
  ○ N-bound glycosylation.
  ○ Cleavage.
  ○ Folding (with the help of chaperone proteins).
  ○ Assembly of multiple subunits into larger proteins.
  ○ Quality checkpoint → misfolded proteins are translocated to cytosol and degraded.

Light Microscopy
A large rER is seen as a basophilic region in the cytoplasm near the nucleus.

MEMO-BOX
Cells with a large production of secretory proteins, e.g., plasma cells, have abundant rER → basophilic cytoplasm in the light microscope.

Smooth Endoplasmic Reticulum

General
- Not associated with ribosomes on its surface:
  - Stains acidophilic like the rest of the cytoplasm
- Sparse in most cells, but characteristically well developed in steroid hormone-producing cells.

Function
- Lipid synthesis, including steroid hormones and membrane lipids
  - Membrane lipids produced in sER are sent to the Golgi apparatus as vesicles (lipids make up vesicle membrane).
- Involved in the breakdown of glycogen
- Detoxification of organic chemicals
- Ca^{2+}-store, e.g., in muscle cells

GOLGI APPARATUS

Structure
- Stack of 3–10 flattened membranous sacs (cisterns).
- Located adjacent to the nucleus, with the ER sandwiched between the nucleus and the Golgi apparatus.
- Sacs are convex towards the nucleus (cis-face) and concave towards the plasma membrane (trans-face).

Function
Modification and sorting of proteins and lipids:
- Receives all proteins and membrane lipids synthesized in ER via transport vesicles
  - Sorts these proteins and membrane lipids
  - Packages and sends them to the right destination with the help of transport vesicles with content-specific surface markers, which target complimentary receptors at the destination
- Proteins and lipids are transported through the Golgi apparatus in cis–trans-direction, with the help of transport vesicles, and are modified during the transit:
  - O-bound glycosylation:
    - For example, of proteoglycans.
    - The glycosylations on the luminal face of membrane proteins and lipids end up as a part of the glycocalyx, as the luminal face of the membranes in ER, Golgi apparatus, and vesicles ends up as the extracellular face of the cell membrane after fusion.
  - Modification of the N-bound glycosylation made in rER:
    - For example, phosphorylation of mannose-tag on lysosomal enzymes

Consist of
See Table 3.1.

Light microscopy
- Normally not seen in the light microscope
- In some cells seen as a pale region in a basophilic cytoplasm (negative Golgi stain), e.g., in plasma cells.

Table 3.1 Golgi Apparatus

Part	Structure	Function	Direction of protein- and lipid transport
Cis-Golgi network	Anastomosing network of tubules	Receives vesicles from ER with proteins and membrane lipids	
Cis-part	Inner cisterns	Glycosylation of proteins and membrane lipids	
Medial part	Medial cisterns		
Trans-part	Outer cisterns		
Trans-Golgi network	Anastomosing network of tubules	• Sorting of proteins and membrane lipids • Detachment of vesicles, containing specific cargo according to their destination	

TRANSPORT VESICLES

General
- Vary in size, shape, and content
- Are formed from and fuse with membranous organelles
- Found in large numbers between:
  - ER and the cis-Golgi network
  - Trans-Golgi network and the cell membrane
  - The different cisterns of the Golgi apparatus

Function
- Transport of molecules (cargo):
  - Within vesicle lumen, e.g., secretory proteins
  - As components of vesicle plasma membrane, e.g., membrane lipids and membrane proteins
- Involved in:
  - Endocytosis: substances enter the cell in vesicles formed from invaginations of the cell membrane.
  - Exocytosis: substances leave the cell as vesicles fuse with the cell membrane.

Light microscopy
Only large vesicles are visible in the light microscope.

ENDOSOMES

Structure
Dynamic system of membranous vesicles and tubes

Function
Sorting of endocytosed material:
1. Endocytosed vesicles fuse with early endosomes.
2. Endocytosed material and receptors are sorted.
3. Sorted material and receptors are dispatched in new vesicles, which either:
   - Return to the cell membrane domain from which it came, often containing receptors, which are thus recycled
   - Are transported through the cell, from one cell membrane domain to the other (transcytosis)
   - Fuse with late endosomes, which mature into lysosomes → endocytosed material is broken down

Divided into
- Early endosomes
  - Receive endocytosed vesicles
- Late endosomes
  - Receive sorted material in vesicles from early endosomes
  - Fuse with vesicles from the Golgi apparatus containing lysosomal enzymes → mature into lysosomes

LYSOSOMES

General
- The digestive organelles of cells
- Formed from late endosomes

Structure
Vesicles, $\oslash \approx 0.5$ µm

Function
Digestion of all types of biological macromolecules:
- Hold multiple hydrolytic enzymes, which are active at low pH.
- H^+ pumps in the lysosomal membrane lower luminal pH → activates the hydrolytic enzymes → break down macromolecules.

Pathways providing material for digestion in lysosomes
Divided into
- Autophagy: the cells own contents
  - Macroautophagy: cellular components, e.g., old organelles, are surrounded by ER membrane → autophagosome → fuse with lysosome.
  - Microautophagy: cytoplasmic proteins are invaginated into lysosome.
  - Chaperone-mediated autophagy: chaperone protein binds cytoplasmic protein and transports it through the lysosome membrane.
- Heterophagy: endocytosed material in late endosomes.
  - Phagocytosis:
    - Larger material in large vesicles, e.g., bacteria
    - Performed by specialized cells, e.g., macrophages
  - Pinocytosis:
    - Fluid with dissolved small molecules, in small vesicles
    - Constitutively performed in all cells
  - Receptor-mediated endocytosis:
    - Specific molecules are selectively endocytosed.
    - Molecules (ligands) bind to cargo receptors on cell surface → ligand–receptor complexes accumulate in lipid rafts → endocytosed in vesicles.

Light microscopy
- Can be seen in some cells, e.g., as azurophilic granules in neutrophils.
- In some cells residual bodies of nondegradable end products from lysosomes are found, e.g., lipofuscin granules in neurons.

MITOCHONDRIA

General
- The organelles, which generate most of the cell's ATP, used as an energy supply.
- The number of mitochondria in a cell reflects its energy demand.
- Contain its own circular mtDNA and protein synthesis machinery:
  - Synthesizes 5 % of the mitochondrial proteins.
  - Remaining 95 % of the mitochondrial proteins are encoded by genes of the nuclear DNA and synthesized by the regular protein synthesis machinery of the cell.

Structure
- Rounded/elongated
- $\oslash$ 1 μm and up to 10 μm long
- Surrounded by two separate plasma membranes

Function
- Energy production:
  - Produce ATP through oxidative phosphorylation (O_2-demanding) fueled by:
    - Breakdown of pyruvate in the citric acid cycle
    - Breakdown of fatty acids by β-oxidation
- Steroid hormone synthesis:
  - Initial part of steroid hormone synthesis
- Initiation of apoptosis:
  - Sense cellular stress: excessive cellular stress → initiation of apoptosis

Consist of
- Outer mitochondrial membrane
  - Large porins make it relatively permeable.
- Intermembrane space
  - 10–20 nm wide
  - Contains fluid with a composition alike that of the cytosol, because of the high permeability of the outer membrane

- Inner mitochondrial membrane:
  - Impermeable
  - Makes multiple folds (cristae) or tubules into the lumen (matrix) → enhances inner surface area
  - Contains multiple F_1–F_0 protein complexes, where the ATP synthesis takes place
- Matrix
  - The mitochondrial inner lumen
  - Contains:
    - Enzymes, e.g., for citric acid cycle
    - The circular mtDNA and protein synthesis machinery

Formation
Growth and division of existing mitochondria give rise to new mitochondria.

PEROXISOMES

General
- Contains oxidative enzymes (O_2-demanding)
- Involved in processes that produce or degrade hydrogen peroxide (H_2O_2)

Structure
Vesicles, $\varnothing \approx 0.5\ \mu m$

Function
- Detoxification:
  - For example, of alcohols and aldehydes
- β-Oxidation of fatty acids → breakdown of lipids

MEMO-BOX
PEROXIsomes produce/degrade hydrogen **PEROXI**de

Nonmembranous Organelles

CYTOSKELETON

Structure

Internal cell skeleton composed of thin filaments.

Function

- Mechanical support, e.g., maintaining:
  - Cell shape
  - Cytoplasmic organization
- Movement of:
  - Intracellular components
  - Cilia
  - The cell itself
- Contraction, e.g., in muscle cells

Consist of

Three types of filaments (Table 3.2):
- Actin filaments
- Microtubules
- Intermediate filaments

Intermediate filament protein subunits

General

The protein subunits, which form the tetramers of intermediate filaments make up a big, heterogeneous group, with different types of subunits being used in different cell types.

Divided into

The subunits are divided into, e.g.:
- Nuclear lamins: in all cells
  - Forms a nuclear lamina, which lines the inner surface of the nuclear envelope
- Keratins: in epithelial cells
- Vimentins: in fibroblasts
- Desmins: in muscle cells
- Glial fibrillary acid proteins (GFAP): in astrocytes
- Neurofilaments: in neurons

Table 3.2 Filaments of the cytoskeleton

	Actin filaments	Microtubules	Intermediate filaments
⊘	≈7 nm	≈25 nm	≈10 nm
Structure	Double spiral of two F-actin strands, made from G-actin monomers	Hollow cylinder of 13 protofilaments, made from chains of α- and β-tubulin dimers	Ropelike cylinder of 8 protofilaments, made from chains of protein tetramers
Polarity	• Plus- and minus-end • Grow fastest by polymerization of G-actin at the plus-end	• Plus- and minus-end • Grow by polymerization of dimers at the plus-end • Minus-end embedded in centrosome	None
Stability	Unstable: Continuous buildup/ breakdown at both ends (dynamic instability)	Unstable: Continuous buildup/ breakdown at plus-end (dynamic instability)	Stable
Energy source for polymerization	ATP	GTP	None, proteins self-assemble spontaneously

Associated proteins	• Actin-binding proteins:
	  ○ Regulate polymerization (buildup vs. breakdown)
	  ○ Cross-link multiple actin filaments into 3D-structures
	• Motor proteins:
	  ○ Myosins attach to actin filaments and move towards plus-end → movement
	• Plaque proteins:
	  ○ Connect actin filaments to cell junctions
		• Microtubule-associated proteins:
		  ○ Affect polymerization and stability of microtubules
		  ○ Anchor microtubules to other structures.
		• Motor proteins:
		  ○ Kinesins and dyneins can move along microtubules.
		  ○ Kinesins move towards the plus-end and dyneins towards the minus-end
			• Intermediate filament-associated proteins:
			  ○ Bind together intermediate filaments with microtubules and actin filaments (connect the cytoskeleton)
			• Plaque proteins:
			  ○ Connect intermediate filaments to cell junctions

Location	• Primarily found underlying the cell membrane • Make up the core of microvilli	• Radiate out from the centrosome • Make up the core in centrioles, basal bodies, cilia, and flagella	• Found throughout the cytoplasm • Form nuclear lamina on the inner surface of the nuclear envelope
Function	• Mechanical support • Contraction (with myosin) • Intracellular movement of components (with myosin) • Maintain and change cell shape • Cell migration	• Mechanical support • Intracellular movement of components (with motor proteins) • Movement of cilia and flagella (with motor proteins) • Make up mitotic spindle • Participate in cell migration	• Mechanical support and strength

RIBOSOMES

Structure
20 nm large molecules made of ribosomal RNA (rRNA) and protein

Function
Translation of mRNA into proteins:
- Ribosomes bound to the rER:
  - Secretory proteins
  - Integral membrane proteins
  - Luminal proteins for membranous organelles
- Free ribosomes in the cytosol:
  - Proteins, which stay in the cytosol (cytoplasmic proteins)
  - Proteins, which are transferred to the nucleus, mitochondria, or peroxisomes

Light microscopy
- Ribosomes bound to the rER are dense enough to stain basophilic.
- Free ribosomes in the cytosol are generally too few and sparse to stain basophilic.
  - In some cells with a large production of cytosolic proteins, e.g., developing red blood cells, the free ribosomes are dense enough to stain basophilic.

PROTEASOMES

Structure
A large multi-subunit protein complex, forming a 15 nm long hollow cylinder

Function
Degradation of ubiquitin tagged proteins.

CENTRIOLES

Structure
- $\oslash$ 0.15 µm and $\approx$ 0 2 µm long.
- Hollow cylinders formed from a ring of nine microtubule triplets.

- Centrioles are found:
  - As a pair, arranged at a right angle to each other, in the centrosome (microtubule-organizing center (MTOC))
  - Individually, as part of basal bodies

Function
- The centrosome forms around the centriole pair:
  - From here microtubules continuously grow out from γ-tubulin rings:
    - The microtubule stability constantly varies → the amount and lengths of the microtubules are in constant change (dynamic instability).
  - Duplicate and form the poles of the mitotic spindle during mitosis.
- Basal bodies develop from newly formed single centrioles:
  - Located under the apical cell membrane.
  - Cilia grow out from the basal bodies.

Cytosol (Cytoplasmic Matrix)

Structure
Aqueous gel, surrounding organelles and inclusions

Function
Site of multiple enzymatic processes, e.g., anaerobic glycolysis of glucose to pyruvate

Consist of
- Centrosome:
  - Confined area near the nucleus, formed around the centriole pair
  - Gel structure
- Endoplasm:
  - Remaining area near the nucleus
  - Fluid structure
- Ectoplasm:
  - The part just underneath the cell membrane
  - Gel structure

Inclusions

General
Dispensable and often temporary components of the cell

Consist of
For example:
- Energy stores
- Pigment granules

Energy Stores

Divided into
- Glycogen (glucose store)
- Lipid inclusions (fat droplets)

Light microscopy
- Glycogen:
  - Leaches out during standard preparation:
    - Can be preserved by using nonaqueous fixatives:
      - Unstained in HE
      - Pink in PAS
- Lipid inclusions (lipid droplets):
  - Leach out during standard preparation:
    - Seen as "empty" white areas in the cell
    - Can be preserved by:
      - Making frozen sections of formalin-fixed specimens
      - Using a fixative that fixes lipids, e.g., osmium tetroxide

Pigments Granules

Divided into
- Exogenous pigment granules:
  - From outside the organism
  - For example, carbon dust

- Endogenous pigment granules:
  - ◦ Formed within the organism
  - ◦ For example, lipofuscin granules (nondegradable waste product of lysosomes)

References

1, 5, 33, 34, 43, 45.

Chapter 4
The Nucleus

Contents

General

- Eukaryotic cells are defined by having a nucleus:
  - Most human cells have one nucleus.
  - Some human cells have multiple nuclei, e.g., skeletal muscle cells, and some lack a nucleus, e.g., erythrocytes.
- The largest organelle of the cell.
- Contains all deoxyribonucleic acid (DNA) of cell, except the mitochondrial DNA.

Structure

- $\oslash$ 5–10 μm
- Variable shape
- Surrounded by the nuclear envelope, formed by two layers of plasma membrane

© Springer International Publishing Switzerland 2017
A. Rehfeld et al., *Compendium of Histology*, DOI 10.1007/978-3-319-41873-5_4

Function
- Contains the main part of the human genome, the nuclear DNA, divided into:
  - 23 homologous chromosome pairs in somatic cells:
    - 22 pairs of autosomes
    - One pair of sex chromosomes
- Gene transcription
  - Production of ribonucleic acid (RNA), using the genes of DNA as templates:
    - For example, mRNA, which are translated into proteins by ribosomes
- Replication of DNA
  - Production of two identical copies of the nuclear DNA, prior to cell division

Consist of
- Nuclear envelope:
  - Formed from two layers of plasma membrane
- Nucleoplasm, containing:
  - Chromatin
    - DNA
    - Associated proteins
  - Nucleolus

NUCLEAR ENVELOPE

General
Separates the nucleoplasm from the cytoplasm

Structure
- Two layers of plasma membrane surrounding the nucleus
- Perforated by nuclear pores:
  - The two layers of plasma membrane are continuous at the nuclear pores.

Consist of
- Outer membrane:
  - Associated with multiple ribosomes on the outer surface
  - Continuous with the membrane of the rough endoplasmic reticulum (rER)
- Perinuclear cistern:
  - 15 nm wide space between the outer and the inner membrane
  - Continuous with the lumen of the rER
- Inner membrane:
  - Inner surface is lined with the nuclear lamina.

Function

Selective permeable barrier:

- Permeable to:
  - Fat-soluble molecules ⎤
  - Small, uncharged water-soluble ⎬ Transverse the membrane
    molecules ⎦ by simple diffusion
- Relatively impermeable to:
  - Large water-soluble molecules ⎤ Only cross the nuclear
  - Charged water-soluble molecules ⎦ envelope via the nuclear
    pore complex (see below)

Light microscopy

- The nuclear envelope is too thin to be visualized in the light microscope.
- It is however often seen as a thin dark line surrounding cells, as it has, e.g., been cut obliquely during preparation.

Nuclear lamina

Structure

Formed from nuclear lamins:

- A type of intermediate filaments
- Organized into a strong orthogonal framework

Function

Provide mechanical support for:

- The inner membrane of the nuclear envelope
- Nuclear pore complexes
- Chromatin structures

Nuclear pores

General

- Holes in the nuclear envelope:
  - Make up 15 % of the nuclear envelope surface area.
- In the circumference of the pores, the outer and inner membranes fuse.

Structure

- ⊘ 70–80 nm.
- Each pore contains a large cylindrical multiunit protein complex, the nuclear pore complex.

Function
Bidirectional transportation of proteins, ribonucleoproteins, and RNAs:
- Large molecules:
  - Are transported through the nuclear pore complex by active transport.
  - Molecules are transported if they are "tagged" with:
    - A nuclear localization sequence → import into the nucleus
    - A nuclear export sequence → export from the nucleus
- Smaller water-soluble molecules <9 Da:
  - Simple diffusion through H_2O-filled channels in the nuclear pore complex

NUCLEOPLASM

Chromatin

General
- Formed from:
  - DNA
  - Associated proteins
- The associated proteins mediate folding and packing of DNA into chromatin:
  - This organizes the long DNA molecules (≈2 m in total) into the nucleus
    (◯ 5–10 µm).

Consist of
- DNA:
  - A double helix of two single-stranded DNA molecules
  - ◯ 2 nm
- Associated proteins:
  - Histone proteins:
    - Assemble into nucleosomes, together with DNA
    - Pack the DNA into compact chromatin fibrils
  - Nonhistone proteins:
    - Pack the chromatin fibrils into chromatin fibers
    - For example, proteins of the nuclear matrix, a protein "scaffold" onto
      which chromatin fibrils are anchored

Divided into (Table 4.1)
In cells not undergoing active cell division, chromatin is found in two forms:
- Heterochromatin
- Euchromatin

Heterochromatin

General
- Condensed chromatin: tightly packed loops of chromatin fibers.
- Gene transcription is inactive.

Divided into
- Constitutive heterochromatin:
  ○ Regions of genetically inactive DNA
  ○ Permanently in the form of heterochromatin
  ○ Similar pattern in all cell types, e.g., the DNA regions near the centromeres and telomeres
- Facultative heterochromatin:
  ○ Regions of genetically active DNA, which is rendered transcriptionally inactive by the packaging into heterochromatin.
  ○ Can be converted into euchromatin.
  ○ Pattern differs between cells, e.g., the DNA regions containing tissue-specific genes.

Light microscopy
- Seen as dense basophilic bodies
- Found in three characteristic locations in the nucleus:
  ○ Marginal chromatin:
    ▪ Heterochromatin located just below the nuclear envelope
  ○ Karyosomes:
    ▪ Discrete heterochromatin bodies in the nucleoplasm
  ○ Nucleolar-associated chromatin:
    ▪ Heterochromatin surrounding the nucleolus

Euchromatin

General
- Extended chromatin: loosely arranged loops of chromatin fibers.
- Gene transcription is active.

Light microscopy
Seen as weakly basophilic (light) areas of the nucleus

Table 4.1 Overview of heterochromatin and euchromatin

	Heterochromatin	Euchromatin
Form	Condensed chromatin: Tightly packed loops of chromatin fibers	Extended chromatin: Loosely arranged loops of chromatin fibers
Gene transcription	Inactive	Active
Association of DNA to histones in nucleosomes	• DNA is tightly associated to histones • DNA is not accessible to gene transcription	• DNA is loosely associated to histones • DNA is accessible to gene transcription
Light microscopy	Densely basophilic clumps	Weakly basophilic (light) areas

MEMO-BOX

The chromatin pattern of a cell resembles its gene transcription activity:
- Low transcriptional activity or transcription of few genes → large regions of DNA in the form of heterochromatin → dark nucleus
- Transcription of multiple genes → large regions of DNA in the form of euchromatin → pale nucleus

MEMO-BOX

Euchromatin: **Extended** chromatin

Nucleosomes

Structure
- Small units of DNA and histones
- ⊘ 10 nm

Function
- Packing of DNA into:
  1. Chromatin filament, ◌ 11 nm:
     - The DNA coils 1.65 times (147 base pairs) around histone core, forming a nucleosome
     - Nucleosomes lie as "beads on a string" on the ◌ 2 nm DNA molecules, separated by stretches of ≈50 base pairs of DNA (called "linker DNA")
  2. Chromatin fibrils, ◌ 30 nm:
     - Formed by coiling of the chromatin filament
- Regulation of gene transcription:
  - The histones are modified, e.g., methylated or acetylated, which makes the DNA more or less accessible to gene transcription

Consists of
- Core of histones:
  - Eight histones, a pair of each: H2A, H2B, H3, and H4
  - Histones are positively charged → adhere strongly to the negatively charged DNA
- DNA:
  - Coils 1.65 times around the histone core

Packing of chromatin

General
Chromatin is highly packed to fit within the nucleus (Table 4.2 and Fig. 4.1).

Epigenetic marks

General
- Chemical modifications of the chromatin
- Do not change the sequence of the DNA (the genetic code)
- E.g.:
  - DNA methylations
  - Histone modifications, e.g., histone methylation or acetylation

Function
Regulation of the gene transcription activity

Table 4.2 Packing of chromatin

⊘	Type	Formation	Approximate packing ratio
2 nm	DNA	A double helix of two single-stranded DNA molecules	–
11 nm	Chromatin filament, "beads on a string"	DNA coils 1.65 times around a histone core forming nucleosomes	6×
30 nm	Chromatin fibril	Coiling of the chromatin filament	40×
300 nm	Chromatin fiber	Loops of chromatin fibril, anchored to the nuclear matrix (flexible protein "scaffold")	1,000×
700 nm	Condensed chromatin fiber	Loops of chromatin fiber kept together by condensins	
1,400 nm	• Fully condensed chromosome • Only formed during mitosis	Tight coiling of the condensed chromatin fiber	10,000×

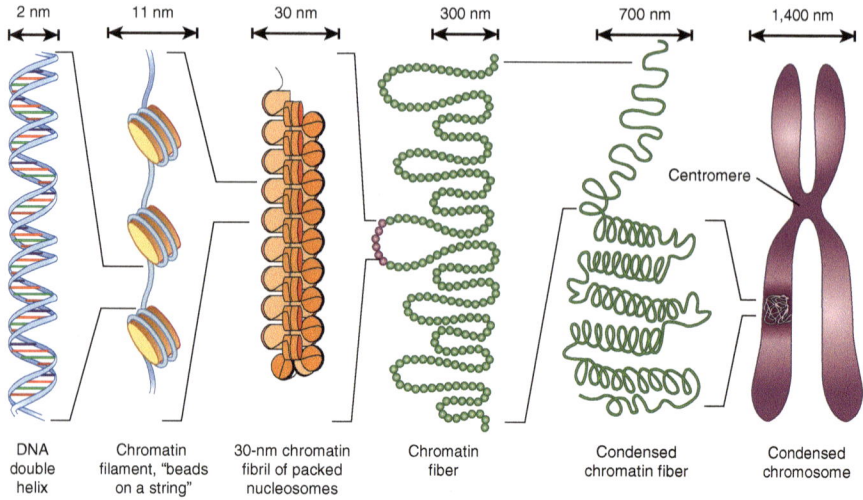

Fig. 4.1 Chromatin packing: the packing of DNA into highly ordered chromatin structures

Formation
- Formed and changed (reprogrammed) during cell differentiation
- Copied in S-phase and transmitted to daughter cells after mitosis, i.e., epigenetic marks are inherited to daughter cells
- Erased to a high degree during meiosis and immediately after fertilization, i.e., epigenetic marks are "reset" in offspring

Nucleolus

General
- Element within the nucleus
- Contains loops of chromatin, which hold DNA regions with ribosomal genes
- One to four nucleoli per nucleus

Structure
- $\varnothing$ up to 1 μm
- Spherical to ovoid

Function
- Transcription of ribosomal RNA (rRNA)
- Site of initial ribosome assembly

> **MEMO-BOX**
> Large protein synthesis requires abundant ribosomes → large nucleolus or multiple nucleoli

Light microscopy
- Seen as a distinct basophilic body within the nucleus
- Surrounded by a basophilic ring of heterochromatin
- Sometimes hidden within areas of heterochromatin

Lifecycle of Cells

General
- Cells arise from preexisting cells through cell division.
- Homeostasis of cell populations is maintained through a balance between cell division and cell death.

Divided into
- Interphase:
  - During this period the cell is not undergoing active cell division.
  - Cells spend most of their time in interphase.
- Cell division:
  - Mitosis:
    - Most common type of cell division
    - Gives rise to two genetically and epigenetically identical daughter cells, containing two copies of each chromosome (diploid, 2n)
  - Meiosis:
    - Specialized type of cell division, only found in germ cells
    - Gives rise to four genetically unique daughter cells, containing only a single copy of each chromosome (haploid, 1n)
- Cell death:
  - Necrosis:
    - Cell death following irreversible damage to the cell, e.g., hypoxia
  - Apoptosis:
    - Regulated cell death

Cell Populations

Divided into
- Somatic cells
- Germ cells

Somatic cells

General
- All non-germ cells
- Can only undergo mitosis
- Diploid cells, i.e., containing two copies of each chromosome (2n)

Divided into
Based on mitotic activity, somatic cells are divided into:
- Static cell population:
  - Cells are permanently in G_0-phase (terminally differentiated, G_{TD})
  - Unable to undergo cell division
  - For example, neurons
- Stable cell population:
  - Cells are in G_0-phase
  - Can be stimulated to reenter G_1-phase and undergo cell division
  - For example, hepatocytes
- Renewing cell population:
  - Cells regularly undergoing cell division
  - For example, the stem cells of epidermis

Germ cells

General
- The only human cell type that undergoes meiosis
- Located in the gonads:
  - Testes in males
  - Ovaries in females

Function
Gives rise to the gametes, i.e., oocytes or sperm cells
- Gametes are:
  - Formed by meiosis
  - Haploid cells, i.e., containing a single copy of each chromosome (1n)

> **MEMO-BOX**
> G_0: "**0**" as in **O**utside cell cycle → not undergoing cell division

CELL CYCLE

General
- A regulated sequence of events that controls cell growth and division
- Lasts about 24 h in cells undergoing cell division (Table 4.3)
- Includes several checkpoints that:
  - Control the transition between stages
  - Respond to internal and external signals

Divided into (Table 4.3, Fig. 4.2)
- Interphase:
  - During this period of the cell cycle, the cell is not in active cell division.
  - Cells spend most of their time in this phase.
- Mitosis:
  - During this period of the cell cycle, the cell is undergoing active cell division.

Table 4.3 Cell Cycle

Principal phase	Phase	Approximate duration
Interphase	G_1-phase	10 h (very variable)
	S-phase	10 h
	G_2-phase	4 h
Mitosis	M-phase	1 h

Fig. 4.2 The phases of the cell cycle

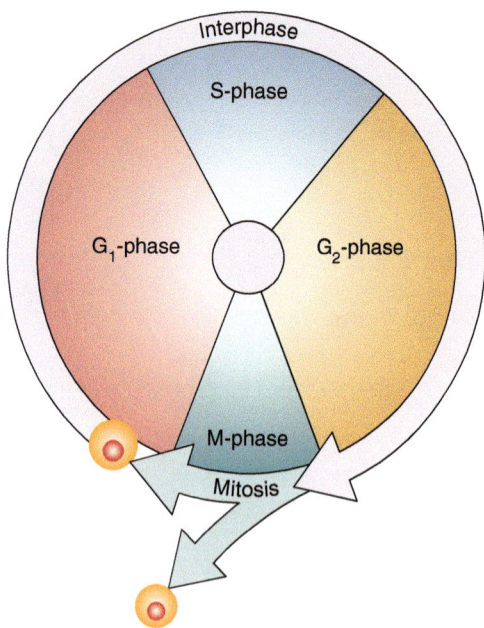

Regulation of cell cycle

Cell cycle is regulated by cyclin–cyclin-dependent kinase (CDK) complexes:

- Different pairs of cyclin–CDK complexes are formed in cyclic levels, corresponding to the stages of the cell cycle.
- Cyclin–CDK complexes control the cell cycle through phosphorylation of regulatory proteins.

> **MEMO-BOX**
> Remember the six **C**s: **C**ell **C**ycle is **C**ontrolled by **C**yclin–**C**DK **C**omplexes.

The Phases of the Cell Cycle

Divided into (Table 4.4)

- Interphase
  - G$_1$-phase
  - S-phase
  - G$_2$-phase
- Mitosis
  - M-phase

Table 4.4 Phases of the cell cycle

Phase	Overall function	Events	Checkpoints

G_1-phase	Growth	Production of cellular components, e.g., RNA and protein needed for DNA replication	• G_1 DNA damage checkpoint:
			  ○ Monitors integrity of DNA
			• Restriction checkpoint:
			  ○ Evaluation of the cells replicative potential
			  ○ Sensitive to
			    ▪ Cell size
			    ▪ Cell state, e.g., its nutritive state
			    ▪ Extracellular signals, e.g., growth factors
			    ▪ Interactions with the extracellular matrix

S-phase	Synthesis of DNA	• Chromatin replication:
		  ○ DNA replication (synthesis of DNA) → two identical copies of DNA
		  ○ Replication of nucleosomes → transmit epigenetic marks on histones to daughter cells (part of the epigenetic inheritance)
		• Centrosome duplication → two centrosomes
			S_1 DNA damage checkpoint:
			• Monitors quality of the replicated DNA

G_2-phase	Growth	• Production of cellular components, e.g., protein needed for cell division
		• Reorganization of organelles
			• G_2 DNA damage checkpoint:
			  ○ Monitors DNA quality
			• Unreplicated DNA checkpoint:
			  ○ Prevents entry into M-phase before DNA replication is complete

M-phase	Mitosis	Mitosis, containing two processes:
		• Karyokinesis: division of the nucleus
		• Cytokinesis: division of the cytoplasm/cell
			• Spindle assembly checkpoint:
			  ○ Prevents entry into anaphase before:
			    ▪ The mitotic spindle has correctly attached to chromosomes
			    ▪ Chromosomes are correctly placed in metaphase plate
			• Chromosome segregation checkpoint:
			  ○ Prevents cytokinesis before chromosomes have been properly separated

MEMO-BOX
- G-phases: "**G**" stands for **G**ap/**G**rowth
- S-phase: "**S**" stands for **S**ynthesis of DNA (replication)
- M-phase: "**M**" stands for **M**itosis
- **C**ytokinesis: Division of the **C**ytoplasm/**C**ell

MITOSIS

General
- Most common type of cell division
- Gives rise to two genetically and epigenetically identical daughter cells, containing two copies of each chromosome (diploid, 2n)

Function
Proliferation of cells, e.g., mediating:
- Growth of tissues
- Maintenance of cell populations
- Repair of injuries

Divided into
- Karyokinesis
  - Division of the nucleus.
  - The two identical copies of chromatin (formed during S-phase) are divided into two newly formed nuclei.
- Cytokinesis:
  - Division of the cytoplasm/cell.
  - Each of the two daughter cells contains one newly formed nucleus.

Consists of (Tables 4.5 and 4.6, Fig. 4.3)
- Prophase
  - Prometaphase (the last part of prophase)
- Metaphase
- Anaphase
- Telophase

Table 4.5 The phases of mitosis

Phase	Begins with	Events
Prophase	Chromosomes condense and become visible	• Chromatin is packed tightly into chromosomes: 　○ Each chromosome consists of two identical sister chromatids: 　　▪ Linked at the centromere 　　▪ Bound together by cohesins • The two centrosomes move towards opposite cell poles • The mitotic spindle forms from the centrosomes: 　○ Polar microtubules: 　　▪ Extend from one cell pole towards the opposite cell pole 　○ Astral microtubules: 　　▪ Radiate out from each centrosome 　　▪ Attach to the inner surface of the plasma membrane 　○ Kinetochore microtubules (see prometaphase)
Prometaphase	Nuclear envelope disappears	• Nuclear lamins are phosphorylated → nuclear lamina disassemble → nuclear envelope disintegrates into vesicles • Polar and astral microtubules move the two centrosomes apart, towards opposite cell poles, using motor proteins • A protein complex called a kinetochore is formed on each sister chromatid opposite to the centromere: 　○ Kinetochore microtubules binds to kinetochores (30–40 microtubules per kinetochore) 　○ Kinetochore microtubules move chromosomes into metaphase/equatorial plate, using motor proteins • The nucleolus disappears
Metaphase	Chromosomes align in the metaphase/equatorial plate	Chromosomes: • Align in the metaphase plate • Are in their most condensed state

(continued)

Table 4.5 (continued)

Phase	Begins with	Events
Anaphase	The initial separation of sister chromatids	• Cohesins are cleaved → centromere of chromosomes split and sister chromatids are pulled towards opposite cell poles: ○ Mediated by the kinetochore microtubules and dynein motor proteins • Cell poles move further apart → elongates the cell ○ Mediated by the polar microtubules and kinesin motor proteins • Organelles are distributed to the two cell poles

Telophase	The nuclear envelopes reappear	• A nuclear envelope is formed at each cell pole
		• Chromosomes decondense within the newly formed nuclei and are no longer visible
		• The nucleoli reappear
		• Cytokinesis (division of cytoplasm):
		 ○ A cleavage furrow between the cell poles is formed by a contractile ring just below the plasma membrane:
		  ▪ Actin filaments
		  ▪ Myosin II filaments
		 ○ Contraction of the ring → division of the cell into two daughter cells

Table 4.6 Overview of mitosis

Phase	Chromosomes	Nuclear envelope	Nucleolus
Prophase	Condensate and become visible	–	–
Prometaphase	–	Disappears	Disappears
Metaphase	Arranged in metaphase plate	–	–
Anaphase	Sister chromatids are separated	–	–
Telophase	Decondensate and are no longer visible	Reappears	Reappears

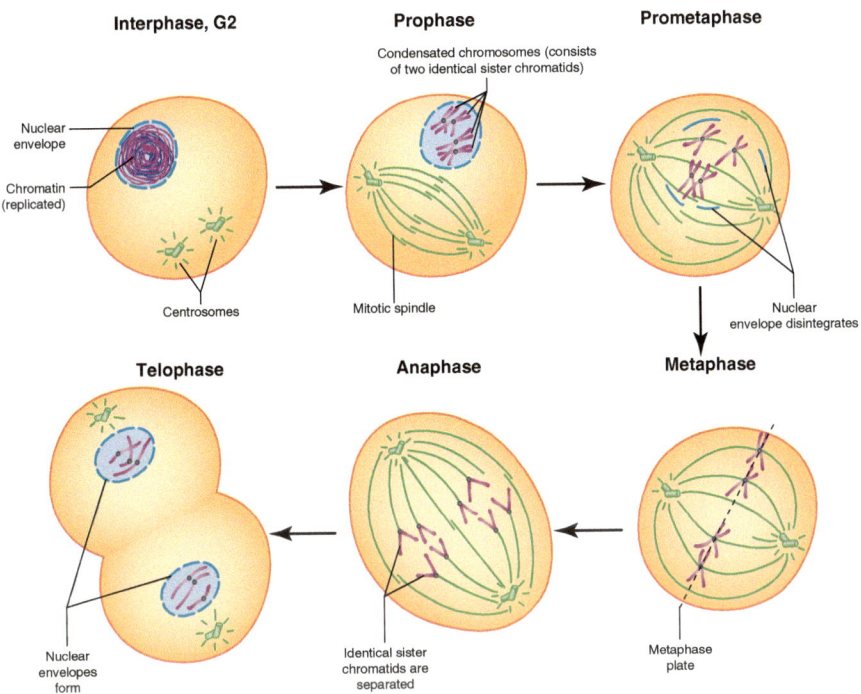

Fig. 4.3 Mitosis: key events taking place during each phase of mitosis

MEMO-BOX
- The phases of mitosis are remembered by:
  - "**I** **P**assed **M**y **A**natomy **T**est," corresponding to **I**nterphase, **P**rophase, **M**etaphase, **A**naphase, **T**elophase
- **Interphase**: Chromosomes are **I**nvisible
- **Prophase**: Chromosomes are **P**erceivable (visible)
- **Metaphase**: Chromosomes in **M**etaphase/**M**iddle plane
- **Anaphase**: Chromosomes move **A**way from each other
- **Telophase**: Cell is split in **T**wo

MEMO-BOX
- **Cohesins**: Named after "**cohes**ion" → **cohere** sister chromatids together
- **Kinetochore microtubules**: attach to **K**inetochores
- **Polar microtubules**: extend from cell **P**ole to cell **P**ole
- **Astral microtubules**: **Astr**on is Greek for star → radiate out from each centrosome like a star

> **MEMO-BOX**
> The cell must first be elongated, before it can be split into two, analogous to when you need an elongated balloon to make balloon animals.

MEIOSIS

General
- Specialized type of cell division, only found in germ cells
- Gives rise to four genetically unique daughter cells, containing only a single copy of each chromosome (haploid, 1n)

Consists of
Two sequential meiotic divisions:
- First meiotic division (meiosis I)
  - Resembles mitosis
  - Preceded by interphase I
    - Includes the S-phase → DNA is replicated
- Second meiotic division (meiosis II)
  - Process identical to mitosis
  - Preceded by interphase II:
    - Lacks the S-phase → no DNA replication

Function
Development of gametes from germ cells:
- Induction of genetic diversity in gametes:
  - Genetic exchange between pairs of homologues (paternal and maternal) chromosomes takes place.
  - Homologues maternal and paternal chromosomes are randomly distributed to daughter cells.
- Reduction of the number of chromosome sets in gamete:
  - The two sequential meiotic divisions, only preceded by a single S-phase, reduce the number of chromosome sets to half from diploid (2n) to haploid (1n).

Divided into
- Interphase I
- First meiotic division
- Interphase II
- Second meiotic division

Genetic exchange during meiosis

General
- Genetic exchange (DNA recombination) between non-sister chromatids of the pairs of homologues (paternal and maternal) chromosomes
- Takes place during the prophase I of the first meiotic division

Divided into
- Recombination without chromosomal crossing-over:
  - Most common
  - Exchange of smaller DNA segments, without crossing-over occurring
- Recombination with chromosomal crossing-over:
  - Exchange of larger DNA segments
  - Chromosomal crossing-over takes place, forming chiasmata

Formation (Fig. 4.4)
1. Formation of double-stranded DNA breaks in chromatids
2. Paring of homologous chromosomes
3. Strand invasion: a bare ended single DNA strand of the broken DNA of a chromatid invades the DNA of the homologous non-sister chromatid.
4. DNA recombination: the invading single DNA strand is elongated by DNA synthesis using the DNA of the non-sister chromatid as a template.
5. The elongated single DNA strand, which now contains DNA segments from the non-sister chromatid, can either do A or B:
   (A) Returns to its origin → crossing-over does not take place.
   (B) Swap place with a single DNA strand of the chromatid that it is invading → crossing-over commonly takes place.

Reduction in number of chromosome sets during meiosis

The number of chromosome sets (ploidy):
- Is reduced during the first meiotic division:
  - From diploid (2n) germ cell:
    - Two sets of chromosomes:
      - One maternal and one paternal set
  - To haploid (1n) gamete, i.e., oocyte or sperm cell:
    - One set of chromosomes
      - With random representation of maternal and paternal chromosomes
- Is restored after fertilization, as fertilization doubles the number of chromosome sets:
  - Oocyte (1n) + sperm cell (1n) = zygote (2n)

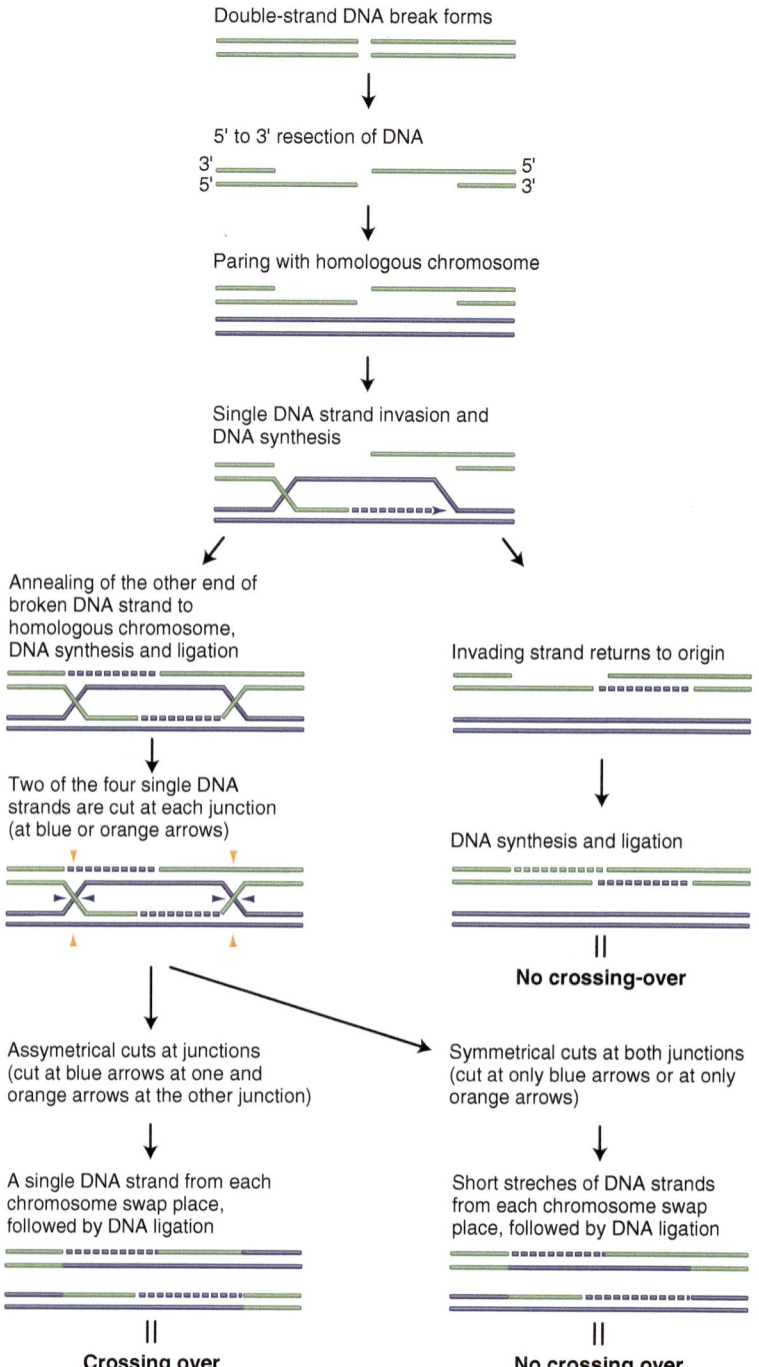

Fig. 4.4 DNA recombination taking place between nonidentical sister chromatids, with and without crossing-over taking place

The Phases of Meiosis

Interphase I
- Similar to the interphase of mitosis.
- DNA is replicated during S-phase.

First meiotic division

General
- Called a reductional division, as the number of chromosome sets is reduced from diploid (2n) to haploid (1n).
- Genetic exchange takes place.
- Homologues maternal and paternal chromosomes are randomly distributed to daughter cells.

Divided into (Tables 4.7 and 4.8, Fig. 4.5)
- Prophase I
  - Leptotene
  - Zygotene
  - Pachytene
  - Diplotene
  - Diakinesis
- Metaphase I
- Anaphase I
- Telophase I

Interphase II
- Short duration
- Lacks S-phase, i.e., no DNA replication takes place

Second meiotic division

General
- Process identical to mitosis
  - Cohesins are cleaved in anaphase II → centromeres of the chromosomes split and sister chromatids are separated.
- Is called an equatorial division, as the sister chromatids are transmitted equally to the two daughter cells (gametes):
  - The two sister chromatids of each chromosome are no longer identical, due to the genetic exchange during the first meiotic division.
  - The four chromatids of each bivalent, of the first meiotic division, are distributed to four gametes:
    - In males: four sperm cells
    - In females: one mature oocyte and two polar bodies, as the firstly formed polar body does not divide any further (Chap. 25)
  - Each gamete then contains a single (haploid), genetically unique set of chromosomes, with random representation of maternal and paternal chromosomes.

Function

Separation of the sister chromatids into two daughter cells (gametes)

Divided into

- Prophase II
- Metaphase II
- Anaphase II
- Telophase II

Table 4.7 The phases of meiosis

Phase	Events	Function
Prophase I:		Genetic exchange
• Leptotene	• The chromosomes condense and become visible • Double-stranded DNA breaks form in chromatids • Pairing of homologous (maternal/paternal) chromosomes → bivalents, each consisting of four chromatids, i.e.: ○ One paternal chromosome, consisting of two identical sister chromatids ○ One maternal chromosome, consisting of two identical sister chromatids	
• Zygotene	• Paired chromosomes attach parallel to each other • Synapsis formation is initiated between the chromosomes, as a synaptonemal complex binds the chromosomes tightly together	
• Pachytene	• Completion of the synapsis • The synaptonemal complex mediates genetic exchange: ○ DNA recombination takes place between the non-sister chromatids of the paired chromosomes (Fig. 4.4)	
• Diplotene	• Separation of the paired chromosomes, as the synaptonemal complex dissolves • Chiasmata are sites where crossing-over has occurred and the paired chromosomes remain attached (Fig. 4.6): ○ At least 1 and commonly 2–3 chiasmata are seen per bivalent	
• Diakinesis	• The nucleolus disappears • The nuclear envelope disintegrates	

(continued)

Table 4.7 (continued)

Phase	Events	Function
Metaphase I	• The paired homologous chromosomes are arranged in the metaphase plane • Kinetochores on sister chromatids are bound together and face the same cell pole	Whole chromosomes are separated

Anaphase I	• Chiasmata are cleaved → maternal and paternal chromosomes separate and are pulled towards opposite cell poles:
	  ○ Homologues maternal and paternal chromosomes are randomly distributed to daughter cells
	• Cohesins are not cleaved → sister chromatids remain together
	• Daughter cells receive 23 single chromosomes, consisting of two sister chromatids:
	  ○ Due to the genetic exchange in prophase I, the sister chromatids are no longer identical	

Telophase I	Similar to that of mitosis	Two genetically unique daughter cells are formed

Table 4.8 Differences between first meiotic division and mitosis

	Meiosis I	Mitosis
Occurs in	Germ cells only	Somatic cells and germ cells
Genetic exchange between homologous chromosomes	+	−
Structures aligned in metaphase plate	Paired homologous chromosomes (bivalents), consisting of four chromatids, i.e.: • One paternal chromosome, consisting of two nonidentical sister chromatids • One maternal chromosome, consisting of two nonidentical sister chromatids	Chromosomes, consisting of two identical sister chromatids
Kinetochores	Kinetochores on sister chromatids are bound together and face the same cell pole	Kinetochores on sister chromatids face opposite cell poles
Cohesins	Not cleaved → sister chromatids remain together	Cleaved → sister chromatids split
Separation of	Whole chromosomes, each consisting of two nonidentical sister chromatids	The two identical sister chromatids of the chromosomes
Distribution of homologous maternal and paternal chromosomes	Randomly distributed	Equally distributed
Number of chromosome sets in daughter cell	One set of chromosomes, i.e., haploid (1n)	Two sets of chromosomes, i.e., diploid (2n)
Daughter cell genotype	Genetically unique	Genetically identical
Epigenetic marks	Not inherited fully to the daughter cells	Inherited to the daughter cells

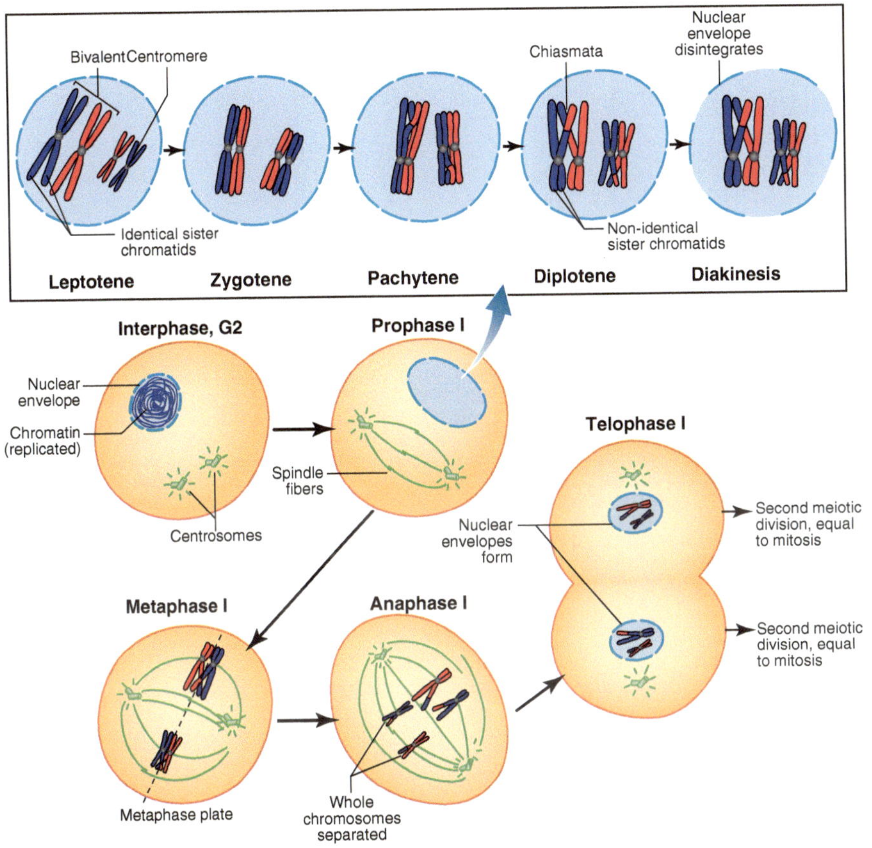

Fig. 4.5 First meiotic division: key events taking place during each phase of the first meiotic division (meiosis I)

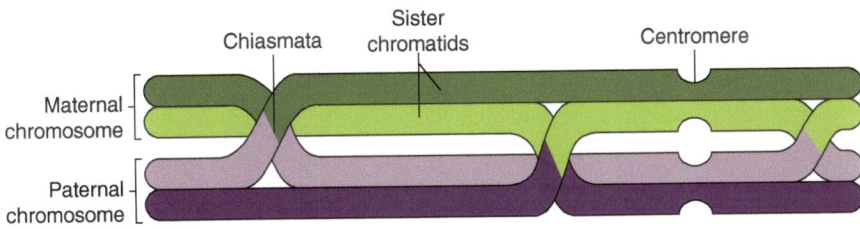

Fig. 4.6 Chromosomal crossing-over in one bivalent: Chiasmata are sites where crossing-over has occurred. Two to four of the chromatids of a bivalent participates in chromosomal crossing-over

CELL DEATH

Divided into (Table 4.9)
- Necrosis
- Apoptosis

Table 4.9 Overview of cell death

	Necrosis	Apoptosis
Initiating cause	Irreversible cell damage, e.g., hypoxia	Various stimuli, e.g., DNA damage
Process	Pathological	Physiological
Plasma membrane	Ruptures → cell contents spread to intercellular space	Intact
Inflammation	Induced in surrounding tissue	No inflammation

Necrosis

General
- Cell death following irreversible damage to the cell, e.g., hypoxia
- A pathological process:
  1. Plasma membrane ruptures
  2. Cellular contents spread to the intercellular space
  3. Inflammation in the surrounding tissue

Apoptosis

General
- Regulated cell death
- A physiological process
  - Regulated by:
    - Internal stimuli, e.g., DNA damage
    - External stimuli, e.g., lack of signals from extracellular matrix
- The plasma membrane remains intact, during the process, why inflammation is avoided.

Function
Removal of cells, e.g.:
- During embryonic development
- Senescent cells

Consist of
Stimulation of apoptosis initiates a suicide program in the cell, consisting of six
steps:
1. Fragmentation of DNA
2. Shrinkage of cell
3. Loss of mitochondrial function and release of cytochrome c from the
   mitochondria to the cytoplasm
4. Initiation of caspase cascade by cytochrome c
5. Formation of numerous blebs in the plasma membrane
6. Separation of cell into large vesicles (apoptotic bodies), which are
   phagocytized by macrophages

References

1, 5, 19, 24, 33, 34, 37.

Part III
Histology of Tissues

Chapter 5
Epithelial Tissue

General
One of the four basic tissue types

Structure
- Closely apposed cells facing free surfaces
- Abundant and well-developed cell junctions → cells adhere to each other
- Avascular
  ○ Nourished from blood vessels in underlying connective tissue
- Rests on basement membrane, which separates epithelial tissue from connective tissue
- Simple epithelia often have polarized cells:
  ○ Cell membrane is divided by tight junctions into:
    ▪ Apical domain: face the free surface
    ▪ Basolateral domain:
      • Lateral domain: communicate with neighboring epithelial cells
      • Basal domain: rests on the basement membrane

© Springer International Publishing Switzerland 2017
A. Rehfeld et al., *Compendium of Histology*, DOI 10.1007/978-3-319-41873-5_5

Divided into
- Surface epithelium
- Glandular epithelium:
  - Forms the secretory portion of glands
  - Described in Chap. 6

Surface Epithelium

General
- Covers outer body surfaces, as the epidermis
- Lines body tubes, which communicate with the exterior, as the epithelium of mucous membranes
- Lines internal closed cavities, e.g.:
  - Blood and lymph vessels, as the endothelium
  - Pericardial, pleural, and peritoneal cavities, as the mesothelium
- Exposed to abundant mechanical stress ⎤
- Fast regeneration via stem cells   ⎦ High cell turnover rate

Divided into (Table 5.1)
Surface epithelium is classified by:
- Number of layers
  - Simple: one layer
  - Pseudostratified: one layer, but appears to have several layers
  - Stratified: multiple layers
- Shape of cells at surface
  - Squamous: height < width
  - Cuboidal: height ≈ width
  - Columnar: height > width

Function
- Simple epithelium:
  - Selective permeable barrier, e.g., in the endothelium
  - Absorption, e.g., in intestinal epithelium
  - Secretion, e.g., in kidney tubules
  - Transport:
    - Along epithelial surface (with the help of cilia), e.g., in respiratory epithelium
    - Across epithelium (transcytosis), e.g., in the endothelium
- Stratified epithelium:
  - Barrier function, e.g., in the epidermis (Chap. 20)
    - Mechanical barrier
    - Selective permeable barrier
    - Against microorganisms, evaporation, and UV radiation
  - Sensation, with the help of sensory receptors, e.g., in the epidermis (Chap. 20)

Light Microscopy
See Table 5.1.

Table 5.1 Surface epithelia and their location

		Squamous	Cuboidal	Columnar
Simple	Light microscopy	• Flat cells (height < width) • Central flattened nucleus	• Height ≈ width • Central round nucleus	• Height > width • Nuclei in same level in neighboring cells (commonly located basally)
	Location	For example, endothelium	For example, kidney tubule epithelium	For example, intestinal epithelium
Pseudostratified	Light microscopy	–	–	• Height > width • All cells touch basement membrane, but only some cells reach apical surface → nuclei in different levels in neighboring cells
	Location	–	–	For example, respiratory tract epithelium
Stratified	Light microscopy	Cells gradually flatten towards the surface: • Basal layer: one layer of basophilic cuboidal/ columnar cells • Middle layers: Polyhedral cells • Superficial layers: Squamous cells	• Multiple cell layers • Superficial cells are cuboidal	• Multiple cell layers • Superficial cells are columnar
	Location	Exists in two forms: • Keratinized: cells in superficial layers have lost their nuclei and are filled up with keratin, e.g., in the epidermis of the skin • Nonkeratinized: superficial cells contain nuclei, e.g., the epithelium the of esophagus	• Rare • For example, epithelium of large ducts of glands	• Rare • For example, epithelium of largest ducts of glands

Urothelium (Transitional Epithelium)

General
- Special stratified epithelium
- Not classified by the shape of cells at surface as other epithelia
- Lines the proximal part of the urinary tract, e.g., the urinary bladder

Structure
- Stratified epithelium.
- Cells of the middle layers have vacuolated cytoplasm and do not gradually flatten towards the surface.
- Superficial cells:
  - Large cells called "umbrella cells" as they cover several of the underlying cells
  - Contains:
    - Apical eosinophilic condensations, caused by many filaments
    - Plaques: areas of thickened apical cell membrane

Function
- Good at distending → found in places where large changes in organ volume occur
- Highly impermeable

Light Microscopy
Changes morphology with degree of distention (Table 5.2)

Table 5.2 Light microscopy of urothelium

		Relaxed state	Distended state
Low magnification		Mucous membrane folded	Mucous membrane smooth
High magnification	Basal layer	Several layers of basophilic cuboidal/ columnar cells	Few layers of basophilic cuboidal cells
	Middle layer	Several layers of pale polyhedral cells	Few/no layers of pale polyhedral cells
	Superficial layer	Large pale rounded cells, convex towards lumen	Large pale cuboidal or flattened cells

Cell Surface Specializations

General
Specializations of the cell surface, mediating various functions

Divided into
- Apical domain specializations:
  - Microvilli
  - Stereocilia
  - Cilia
  - Flagellum
- Lateral domain specializations:
  - Cell-to-cell junctions:
    - Occluding: tight junctions
    - Anchoring:
      - Zonulae adherentes
      - Fasciae adherentes (only in cardiac muscle cells)
      - Desmosomes
    - Communicating: gap junctions
- Basal domain specializations:
  - Basement membrane
  - Cell-to-extracellular matrix (ECM) junctions:
    - Anchoring:
      - Focal adhesions
      - Hemidesmosomes

APICAL DOMAIN SPECIALIZATIONS

Microvilli

General
Thin, small immotile extensions of the cell

Structure
- $\oslash$ 0.1 μm and 1–3 μm long
- Core made from bundle of 20–30 actin filaments, connected to cytoskeleton, and cross-binding proteins

Function

Increase apical surface area up to 20 times → improve absorption from and secretion to the free surface, e.g., in intestinal epithelium

Light Microscopy

- Single microvilli are too thin to be resolved in light microscope.
- Multiple microvilli are seen in the light microscope as a light refracting "striated/brush border."

Stereocilia

General

Thin, long immotile extensions of the cell

Structure

Long bendable microvilli of variable length

Function

- Increase apical surface area → improve absorption from the free surface, e.g., in the epididymis
- Special functions, e.g., in hair cells of the inner ear

Light Microscopy

Stereocilia are seen as long thin extensions in small bundles (resembling hairs of a paint brush) in the light microscope.

Cilia (Kinocilia)

Structure

$\oslash$ 0.25 µm and 5–10 µm long

Consist of (Fig. 5.1)

- Core (axoneme):
  - Cylinder of nine microtubule doublets surrounding a center of two microtubules (9 + 2 structure)
  - Attached to a basal body
- Basal body:
  - Forms basis of cilium
  - Cylinder of nine microtubule triplets

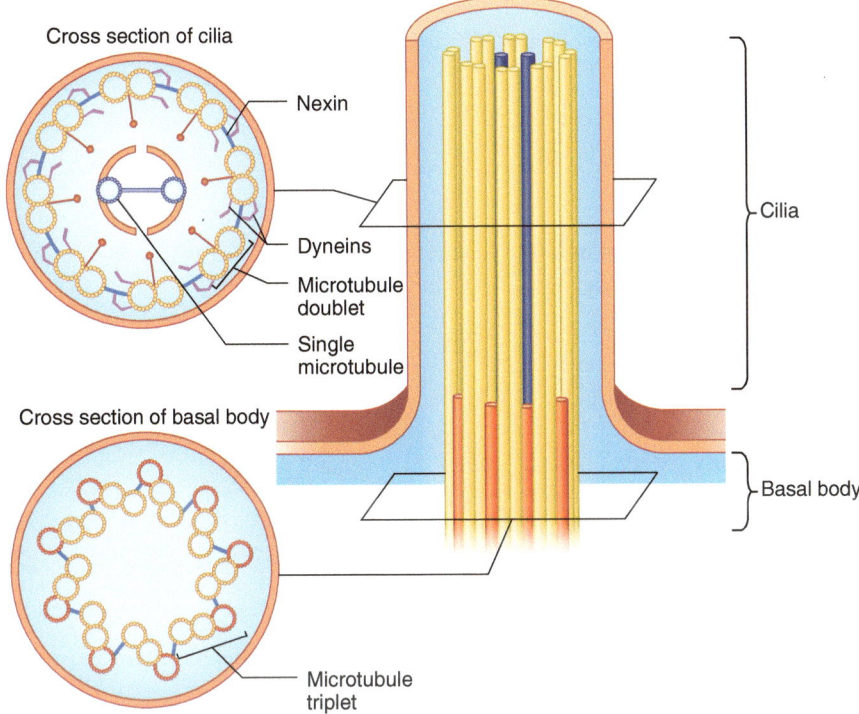

Fig. 5.1 Structure of the cilium: two cross sections, one of the axoneme and one of the basal body, show the structure of the cilium

Formation
- A basal body is formed from a centriole underneath the apical cell membrane.
- Microtubule doublets grow out from the microtubule triplets in the basal body to form the axoneme.

Function
Movement of fluid/mucous on cell surface in one direction, e.g., in the respiratory tract:
- Occurs via coordinated movements of cilia

Movement of cilia
- Microtubule doublets of axoneme are connected to each other with nexin.
- Two motor proteins (dyneins) are attached to each microtubule doublet → can bind to and move along the next microtubule doublet.
- When activated, the dyneins will try to slide one microtubule doublet relative to the other.
- As the microtubule doublets are connected to each other by nexin, the resulting movement is instead a bending of the whole axoneme → cilia bends.

Light Microscopy
Single cilia can be resolved in the light microscope as thin extensions of the apical cell surface.

Primary Cilia

General
Most cells contain one immotile and short primary cilia (9 + 0 structure), which function as a sensor of the extracellular environment.

Flagellum

General
In humans only present on sperm cells

Structure
A single long cilia

Function
Movement of the sperm cell, by undulating movements of the flagellum

LATERAL DOMAIN SPECIALIZATIONS

Light Microscopy
Lateral domain specializations as a group can sometimes be seen as a "terminal bar" in the light microscope, located at the most apical part of the lateral surface.

Occluding Cell Junctions (Tight Junctions, Zonulae Occludentes)

General
Cell junctions, which mainly act to seal off the intercellular space

Structure
- Most apically placed cell junction (Fig. 5.2)
- Form a 0.2 μm-wide belt (zonula) apically around the cell, analogous to the six-pack rings of beverage cans

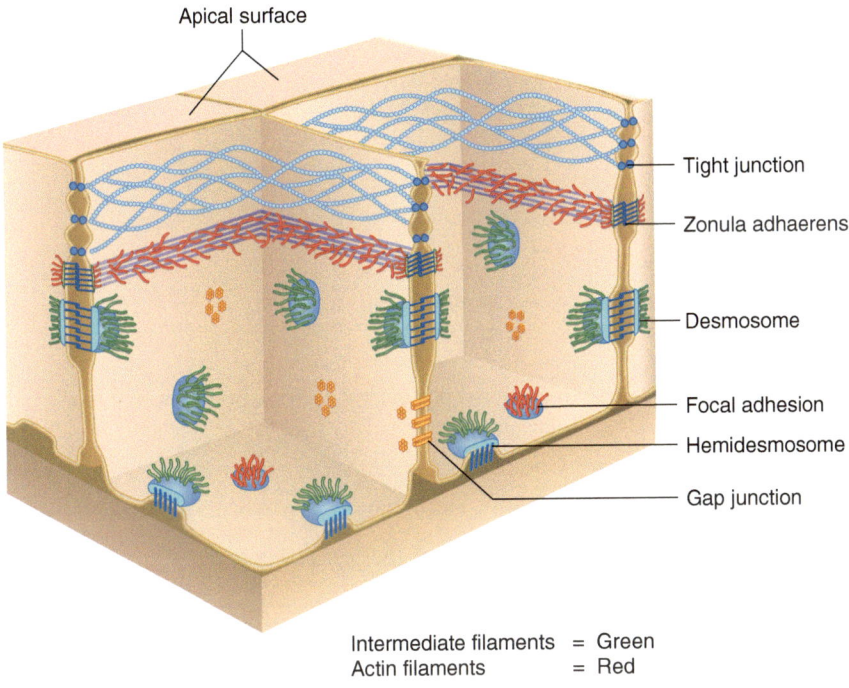

Fig. 5.2 Cell junctions: the cell junctions on the lateral and basal domains

Function
- Barrier of the intercellular space (paracellular pathway) between the cells: permeability depends on composition and amount of strands.
- Polarize cells: divides the cell membrane into an apical and basolateral domain → lateral diffusion of membrane lipids and membrane proteins is confined to each domain.

Consists of
- Transmembrane proteins:
  - Form strands in the plasma membrane
  - Connected intracellularly to the actin cytoskeleton
  - For example, occludins and claudins
- Strands from neighboring cells come together and seal off the intercellular space between the cells.

MEMO-BOX
OCCLUDing cell junction: zonula OCCLUDens
Zonula ocCLudens: formed from ocCLudins and CLaudins

Anchoring Cell Junctions

General
Cell junctions, which mainly act to adhere cells together

Function
Add mechanical strength to tissues: links cytoskeleton in neighboring cells together or to the extracellular matrix

Consist of
- Filaments:
    - Form the intracellular attachment to the cytoskeleton
    - Divided into:
        - Actin filaments
        - Intermediate filaments:
            - Cell junctions with intermediate filaments are stronger than those with actin filaments.
- Plaque:
    - Group of proteins, which form the connection between the filaments and cell adhesion molecules
- Cell adhesion molecules:
    - Transmembrane proteins, which form the contact to other cells or the extracellular matrix
    - Divided into:
        - Cadherins:
            - In cell–cell junctions
            - Form contact with cadherins in neighboring cells
            - Ca^{2+} dependent
        - Integrins:
            - In cell–extracellular matrix junctions
            - Form contact with multiadhesive glycoproteins, e.g., laminins and fibronectin

MEMO-BOX
Cadherins form Cell–Cell junctions and are Ca^{2+} dependent

Divided into
- Cell–cell junctions
  - Zonula adherens
  - Fascia adherens (only in cardiac muscle cells)
  - Desmosome (macula adherens)
- Cell–extracellular matrix junctions (located in basal domain, but described with the other anchoring cell junctions here)
  - Focal adhesion
  - Hemidesmosome

MEMO-BOX
ADHEring contacts: almost all contain **ADHE**sion/**ADHE**rens in their name.

Zonula adherens

General
Forms a belt (zonula) around cells, basal to the tight junction belt (Fig. 5.2)

Consist of
- Actin filaments
- Plaque
- Cadherins

Fascia adherens

General
- Similar to zonula adherens, but only forms a sheet (fascia) in a part of the membrane and not a belt around the entire cell
- Only found in the intercalated discs of cardiac muscle cells

Consist of
- Actin filaments
- Plaque
- Cadherins

Desmosome (macula adherens)

Structure
Point-shaped contact, ⊘ 0.1–0.2 μm (Fig. 5.2)

Consist of
- Intermediate filaments
  - ○ Intermediate filaments are looping through the plaque.
- Plaque
- Cadherins

Focal adhesion

General
- Point-shaped contact at the basal domain (Fig. 5.2).
- Assembly and disassembly of focal adhesions provide basis for cell migration.

Consist of
- Actin filaments
- Plaque
- Integrins

Hemidesmosome

Structure
- Point-shaped contact, ⊘ 0.1–0.2 μm (Fig. 5.2)
- Resembles the desmosome

Consist of
- Intermediate filaments
  - ○ Intermediate filaments are ending in the plaque.
- Plaque
- Integrins

Communicating Cell Junctions (Gap Junctions, Nexuses)

General
Cell junctions, which form channels for transport of small molecules between cells (Fig. 5.2)

Structure
- Group of channels between adjacent cells.
- Each channel is formed from two connexones, one from each cell, which align in the intercellular space.
- Connexones are formed from six circularly arranged connexins.

Function
- Channels for small molecules, e.g., ions.
  - Opening/closing of channels is regulated.
- Allows coordination of adjacent cells, e.g., contraction in cardiac muscle cells.

MEMO-BOX
NEXus consists of six con**NEX**ins, which form one con**NEX**one.

Intercellular Space

General
Spaces between cells

Structure
Intercellular spaces between neighboring cells are formed, as the glycocalyx (negatively charged) on each cell repels each other.

Function
- Site of fluid transfer
- Space for free nerve endings and leukocytes

Lateral surface folds
General
In some epithelial cells, lateral surface folds are found, e.g., in some cells of the intestinal epithelium.

Function
Increase the lateral surface area → improve absorption from and secretion to the intercellular space

BASAL DOMAIN SPECIALIZATIONS

Basement Membrane

Function
- Anchors epithelia to underlying connective tissue
- Passive filter for molecules and cells, e.g., leucocytes
- Affects organization, polarization, and differentiation of epithelial cells
- Forms a structural basis for regeneration of epithelium

Consist of
- Basal lamina (similar to external lamina in non-epithelial tissues)
  - Lamina lucida (preparation artifact)
  - Lamina densa
    - Type IV collagen ($\approx$50 % of protein in basal lamina)
    - Proteoglycans
    - Multiadhesive glycoproteins, e.g., laminins and fibronectin, which bind to both integrins of cell-to-extracellular matrix junctions and collagen → anchors cells to the extracellular matrix
  - Epithelial cells produce the contents of the basal lamina.
- Reticular lamina (lamina reticularis):
  - Reticular fibers in ground substance
  - Anchoring fibrils from the basal lamina loop around the reticular fibers → attach basal lamina to underlying connective tissue.
  - Fibroblasts produce the contents of the reticular lamina, which is a part of the underlying connective tissue.

Light Microscopy
- Rarely seen in HE stain
- Stained with PAS and silver stains → visible in the light microscope

Anchoring Cell Junctions

General
Hemidesmosomes and focal adhesions are described together with the other anchoring cell junctions, under lateral domain specializations (see above).

Basal surface infoldings
General
In some epithelial cells, basal surface infoldings are found, e.g., in kidney tubule epithelium.

Function
Increase the basal surface area → improve absorption and secretion across basal domain of the plasma membrane

Guide to Practical Histology: Surface Epithelium

General
- Avascular
- The cells are densely packed.
- Line "free" surfaces, i.e., always face a lumen or an exterior surface.

Simple Squamous Epithelium

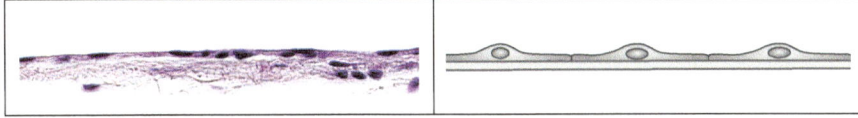

Left: photomicrograph of simple squamous epithelium. Magnification: high. Stain: HE (Courtesy of professor Jørgen Tranum-Jensen, University of Copenhagen). *Right*: simplified illustration of simple squamous epithelium

Characteristics
- Flat cells.
- Height < width.
- Sometimes a small central prominence is seen, containing the flattened nucleus.

Location
For example, endothelium of blood vessels

Simple Cuboidal Epithelium

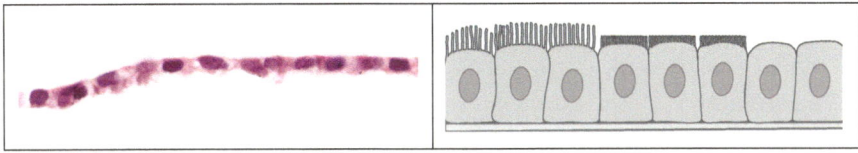

Left: photomicrograph of simple cuboidal epithelium. Magnification: high. Stain: HE (Courtesy of professor Jørgen Tranum-Jensen, University of Copenhagen). *Right*: simplified illustration of simple cuboidal epithelium with apical cilia (left), apical brush border (microvilli) (middle), and without apical specializations (right).

Characteristics
- Height ≈ width
- Central round nucleus, which fills up most of the cell

Location
- Without apical specializations, e.g., in small ducts of glands
- With an apical brush border, e.g., in the kidney tubules
- With apical cilia, e.g., as the ependymal cells of the central nervous system

Can be mistaken for
Low simple columnar epithelium:
- There is a smooth transition between the two types of epithelium.

Simple Columnar Epithelium

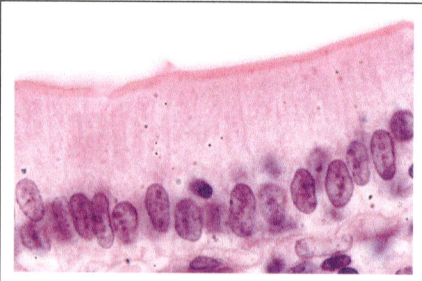 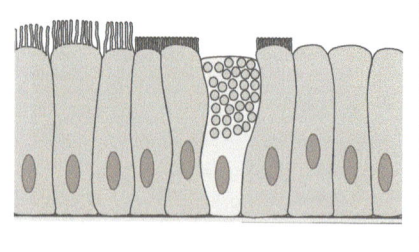

Left: photomicrograph of simple columnar epithelium with a brush border. Magnification: high. Stain: PAS-hematoxylin (Courtesy of professor Jørgen Tranum-Jensen, University of Copenhagen). *Right*: simplified illustration of simple columnar epithelium with apical cilia (left), apical brush border (microvilli) and an interspersed goblet cell (middle), and without apical specializations (right).

Characteristics
- Height > width
- Nuclei in same level in neighboring cells (commonly basally located)

Location
- Without apical specializations, e.g., in smaller ducts of glands
- With an apical brush border and interspersed goblet cells, e.g., in intestinal epithelium
- With apical cilia, e.g., in the uterine tubes

Can be mistaken for
- Pseudostratified columnar epithelium:
  - Cells are normally taller
  - Nuclei in different level in neighboring cells
- High simple cuboidal epithelium:
  - There is a smooth transition between the two types of epithelium.

Pseudostratified Columnar Epithelium

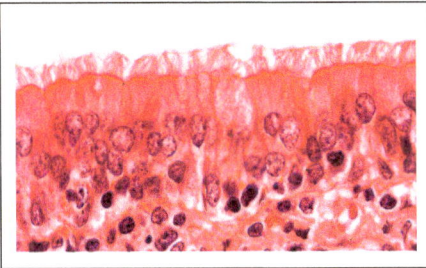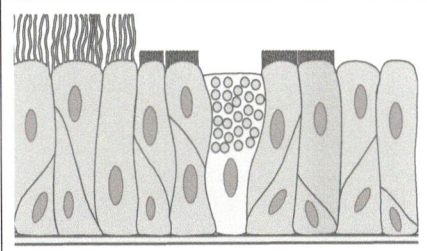

Left: photomicrograph of pseudostratified columnar epithelium with cilia. Magnification: high. Stain: HE (Courtesy of professor Jørgen Tranum-Jensen, University of Copenhagen). *Right*: simplified illustration of pseudostratified columnar epithelium with apical cilia (left), apical brush border (microvilli) and an interspersed goblet cell (middle), and without apical specializations (right).

Characteristics
- Height > width
- All cells touch the basement membrane.
- Only some of the cells reach the apical surface.
- Nuclei are located in different levels in neighboring cells.

Location
- Without apical specializations, e.g., in part of the penile urethra
- With apical cilia and interspersed goblet cells, e.g., in the upper respiratory tract
- With apical stereocilia, e.g., in the ductus epididymidis

Can be mistaken for
- Simple columnar epithelium:
  - Cells are normally shorter.
  - Nuclei are located in the same level in neighboring cells (commonly basally located).
- Stratified columnar epithelium:
  - Not all cells touch the basement membrane.
  - Do not have apical cilia or stereocilia.

Stratified Squamous Epithelium

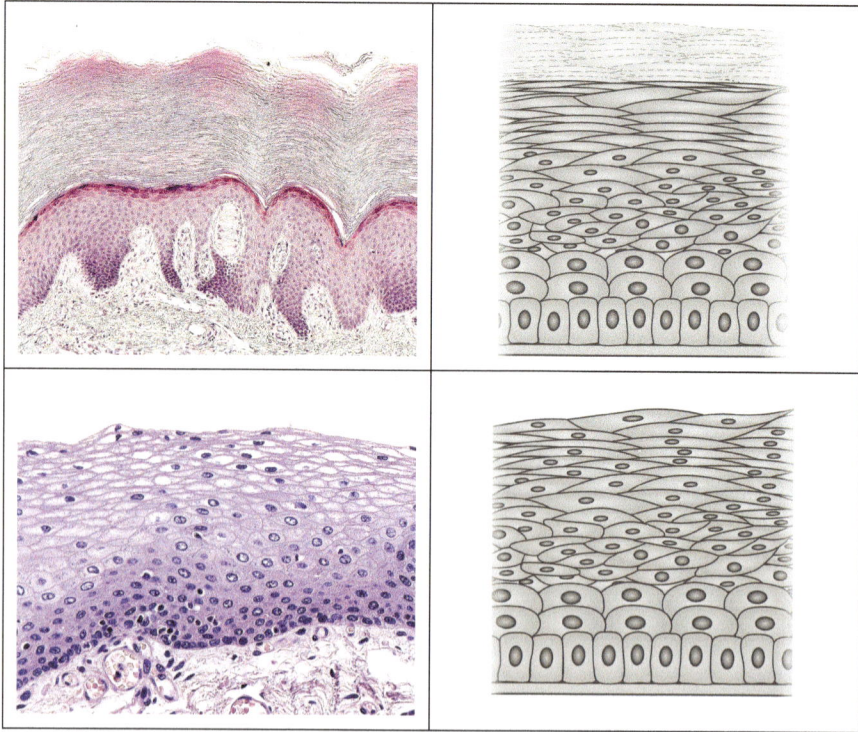

Top left: photomicrograph of stratified squamous keratinized epithelium. Magnification: low. Stain: HE (Courtesy of associate professor Steen Seier Poulsen, University of Copenhagen). *Top right*: simplified illustration of simple squamous keratinized epithelium. *Bottom left*: photomicrograph of stratified squamous nonkeratinized epithelium. Magnification: high. Stain: HE (Courtesy of associate professor Steen Seier Poulsen, University of Copenhagen). *Bottom right*: simplified illustration of simple squamous nonkeratinized epithelium

Characteristics
- Cells gradually flatten towards the surface:
  - Basal layer: one layer of basophilic cuboidal/columnar cells
  - Middle layers: polyhedral cells
  - Superficial layers: squamous cells
- Can be keratinized or nonkeratinized:
  - Keratinized:
    - Cells in the superficial layers:
      - Have lost their nuclei
      - Are filled up with keratin → stain eosinophilic
      - Have unclear cell borders
    - Seen as a homogenous mass of parallel eosinophilic cell layers
      - The mass sometimes detaches from the underlying cell layers in specimens.
  - Nonkeratinized:
    - Superficial cells contain nuclei

Location
- Keratinized, e.g., in the epidermis of the skin
- Nonkeratinized, e.g., the epithelium of the esophagus

Can be mistaken for
Urothelium:
- Cells do not gradually flatten towards the surface.
  - Only a single superficial layer of flattened cells can be seen.
- Middle and superficial layers contain pale cells with a vacuolated cytoplasm.

Stratified Cuboidal/Columnar Epithelium

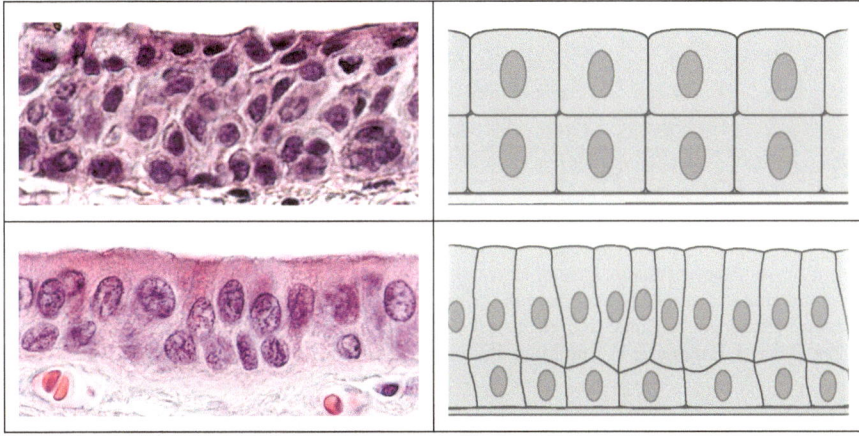

Top left: photomicrograph of stratified cuboidal epithelium. Magnification: high. Stain: HE (Courtesy of professor Jørgen Tranum-Jensen, University of Copenhagen). *Top right*: simplified illustration of stratified cuboidal epithelium. *Bottom left*: photomicrograph of stratified columnar epithelium Magnification: high. Stain: HE (Courtesy of professor Jørgen Tranum-Jensen, University of Copenhagen). *Bottom right*: simplified illustration of stratified columnar epithelium

Characteristics
- Multiple cell layers.
- Superficial cells are cuboidal/columnar.

Location
- Without apical specializations, e.g., in larger ducts of glands
- With interspersed goblet cells, e.g., in the conjunctiva

Can be mistaken for
Pseudostratified columnar epithelium:
- All cells touch the basement membrane.
- Often found with apical cilia or stereocilia, which are not seen in stratified epithelium.

Urothelium (Transitional Epithelium)

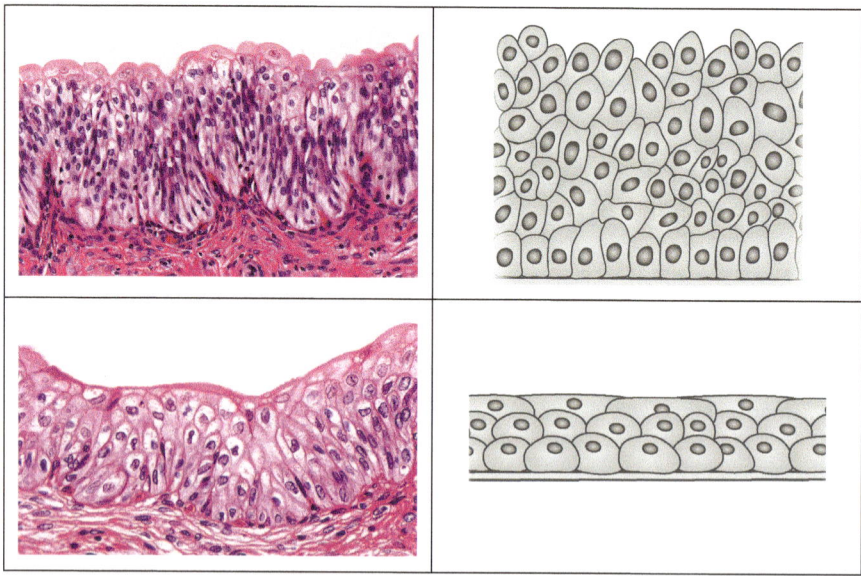

Top left: photomicrograph of urothelium in relaxed state. Magnification: high. Stain: HE (Courtesy of professor Jørgen Tranum-Jensen, University of Copenhagen). *Top right*: simplified illustration of urothelium in relaxed state. *Bottom left*: photomicrograph of urothelium in distended state. Magnification: high. Stain: HE (Courtesy of professor Jørgen Tranum-Jensen, University of Copenhagen). *Bottom right*: simplified illustration of urothelium in distended state

Characteristics
- Cells do not gradually flatten towards the surface:
  - Basal layers: basophilic cells
  - Middle layers: pale polyhedral cells with a vacuolated cytoplasm
  - Superficial layer:
    - A single layer of large pale cells
    - Each cell covers several underlying cells.
    - Cells change morphology with the degree of distension:
      - Relaxed state: a single layer of rounded cells, convex towards lumen
      - Distended state: a single layer of cuboidal or flattened cells
- Changes morphology with degree of distention (Table 5.3)

Table 5.3 Microscopic characteristics of urothelium

		Relaxed state	Distended state
Low magnification	Mucous membrane	Folded	Smooth
	Underlying layers of smooth muscle tissue	Thick	Thin
High magnification	Superficial layer of large, pale cells	Rounded cells, convex towards lumen	Cuboidal or flattened cells
	Middle layers of pale polyhedral cells	Several layers	Few/no layers
	Basal layers of basophilic cells	Several layers	Few layers

Location

Only found lining the proximal part of the urinary tract, e.g., the ureters and the urinary bladder

Can be mistaken for

Stratified squamous nonkeratinized epithelium:
- Cells gradually flatten towards the surface
- Several layers of superficial flattened cells.

References

5, 33, 34.

Chapter 6
Glandular Epithelium and Glands

Contents

Glandular Epithelium

Function
- Epithelial cells that are highly specialized for secretion:
  - Secretion is the release of specific products synthesized within the cell
- Other cell types also secrete products, e.g.:
  - Fibroblasts: secrete extracellular matrix components
  - Plasma cells: secrete antibodies

© Springer International Publishing Switzerland 2017   101
A. Rehfeld et al., *Compendium of Histology*, DOI 10.1007/978-3-319-41873-5_6

Formation

Glandular epithelium is formed from an ingrowth of surface epithelium:
- Exocrine glandular tissue
  - Maintains a connection to the surface epithelium during development, i.e., has a duct system
- Endocrine glandular tissue
  - Does not maintain a connection to the surface epithelium during development, i.e., lacks a duct system

Mechanisms of secretion

Divided into
- Constitutive secretion, found in all cell types
  - Unregulated exocytosis of small vesicles
  - Vesicles are not visible in the light microscope
  - This is the standard route out of the trans-Golgi network for proteins not sorted to other destinations, e.g., growth factors and procollagen
- Regulated secretion, only found in specialized cells, e.g., glandular epithelial cells
  - Exocytosis of large stored vesicles in response to a stimulus.
  - Vesicles are normally visible in light microscope.
  - Only specific protein products are sorted to this pathway out of the trans-Golgi network.
  - Regulated by:
    - The autonomous nervous system
    - The endocrine system

Glands

General

Cell or organ specialized for secretion of products that are used in another location

Divided into
- Exocrine glands
- Endocrine glands

Consist of

Most multicellular glands consist of:

- Parenchyma of epithelial tissue
  - Glandular epithelium
    - Forms the secretory part
  - Surface epithelium
    - Forms the duct system
    - Only in exocrine glands
- Stroma of connective tissue
  - Supports and organizes epithelial tissue parts

Exocrine Glands

General

- Secretory cells that secrete products to the free apical cell surface.
- Glandular epithelium is connected to the surface epithelium directly or via a duct system.
  - Products are secreted either directly or transported to a surface epithelium through the duct system.

Divided into

Exocrine glands are classified by:

- Number of gland cells
  - Unicellular exocrine glands
  - Multicellular exocrine glands
- Secretory product
  - Mucous
  - Serous
  - Mixed mucoserous
- Structure of gland
  - Duct system organization
  - Shape of end pieces
- Method of secretion
  - Merocrine secretion
  - Apocrine secretion
  - Holocrine secretion

Number of Gland Cells

Unicellular Exocrine Glands (Goblet Cells)

General
- Virtually the only unicellular exocrine gland in humans
- Found dispersedly in, e.g., respiratory and intestinal epithelium

Light Microscopy
- Flask-shaped cell, with nucleus placed in the narrow basal part of the cell.
- Apical broad cell part is filled with mucin-containing vesicles.

Multicellular Exocrine Glands

Divided into
- Exocrine glands within surface epithelium:
  - Secreting epithelial surface
    - Looks like an epithelium composed solely of goblet cells
    - Only found in the epithelium of the stomach
  - Intraepithelial glands
    - Invagination of glandular epithelium within a normal surface epithelium
    - For example, in the male urethra and on the internal surface of the eyelid
- Exocrine glands within connective tissue:
  - Most common multicellular gland type, e.g., parotid gland.
  - Glandular epithelium is arranged in end pieces, connected to the surface epithelium via a duct system.

Secretory Product

General
Glands are named after their secretory product:
- Glands with purely mucous or serous secretions are called mucous glands or serous glands, respectively.
- Mixed glands are called mucoserous or seromucous glands, depending on the major content.

Divided into
- Mucous product: viscous secretion, made from mucin and H_2O
- Serous product: thin, aqueous secretion, containing various enzymes
- Mixed product: mixed mucous/serous secretion

Structure of Gland

General
Glands are named after structure:
- Depending on the organization of the duct system, the glands are named simple straight, simple coiled, or compound.
  - When a single duct has >1 end pieces, it is named simple branched.
- Depending on the shape of the end pieces, the glands are called tubular, alveolar, or acinar.
  - Glands with end pieces of different shapes are named tubuloacinar or tubuloalveolar.

Divided into (Fig. 6.1)
- Duct system organization
  - Simple (unbranched) duct
    - Straight
    - Coiled
  - Compound (branched) duct
- End piece
  - Shape:
    - Tubular
      - Tube-shaped lumen and outer surface
      - For example, in eccrine sweat glands
    - Alveolar
      - Sac-shaped lumen and outer surface
      - For example, in mammary glands
    - Acinar
      - Tube-shaped lumen and sac-shaped outer surface → cone-/pyramid-shaped cells
      - Most common type, e.g., in parotid glands
  - Organization:
    - Single: a single end piece at the end of the duct
    - Branched: several end pieces on a simple (unbranched) duct
    - Coiled (only tubular end pieces)

Type of Secretory Method

General
Glands are named after their type of secretory method.
- Merocrine glands: most glands
- Apocrine glands: primarily in the lactating mammary glands (Chap. 27)
- Holocrine glands: only sebaceous and modified sebaceous glands (Chap. 20)

Duct system and end piece organization

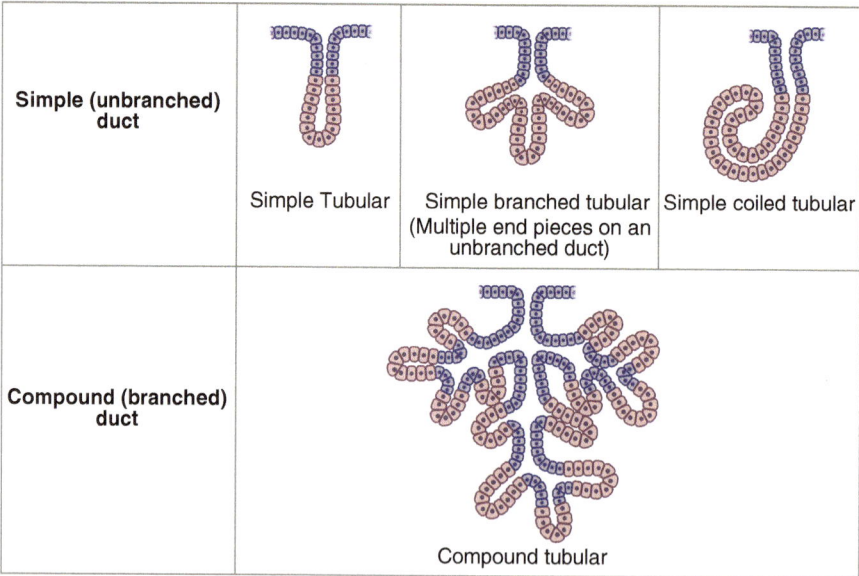

End piece shape

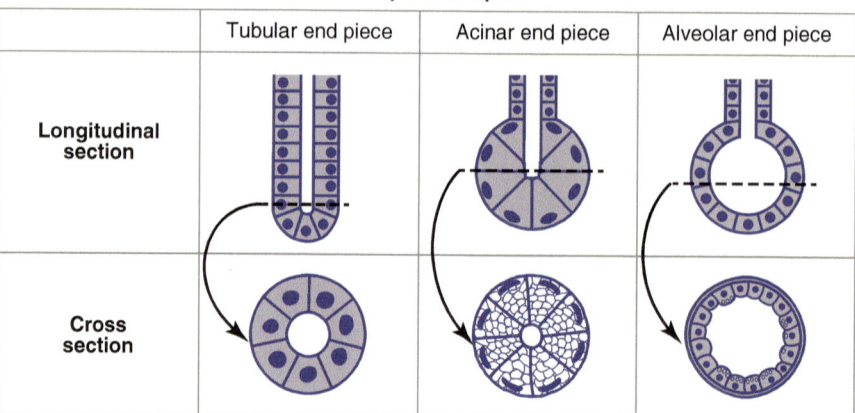

Fig. 6.1 Duct system and end pieces: the different types of duct system organizations and end piece shapes

Divided into
- Merocrine secretion
  ○ Exocytosis of vesicles
  ○ Most common type, e.g., in parotid gland
- Apocrine secretion
  ○ Ligation of an apical cell part, containing the secretory product (e.g., lipid droplets) and a surrounding envelope of cytoplasm and cell membrane
  ○ Primarily found in the lactating mammary gland (Chap. 27)
- Holocrine secretion
  ○ Extrusion of the whole cell, containing secretory product
  ○ Only found in sebaceous glands and modified sebaceous glands (Chap. 20)

MEMO-BOX
- MErocrine secretion: secretion by Exocytosis
- Apocrine secretion: secretion by ligation of Apical cell part
- Holocrine secretion: secretion by extrusion of wHole cells

Exocrine Glands Within Connective Tissue

General
Most common type of multicellular exocrine gland

Consists of (Fig. 6.2)
- Parenchyma
  ○ Secretory end pieces
  ○ Duct system (by some considered a part of the stroma)
- Stroma

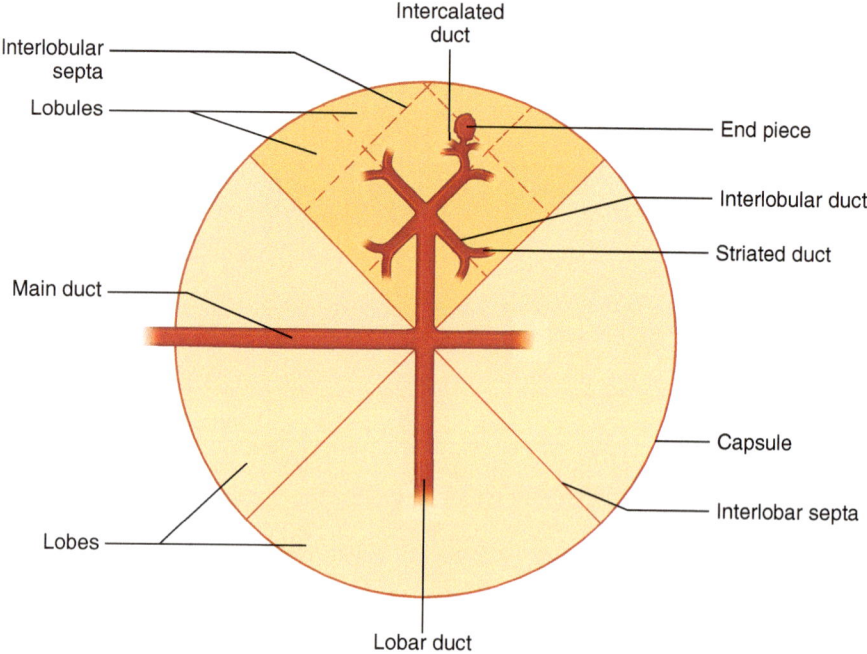

Fig. 6.2 Organization of a multicellular exocrine gland within connective tissue

PARENCHYMA

Secretory End Pieces

Structure
- Glandular epithelial cells in end pieces.
- End pieces form the blind ends of the duct system.

Function
Secretory (functional) part of gland

Light Microscopy
- End pieces are seen in cross sections as small rounded units (Fig. 6.1).
- Morphology of end pieces varies with type of secretory product (Table 6.1).

Table 6.1 Microscopic characteristics of serous, mucous, and mixed acinar end pieces

	Mucous end piece	Serous end piece	Mixed end piece
Illustration of cross section			
End piece morphology	• Large and irregular • Distinctly separated	• Small and rounded • Hard to distinguish from each other	Same as mucous end piece, but with clumps of serous cells located peripherally
Cells			
• Nucleus	Flat and basal	Round and basal	• Mixture of mucous and serous cells
• Cytoplasm	• Filled with mucin vesicles • Mucin is lost during routine preparation → weakly stained cytoplasm with a vacuolated appearance	• Well-developed rER → basophilic near nucleus • Apical vesicles, often acidophilic	• Artifact during preparation → serous cells swell and displace to the outside of the mucous cells the in end piece as "demilunes"
• Vesicles	Visible	± Visible	• Visible in mucous cells • ±Visible in serous cells
Cell borders	Visible	Indistinct	Visible between mucous cells
Lumen	Large, normally visible in the light microscope	Small, normally not visible in the light microscope	Large, normally visible in the light microscope
Location	For example, in sublingual glands	For example, in parotid glands	For example, in glands of epiglottis

MEMO-BOX
- **S**erous acinar end pieces look like "**S**alami pizzas" with their round nuclei (salami slices).
- **M**ucous acinar end pieces look like "**M**agnolia flowers" with their large lumen (green center of flower) and light cells, with visible borders (petals).

Myoepithelial cells

General

- Thin layer of contractile cells found between:
  - Glandular epithelial cells and their basal lamina in end pieces
  - Surface epithelium and their basal lamina of some ducts
- Found in sweat, tear, mammary, and salivary glands

Structure

- Flat cells with long cell extensions
- Surround end pieces and ducts

Function

Contraction → assist in squeezing out the secretory products from gland

Duct System

Structure (Table 6.2)
- Composed of surface epithelium.
- Epithelium changes with the ⊘ of the duct.

Function
- Transports secretory products from end pieces to the surface.
- The duct epithelium of some glands modifies the secretory product during the passage, e.g., in the salivary glands.

Light Microscopy
See Table 6.2.

STROMA

Structure (Table 6.3)
Connective tissue containing blood vessels and nerves

Function
Supports and organizes the parenchyma

MEMO-BOX
- "Inter" means between: **INTER**lobular ducts runs in the **INTER**lobular septae, between lobuli.
- "Intra" means within: intralobular ducts runs within lobuli.
- End pieces: the pieces at the very end of the duct system.

Table 6.2 Duct system

Duct part	Path	⊘	Epithelium
Main duct ↓	Transverse capsule of gland, ends at epithelial surface	Large	Stratified cuboidal/columnar with multiple layers
Lobar ducts ↓	Run in lobes		Fewer layers
Interlobular ducts ↓	Run in interlobular septae		Fewer layers
Intralobular ducts: • Striated ducts ↓	Run in lobules		Simple columnar
• Intercalated ducts	Run in lobules and connect directly with end pieces	Small	Simple cuboidal

Table 6.3 Stroma of glands

Connective tissue part	Location
Capsule ↓	Surrounds the gland
Interlobular septa ↓	Divide the gland into lobes
Interlobular septa ↓	Divide the lobes into lobules
Reticular connective tissue	Surrounds intralobular ducts and end pieces

Endocrine Glands

General
- Contain no duct system or secretory end pieces.
- Cells secrete their products (hormones) to intercellular space, from where they diffuse into the blood stream of adjacent capillaries.
- The tissue is densely vascularized, commonly with fenestrated capillaries.

Function
Secretion of hormones:
- Hormones can, via distribution through the blood circulation, affect target cells in the whole body.
  - Hormones act via receptors in target cells.
- Secretion is regulated by negative and positive feedback mechanisms (Chap. 24).

Divided into

Endocrine glands are classified by:

- Number of cells
  - ○ Unicellular endocrine glands, e.g., the enteroendocrine cells of the gastrointestinal tract
  - ○ Multicellular endocrine glands, e.g., the adrenal gland
- Histology
  - ○ Trabecular endocrine tissue.
    - ▪ Anastomosing plates/strings of cells, separated by densely vascularized loose connective tissue.
    - ▪ Unlike normal epithelial cells, the cells lack an apical free surface (named epithelioid cells).
    - ▪ Make up all endocrine tissues, except in the thyroid gland.
  - ○ Follicular endocrine tissue
    - ▪ Simple (one layered) epithelium, surrounding fluid-filled cavities (follicles).
    - ▪ Epithelial height varies with secretory activity.
      - • Passive gland: squamous/cuboidal epithelium
      - • Active gland: columnar epithelium
    - ▪ Only found in the thyroid gland
- Secretory product
  - ○ Peptide hormones
    - ▪ For example, insulin
    - ▪ Secreted by merocrine secretion
  - ○ Steroid hormones
    - ▪ For example, testosterone and estrogens
    - ▪ Diffuse freely out of the cells after production
  - ○ Amine hormones
    - ▪ For example, adrenalin and thyroxin.
    - ▪ Thyroid hormones are transported across the cell membrane by carrier proteins.
    - ▪ Remaining amine hormones are secreted by merocrine secretion.

Endocrine Cells

Structure

Morphology varies with the type of hormones produced:

- Peptide/amine hormone-producing cells commonly contain:
  - ○ Well-developed rER, Golgi apparatus, and multiple secretory vesicles
- Steroid hormone-producing cells contain:
  - ○ Well-developed organelles and inclusions needed for the synthesis of steroid hormones
    - ▪ Abundant sER
    - ▪ Mitochondria with tubular cristae
    - ▪ Abundant lipid droplets
      - ○ Contain precursor molecules for steroid hormone synthesis, e.g., cholesterol
      - ○ Seen as cytoplasmic vacuoles in the light microscope

Guide to Practical Histology: Glandular Epithelium

EXOCRINE GLANDS WITHIN SURFACE EPITHELIUM

Secreting Epithelial Surface

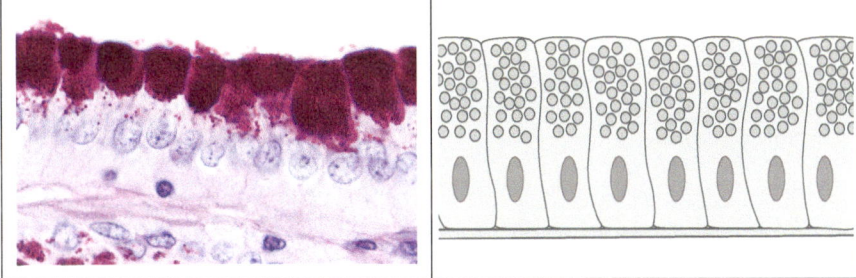

Left: photomicrograph of secreting epithelial surface. Magnification: high. Stain: PAS, hematoxylin and aurantia (Courtesy of associate professor Steen Seier Poulsen, University of Copenhagen). Right: Simplified illustration of secreting epithelial surface

Characteristics

Epithelium of mucous secreting cells:
- Epithelial cells resemble goblet cells.

Location

Only found in the epithelium of the stomach

Intraepithelial Glands

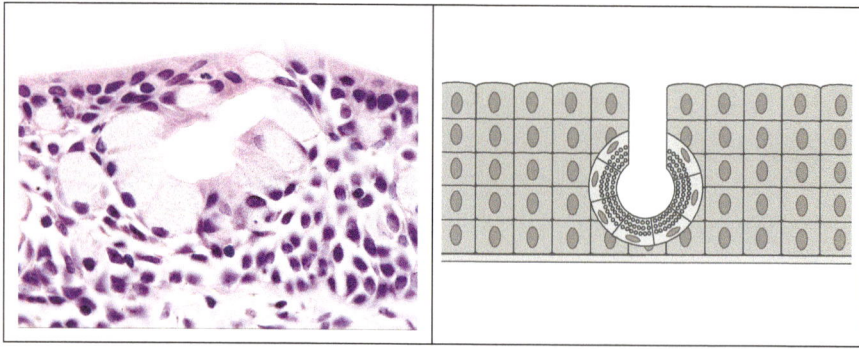

Left: photomicrograph of intraepithelial glands. Magnification: high. Stain: HE (Courtesy of professor Jørgen Tranum-Jensen, University of Copenhagen). *Right*: simplified illustration of intraepithelial glands

Characteristics
A small invagination of glandular epithelium, within "normal" surface epithelium

Location
For example, in the conjunctiva of the internal surface of the eyelid

EXOCRINE GLANDS WITHIN CONNECTIVE TISSUE

Characteristics
- Cross sections of:
  - Secretory end pieces
  - Ducts
- Shape of secretory end pieces differs between glands (Table 6.4):
  - Tubular
  - Alveolar
  - Acinar, the most common type

Divided into
- Merocrine glands, the most common type
- Apocrine glands
- Holocrine glands

Table 6.4 Microscopic characteristics of tubular, alveolar, and acinar end pieces

	Tubular end piece	Alveolar end piece	Acinar end piece
Illustration of cross section			
Photomicrograph of cross section			
Location	For example, in sweat glands	For example, in mammary glands	For example, in the parotid gland

Top left: simplified illustration of tubular end piece. Top center: simplified illustration of alveolar end piece. Top right: simplified illustration of acinar end piece. Middle left: photomicrograph of tubular end piece. Magnification: high. Stain: HE (Courtesy of associate professor Steen Seier Poulsen, University of Copenhagen). Middle center: photomicrograph of alveolar end piece. Magnification: high. Stain: HE (Courtesy of associate professor Steen Seier Poulsen, University of Copenhagen). Middle right: photomicrograph of acinar end piece. Magnification: high. Stain: HE (Courtesy of professor Jørgen Tranum-Jensen, University of Copenhagen)

Merocrine Glands

Characteristics
- Cross sections of secretory end pieces:
  - Commonly numerous and densely packed
  - Can be tubular, alveolar, or acinar (Table 6.4)
  - Morphology differs according to secretory product (Table 6.5):
    - Serous
    - Mucous
    - Mixed
- Cross sections of ducts
  - Seen scattered within the cross sections of secretory end pieces
  - Lined with simple/stratified, cuboidal/columnar epithelium
  - Visible lumen

Table 6.5 Microscopic characteristics of serous, mucous, and mixed acinar end pieces

	Mucous end piece	Serous end piece	Mixed end piece
Illustration of cross section			
Photo-micrograph of cross section			
End pieces	• Large and irregular • Distinctly separated	• Small and rounded • Hard to distinguish from each other	As the mucous end piece, but with clumps of serous cells located peripherally
Cells:			
• Nucleus	Flat and basal	Round and basal	Mixture of mucous and serous cells
• Cytoplasm	Light and vacuolated → light cells	• Basophilic basally → dark cells • Apical vesicles, often acidophilic	
• Vesicles	Visible	± Visible	• Visible in the mucous cells • ± Visible in serous cells
Cell borders	Visible	Indistinct	Visible between mucous cells
Lumen	Large, normally visible in the light microscope	Small, normally not visible in the light microscope	Large, normally visible in the light microscope
Location	For example, duodenal glands	For example, parotid gland	For example, glands of epiglottis

Top left: simplified illustration of mucous end piece. *Top center*: simplified illustration of serous end piece. *Top right*: simplified illustration of mixed end piece. *Second row left*: photomicrograph of mucous end piece. Magnification: high. Stain: HE (Courtesy of associate professor Steen Seier Poulsen, University of Copenhagen). Second row center: photomicrograph of serous end piece. Magnification: high. Stain: HE (Courtesy of associate professor Steen Seier Poulsen, University of Copenhagen, University of Copenhagen). Second row right: photomicrograph of mixed end piece. Magnification: high. Stain: HE (Courtesy of professor Jørgen Tranum-Jensen, University of Copenhagen)

Location

Merocrine glandular tissue makes up most multicellular exocrine glands:
- Shape of end pieces differs between glands:
  - ○ Tubular end pieces, e.g., sweat glands
  - ○ Alveolar end pieces, e.g., prostate gland
  - ○ Acinar end pieces, e.g., parotid glands
- The product of most glands is mixed, i.e., the glands contain both serous, mucous, and mixed end pieces, in varying ratios.
  - ○ Exceptions:
    - ▪ Pure serous glands, e.g., the parotid glands
    - ▪ Pure mucous glands, e.g., the Brunner glands of the duodenum

Apocrine Glands

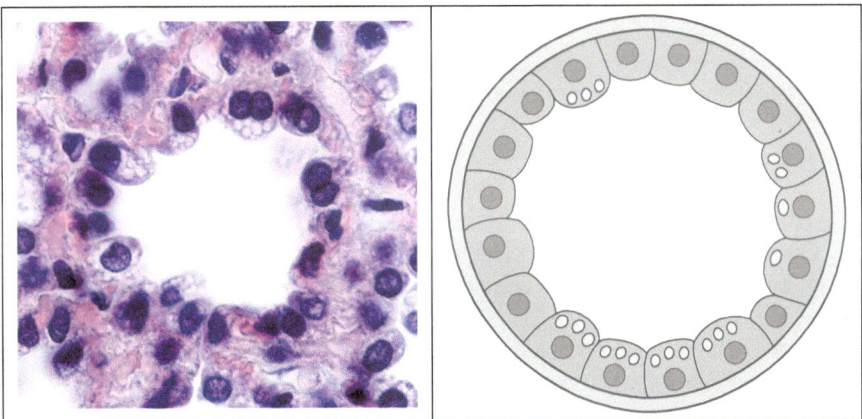

Left: photomicrograph of alveolar end piece of a lactating mammary gland. Magnification: high. Stain: toluidine blue (Courtesy of associate professor Steen Seier Poulsen, University of Copenhagen) *Right*: simplified illustration of alveolar end piece of a lactating mammary gland

Characteristics

- Cross sections of secretory end pieces
  - ○ Numerous and densely packed alveolar end pieces with:
    - ▪ Simple cuboidal epithelium
    - ▪ Large lumen, often containing eosinophilic secretions
  - ○ The cells of the end pieces
    - ▪ Are convex towards lumen
    - ▪ Often contain apical lipid droplets
- Cross sections of ducts
  - ○ Seen scattered within the cross sections of secretory end pieces
  - ○ Lined with simple/stratified, cuboidal/columnar epithelium
  - ○ Visible lumen

Location
- Apocrine secretion is primarily seen in the lactating mammary glands
- Apocrine sweat glands (apocrine secretion here is debated)

Holocrine Glands

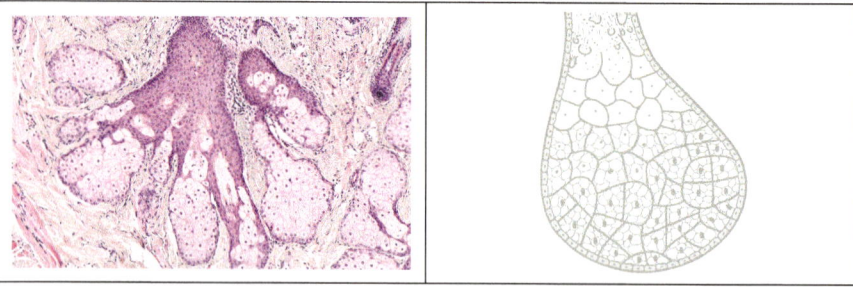

Left: photomicrograph of sebaceous gland. Magnification: High. Stain: HE (Courtesy of associate professor Steen Seier Poulsen, University of Copenhagen). Right: simplified illustration of sebaceous gland

Characteristics
- One to several large acinar end pieces
  - End pieces are seen as a large aggregation of cells, which resembles a "grape cluster."
  - Basal layer
    - Smaller cuboidal basophilic cells
  - Middle layers
    - Pale polyhedral cells with a vacuolated cytoplasm and gradually smaller nuclei (cells resemble fish eyes)
  - Luminal layers
    - Pale cells breaking into pieces
- Ducts are often not seen.
- Often seen adjacent to a hair follicle, i.e., in dermis of the skin.

Location
Only found as the sebaceous glands and modified sebaceous glands, e.g., in the skin

ENDOCRINE GLANDULAR TISSUE

General
- Without cross sections of secretory end pieces and ducts
- Cells in cords/groups/follicles
- Contains multiple capillaries
  - Seen as narrow white spaces with multiple eosinophilic erythrocytes

Follicular Endocrine Tissue

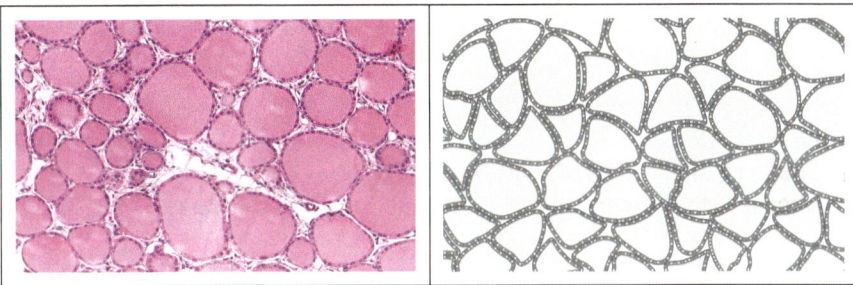

Left: photomicrograph of follicular endocrine tissue. Magnification: low. Stain: HE (Courtesy of professor Jørgen Tranum-Jensen, University of Copenhagen). *Right*: simplified illustration of follicular endocrine tissue

Characteristics
- Consists of multiple follicles
  - Rings of simple epithelium
  - Epithelium surrounds a lumen with homogenous eosinophilic material (colloid).
- Connective tissue with capillaries is seen between the follicles.

Location
Only found in the thyroid gland

Trabecular Endocrine Tissue

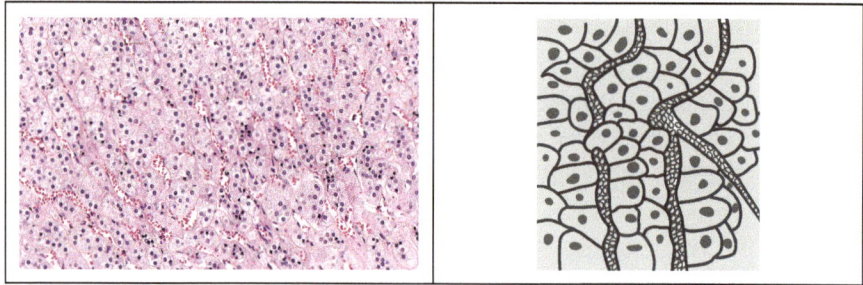

Left: photomicrograph of trabecular endocrine tissue. Magnification: low. Stain: HE (Courtesy of professor Jørgen Tranum-Jensen, University of Copenhagen). *Right*: simplified illustration of trabecular endocrine tissue

Characteristics
- Anastomosing strands of cells forming a disorganized network
- Separated by loose connective tissue with numerous capillaries
- Morphology differs depending on hormonal product:
  - Steroid hormone-producing tissue
    - Cells are large and pale.
    - Contain many small lipid droplets, seen as empty vacuoles →
      "popcorn-/foam"-like cells.
  - Peptide/amine hormone-producing tissue
    - Cells are small and dark.

Location
Areas of both types are found, e.g., in the adrenal gland.
- Cortex: steroid hormone-producing endocrine tissue
- Medulla: peptide/amine hormone-producing endocrine tissue

Can be mistaken for
Brown fat
- Cells in aggregations, not in strands.
- Cells contain larger lipid droplets.
- Not divided into morphologically different areas, as many trabecular endocrine tissues are.

References
5, 12, 20, 33, 34.

Chapter 7
Connective Tissue

Contents

General
- One of the four basic tissue types.
- Connective tissue is separated from the other basic tissue types.
  - From epithelial tissue by a basal lamina
  - From muscle and nerve tissue by an external lamina (similar to basal lamina)

Structure
Separated cells in abundant extracellular matrix

Function
- Connective tissue proper fills out the spaces between the other tissue types, carrying out specific functions, e.g.:
  - Connects tissues, e.g., muscles to bone as tendons
  - Encloses and separates tissues, e.g., as fascia

© Springer International Publishing Switzerland 2017
A. Rehfeld et al., *Compendium of Histology*, DOI 10.1007/978-3-319-41873-5_7

- Supports tissues, e.g., epithelial parenchyma in organs as the stroma
- Nourishes avascular tissues, e.g., epithelia as the underlying vascularized loose connective tissue
- Additional specific functions vary between the different types of connective tissue, e.g.:
  - Loose connective tissue: primary site of inflammation
  - Dense elastic tissue: highly elastic

Consist of
- Extracellular matrix
  - Ground substance
  - Fibers
  - Multiadhesive glycoproteins
- Cells
  - Resident (fixed) cell population
  - Transient (wandering) cell population

Divided into
- Connective tissue proper
  - Loose (areolar) connective tissue
  - Dense connective tissue
    - Regular
    - Irregular
    - Elastic
- Embryonic connective tissue
  - Mesenchyme
  - Mucous connective tissue
- Specialized connective tissue
  - Reticular connective tissue
  - Cartilage (Chap. 8)
  - Bone (Chap. 9)
  - Bone marrow (Chap. 10)
  - Adipose tissue (Chap. 11)
  - Blood (Chap. 12)
  - Lymphatic tissue (Chap. 19)

Extracellular Matrix

General
The noncellular component of tissues

Consist of
- Ground substance
- Fibers
- Multiadhesive glycoproteins

GROUND SUBSTANCE

Consist of (Fig. 7.1)

Proteoglycans:
- Single proteoglycans (shape resembles a bottle brush)
  ○ One core protein.
  ○ Multiple glycosaminoglycans, long polysaccharide chains of disaccharide repeats, bound covalently to the core protein (like bristles of a bottle brush).
- Proteoglycan aggregates (shape resembles a bottle brush)
  ○ Hyaluronan, a large 2.5 μm long glycosaminoglycan, which functions analogous to a core protein.
  ○ Multiple proteoglycans bound non-covalently to hyaluronan via linker proteins (like bristles of a bottle brush).

Structure

Viscous gel:
- Multiple negative charges from SO_4^{2-} and COO^- groups on the glycosaminoglycans attract cations and $H_2O \rightarrow$ form a viscous gel.
- The network of proteoglycans forms a molecular filter within the gel.

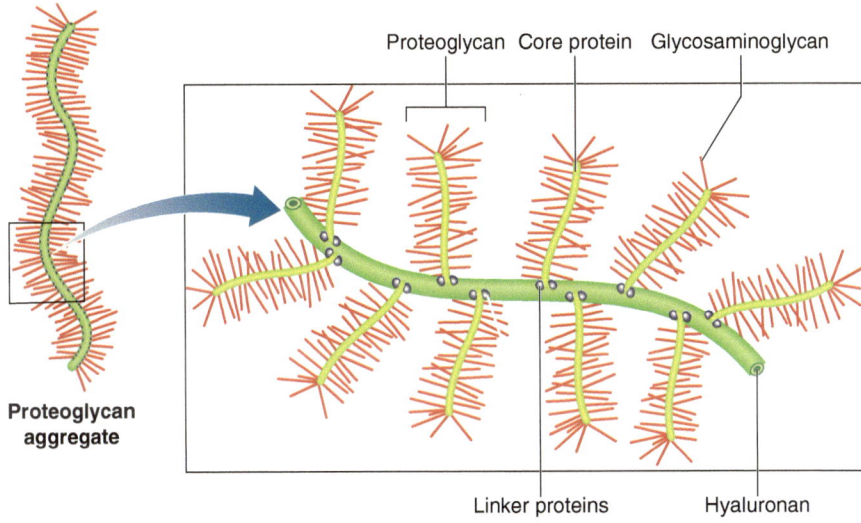

Fig. 7.1 Structure of a proteoglycan aggregate

Function
- Viscous gel:
  - ○ Diffusion media for water-soluble substances
  - ○ Resists compression and absorbs shocks (analogous to a wet sponge)
- Molecular filter:
  - ○ The network of proteoglycans impairs the passage of large molecules and microorganisms.
  - ○ Small molecules can diffuse freely through the network of proteoglycans.
- Specific function varies with the composition of the ground substance, i.e., the types of proteoglycans and glycosaminoglycans.

Light microscopy
- Leaches out during routine preparation
- Is contained in cartilage, where it stains basophilic/metachromatic

FIBERS

Divided into (Table 7.1)
- Collagen fibers
- Reticular fibers
- Elastic fibers

Collagen molecules

General
- The molecular units of collagen and reticular fibers.
- Collagen fibrils are often formed from more than one type of collagen molecules
- Certain types of collagen molecules are primarily used in the collagen fibers of some tissues, e.g., type II collagen in cartilage

Divided into
Twenty-nine types of collagen molecules exist, e.g.:
- Fibrillar collagens (assemble into collagen fibrils), e.g.:
  - ○ Collagen type I
    - ▪ Most common type, which makes up 90% of all collagen
    - ▪ Found in, e.g., dermis, tendons and bone
  - ○ Collagen type II
    - ▪ Found in cartilage
  - ○ Collagen type III
    - ▪ Form reticular fibers
- Basement membrane-forming collagens, e.g.:
  - ○ Collagen type IV
    - ▪ Only found in the basal lamina.
    - ▪ Type IV collagen molecules do not form collagen fibrils but assemble into a 3D network.

Table 7.1 Fibers of the extracellular matrix

	Collagen fibers	Reticular fibers	Elastic fibers
Structure	Wavy fibers of variable width, $\oslash$ 1–20 µm	• Thin fibers • Branch to form a meshwork (reticulum)	• Thin fibers, $\oslash$ 0.2–1 µm • Branch to form a 3D network

Consists of	Collagen molecules polymerized into collagen fibrils:
	• Collagen fibrils are often formed from more than one type of collagen molecules
		Fibrils of type III collagen, $\oslash$ ≈20 nm, which are heavily glycosylated:
		• Fibrils do normally not bundle, when forming the reticular fibers, i.e., reticular fibers are often individual fibrils of type III collagen
			• Elastin (>90 % of fiber):
			  ○ Coiled molecules cross-linked into a 3D network
			  ○ Forms the core of the fiber
			• Fibrillin

Formation	1. Procollagen molecules are synthesized (requires vitamin C)
	  ↓ Exocytosed and cleaved extracellularly
	2. Collagen molecules, 300 nm long, $\oslash$ 1.5 nm
	  ↓ Polymerize (self-assemble) into
	3. Collagen fibrils, $\oslash$ 20–300 nm
	  ↓ Bundle into
	4. Collagen fibers, $\oslash$ 1–20 µm
		1. Procollagen molecules are synthesized (requires vitamin C)
		  ↓ Exocytosed and cleaved extracellularly
		2. Type III collagen molecules, 300 nm long, $\oslash$ 1.5 nm
		  ↓ Polymerize (self-assemble) into
		3. Collagen fibrils of type III collagen, $\oslash$ ≈20 nm
			Proelastin and profibrillin molecules are exocytosed and cleaved extracellularly to form elastin and fibrillin:
			• Elastin polymerize (self-assemble) into a 3D network
			• Fibrillin forms microfibrils, which surround a core of elastin (absent in elastic lamellae)

Function	Flexible fibers with high tensile strength	Provides a supporting framework for cells.	Elasticity: • Fibers can stretch to 150 % of length and return to the original state • Mechanism of the elasticity is the stretching of the coiled elastin fibers followed by complete recoil
Location	Most abundant fiber type of connective tissue	Located in: • Near relation to cells, just below the basal/external laminae • Reticular connective tissue, where reticular cells produce the fibers	• Found in many connective tissues • In dense elastic connective tissue: Fibers are coarser, $\oslash$ 5–15 µm, and arranged in parallel, e.g., as elastic lamellae of arteries

Light microscopy	Seen as wavy fibers of variable width (often thick):
	• HE: stains collagen fibers pink
	• Van Gieson: stains collagen fibers red
	• Mallory: stains collagen fibers blue
		• Thin fibers, not visible in routine stains
		• Special stains:
		  ○ Silver: stains reticular fibers black/brown
		  ○ PAS: stains reticular fibers pink
			Thin wavy fibers:
			• Weakly stained, but strongly refractive in routine stains
			• Special stains:
			  ○ Orcein: stains elastic fibers red/brown
			  ○ Resorcin-fuchsin: stains elastic fibers blue/black

MEMO-BOX

I, II, III, IV → A, B, C, D
- Collagen type I: in nearly **A**ll connective tissue types (makes up 90 % of collagen)
- Collagen type II: **B**oth in hyaline and elastic cartilage
- Collagen type III: Form reti**C**ular fibers
- Collagen type IV: Only in lamina **D**ensa (part of the basal lamina)

MEMO-BOX

ELASTIc fibers: consist of >90 % **ELASTI**n

MULTIADHESIVE GLYCOPROTEINS

General

Abundant proteins, which stabilize the extracellular matrix

Structure

Glycoproteins with multiple binding domains, e.g.:
- Fibronectin: most abundant type in connective tissue
- Laminin: found only in basal/external laminae

Function
- Stabilize the extracellular matrix
  - Bind to multiple extracellular matrix components, e.g., collagens and proteoglycans
- Anchor cells to the extracellular matrix
  - Bind to integrins of cell surface receptors
- Control cell migration within connective tissue

MEMO-BOX

LAMINin: only found in basal/external **LAMIN**ae

Connective Tissue Cells

Divided into
- Resident (fixed) cell population
  - Fibroblasts
  - Macrophages
  - Mast cells
  - Plasma cells
  - White adipocytes
  - Mesenchymal stem cells
  - Reticular cells
- Transient (wandering) cell population
  - Monocytes
  - Lymphocytes
  - Neutrophils
  - Eosinophils
  - Basophils
  - Dendritic cells

RESIDENT CELL POPULATION

General
- Permanent cells of connective tissue.
- Relatively stable cell population.
- Cells commonly have low motility.

Fibroblasts

General
- Most common cell in connective tissue.
- Fibroblasts involved in wound healing develop contractile function and are called myofibroblasts.

Function
Production of all components of extracellular matrix

Light microscopy
- Large flattened cell with thin cell extensions
- Elongated nucleus
- The appearance changes depending on the activity of the cell:
  - Inactive: dark (heterochromatic) nucleus and a pale cytoplasm due to low amount of rER → only nucleus is visible in routine stains
  - Active: light (euchromatic) nucleus with visible nucleoli and a basophilic cytoplasm due to a well-developed rER

Macrophages

General (Table 7.3)
- Are derived from monocytes, which migrate to connective tissue from the blood
- Life span ≈ 2 months
- Can be activated by cytokines and pathogens → cell grows larger and increases capacity for phagocytosis

Function
Important roles in innate immune system:
- Phagocytosis
  - Engulfment of, e.g., small particles, microorganisms, damaged/dead cells → phagosome.
  - Phagosome fuses with lysosomes → material is broken down.
- Antigen presentation
  - Antigens (short polypeptides) from degraded phagocytized material are presented to lymphocytes on cell surface.
- Cytokine secretion
  - Regulate immune system

Light microscopy
- Rounded/spindle-shaped cell, ⊘ 10–30 μm
- Indented/C-shaped dark (heterochromatic) nucleus
- Pale cytoplasm with many lysosomes, which are only visible with specific staining:
  - Only the nucleus is clearly visible in routine stains.

Mononuclear phagocyte system
General (Table 7.2)
- Family of macrophage-like cells.
- All are derived from monocytes/monocyte progenitor cells.

Table 7.2 Cells of the mononuclear phagocyte system

Name	Location	Main function
Monocyte	Blood	Precursor cell
Macrophage	• Connective tissue • Bone marrow • Lymphatic tissue	• Phagocytosis • Antigen presentation • Cytokine secretion
Kupffer cell	Liver	
Alveolar macrophage	Lungs	
Microglia	Central nervous system	
Langerhans cell (dendritic cell of the skin)	Epidermis	Antigen presentation
Dendritic cell	• Connective tissue • Lymphatic tissue	
Osteoclast	Bone	Breakdown of bone tissue

Mast Cells

General (Table 7.3)
• Derived from immature mast cells, which migrate to connective tissue from blood
• Related to, but distinct from basophils (share common basophil/mast cell progenitor cell, located in the bone marrow)
• Located close to small blood vessels, especially in the connective tissue of the skin and gastrointestinal tract

Function
• Role in innate immune system:
  ○ Binds IgE antibodies to surface
    ▪ Antigen/allergen binds to IgE → exocytosis of granules containing mediators of inflammation, e.g.:
      • Histamine: increase permeability of blood vessels
      • Heparin: anticoagulative effect
      • Neutrophil/eosinophil chemotactic factors: attract neutrophils/eosinophils
• Associated with allergic reactions and chronic inflammation

Light microscopy
• Ovoid cell, ⊘ 20–30 μm
• Small spherical nucleus
• Multiple large, ⊘ 0.5 μm, intensely basophilic/metachromatic granules, only preserved with special fixatives

Table 7.3 Overview of immune cells in connective tissue

	Macrophage	Mast cell	Plasma cell	Monocyte	B/T lymphocyte	Neutrophil	Eosinophil	Basophil	Dendritic cell
Ø	10–30 µm	20–30 µm	10–20 µm	12–18 µm	≈7 µm	10–15 µm	10–15 µm	10–15 µm	≈15 µm
Shape	Rounded/spindle-shaped	Ovoid	Ovoid	Round	Round	Round	Round	Round	Many highly branched cell extensions
Nucleus	Indented/C-shaped	Small, spherical	Round/ovoid with clumps of heterochromatin like a clock face	Indented/C-shaped	Large, round, and dark	2–4 lobes	2 lobes	2–3 lobes	Large and light
Cytoplasm	Weakly stained with lysosomes	Many basophilic granules	Basophilic	Weakly stained with lysosomes	Thin basophilic rim	Many weakly stained granules	Many eosinophilic granules	Many basophilic granules	Weakly stained
Function	• Phagocytosis • Antigen presentation • Cytokine secretion	Role in innate immune system	Produce antibodies	Differentiates to macrophages	Role in both innate and adaptive immune system	Phagocytosis	Fight parasitic infections	• Role in innate immune system • Closely related to that of mast cells	Antigen presentation
Cell population	Resident (fixed) cell population			Transient (wandering) cell population					

Plasma Cells

General (Table 7.3)
- Differentiate from activated B lymphocytes
- Life span 10–30 days
- Abundant in loose connective tissue, especially in the mucous membranes of the gastrointestinal and respiratory tracts

Function
- Secretes immunoglobulins (antibodies)
- A part of the adaptive immune system

Light microscopy
- Ovoid cell, ⊘ 10–20 μm.
- Basophilic cytoplasm due to a well-developed rER.
- Pale area in cytoplasm corresponds to the Golgi apparatus (negative Golgi stain).
- Eccentric round/ovoid nucleus with clumps of heterochromatin arranged like a clock face, i.e., clumps of chromatin are seen in the periphery of the nucleus, as the numbers on a clock face.

White adipocytes

General
- Found in loose connective tissue both as individual cells and in groups.
- Large groups of white adipocytes are called adipose tissue (Chap. 11).

Function
- Lipid storage
- Endocrine function
  - Secrete, e.g.:
    - Hormones, e.g., leptin, which regulates the appetite
    - Growth factors
    - Cytokines

Light microscopy
- Rounded/polyhedral cell
- ⊘ 15–150 μm
- Peripheral flattened nucleus
- Surrounded by an external lamina (similar to a basal lamina)
  - Only type of connective tissue cell, which has an external lamina
- Contains a single large lipid inclusion (lipid droplet), which fills up almost all of the cytoplasm

Staining
- Lipid leaches out during routine preparation
  - Only the nucleus and a thin rim of cytoplasm remain
    - A single adipocyte looks like a signet ring.
    - Groups of adipocytes form a polygonal meshwork (resembles chicken wire).
- Lipid can be preserved using frozen sections or fixed and stained, e.g., with osmium tetroxide which stains the cell black/brown.

Mesenchymal Stem Cells

General
Mainly found as pericytes surrounding capillaries and venules

Function
Stem cell, capable of differentiating into, e.g., smooth muscle cells, endothelial cells, and fibroblasts

Light microscopy
Smaller than fibroblasts but difficult to distinguish from these in the light microscope

Reticular Cells

General
Only present in reticular connective tissue, which forms the stroma of the bone marrow and lymphatic tissues (except in the thymus)

Function
Production of reticular fibers

Light microscopy
- Star-shaped cell.
- Large ovoid euchromatic nucleus.
- Weakly basophilic cytoplasm.
- Cell extensions from the reticular cells ensheath the produced reticular fibers completely → 3D cellular network.

TRANSIENT CELL POPULATION

General (Table 7.3)
- Are all leukocytes (white blood cells)
- Motile cells
- Temporary visitors in connective tissue
  - Migrate from the blood to the connective tissue only in response to specific stimuli, e.g., inflammation
  - Do not stay permanently, as they either:
    - Differentiate, e.g. monocytes → macrophages
    - Recirculate into lymph
    - Have short life spans
- Become functional as they enter the connective tissue

Monocytes

General
- Recruited to connective tissue during inflammation
- Arrive at the site of inflammation ≈ 24 h after neutrophils

Function
Migrate from blood to connective tissue, where they differentiate into cells of the mononuclear phagocyte system, e.g., macrophages

Light microscopy
- Rounded cell
- ⊘ 12–18 μm
- Indented/C-shaped nucleus
- Weakly stained cytoplasm with many lysosomes, which are only visible when stained specifically, e.g., with azure dyes (stain dark blue/purple)

Lymphocytes

General
- Normally sparse in connective tissue but increase in number at sites with inflammation
- Under normal conditions present in the connective tissue of the mucous membranes of gastrointestinal and respiratory tract

Function
- The main functional cell of the immune system
- Have a role in both the innate and adaptive immune system

Divided into
- B lymphocytes
  - ≈25 %
  - Facilitate humoral (antibody-mediated) immunity
- T lymphocytes
  - ≈70 %
  - Facilitate cell-mediated immunity
  - Participate in humoral (antibody-mediated) immunity
- Natural killer (NK) cells
  - ≈5 %
  - Destroy virus-infected cells

Light microscopy
- B/T lymphocytes
  - Small round cell, $\varnothing \approx 7$ μm
  - Spherical dark (heterochromatic) nucleus
  - Surrounded by a thin rim of cytoplasm, which stains basophilic due to abundant free ribosomes
- NK cells
  - Large round cell, $\varnothing \approx 15$ μm
  - Kidney-shaped nucleus
  - Cytoplasm with many granules, which are only visible when stained specifically, e.g., with azure dyes (stain dark blue/purple)

Neutrophils

General
- Under normal conditions, neutrophils are absent in connective tissue.
- Usually the first cells to be recruited to connective tissue during inflammation.
- After migrating out of blood, neutrophils live for 1–2 days.
  - After death they form pus, with other dead cells and microorganisms.
  - Pus is phagocytized by macrophages, which arrive to the site of inflammation ≈ 24 h later.
- A large reserve pool of neutrophils exists in the blood and bone marrow.

Function

Role in the innate immune system:
- Phagocytosis
  1. Engulfment of, e.g., microorganisms → phagosome.
  2. Phagosome fuses with granules.
     - Microorganisms are killed via either:
       - O_2-dependent mechanism (most efficient): by highly reactive O_2 intermediates, e.g., O_2-, made in the cell during a "respiratory burst"
       - O_2-independent mechanism: by antimicrobial proteins and peptides
     - Material is digested by enzymes.
- Cytokine secretion, e.g., the fever-causing interleukin-1.

Light microscopy
- Round cell, ⊘ 10–15 μm
- Multilobular nucleus, 2–4 lobes
- Cytoplasm with abundant granules
  - Primary granules (lysosomes)
    - Few, large, ⊘ 0.5 μm
    - Contain enzymes that can generate highly reactive bactericidal substances
    - Only visible when specifically stained, e.g., with azure dyes (stain dark blue/purple) and are thus called azurophilic granules
  - Secondary, specific granules
    - Many fine, weakly stained → barely visible in light microscope
    - Contain enzymes and antimicrobial peptides

Eosinophils

General
- Recruited to connective tissue during inflammation
- In normal conditions present in the connective tissue of the mucous membranes of the gastrointestinal and respiratory tracts

Function
- Role in the innate immune system
  - Exocytosis of granules, containing:
    - Cytotoxic proteins → fight parasitic infections
    - Cytokines → modulate inflammatory response
- Associated with allergic reactions and chronic inflammation

Light microscopy
- Round cell, ⃠ 10–15 μm
- Bilobed nucleus (two lobes, resembles a pair of sunglasses)
- Cytoplasm with abundant granules
  - Primary granules (lysosomes):
    - Few large, ⃠ 0.5 μm
    - Only visible when specifically stained, e.g., with azure dyes (stain dark blue/purple) and are thus called azurophilic granules
  - Secondary, specific granules
    - Many large refractive acidophilic (eosinophilic) specific granules, ⃠ 0.5–1 μm
    - Contain proteins with cytotoxic effect on parasites

Basophils

General
Related to but distinct from mast cells (share common basophil/mast cell progenitor cell, located in the bone marrow)

Function
Role in innate immune system:
- Bind IgE antibodies to surface
  - Antigen/allergen binds to IgE → exocytosis of granules containing mediators of inflammation, e.g.:
    - Histamine: increase permeability of blood vessels
    - Heparin: anticoagulative effect
- Associated with allergic reactions and chronic inflammation

Light microscopy
- Round cell, ⃠ 10–15 μm
- Irregular, lobed nucleus, 2–3 lobes, usually obscured by the densely stained granules in light microscope
- Cytoplasm with abundant granules
  - Primary granules (lysosomes):
    - Few large, ⃠ 0.5 μm
    - Only visible when specifically stained, e.g., with azure dyes (stain dark blue/purple) and are thus called azurophilic granules
  - Secondary, specific granules
    - Many large basophilic/metachromatic granules, ⃠ 0.5 μm
    - Contain, e.g., histamine and heparin

MEMO-BOX
Granulocytes: contain numerous granules in their cytoplasm
- **NEUTR**ophils: Contain many "**NEUTR**ally" (weakly) stained granules
- **EOSINOPHIL**s: Contain many acidophilic (**EOSINOPHIL**ic) granules
- **BASOPHIL**s: Contain many **BASOPHIL**ic granules

Dendritic cells

General
Located in small numbers in the connective tissue of all organs.

Function
Antigen presentation:
- Take up antigens from the extracellular environment by endocytosis
- Leave the connective tissue via blood and lymph → Lymphatic tissue, where they present the antigens to T lymphocytes

Light microscopy
- $\varnothing \approx 15$ μm, with many highly branched cell extensions
- Large and light nucleus
- Weakly stained cytoplasm → Only the nucleus is clearly visible in routine stains.

MEMO-BOX
Dendron is Greek for "tree": Dendritic cells have highly branched "treelike" cell extensions.

Connective Tissue Types

Structure (Table 7.4 and 7.5)
Based on composition most connective tissue types can be described as:
- Loose: more cells than fibers
- Dense: more fibers than cells

MEMO-BOX
- **LOOSE** connective tissue: **LOOSE**ly arranged fibers (irregular pattern)
- Dense **IRREGULAR** connective tissue: dense fibers in **IRREGULAR** pattern
- Dense **REGULAR** connective tissue: dense fibers in **REGULAR** (parallel) pattern

Table 7.4 Structure of connective tissue proper

	Loose (areolar) connective tissue	Dense connective tissue		
		Irregular	Regular	Elastic
Extracellular matrix	Few, loosely arranged fine fibers in an irregular pattern	Thick bundles of collagen fibers in an irregular pattern	Thick bundles of parallel collagen fibers	Bundles of collagen fibers and thick parallel elastic fibers
Cells	Abundant cells of many types, typically transient cells	Few scattered fibroblasts	Few fibroblasts with flattened nuclei in rows between the fiber bundles	• In elastic ligaments: Dispersed fibroblasts • In elastic lamellae of arteries: Dispersed smooth muscle cells
Blood vessels and nerves	Generally many blood vessels and nerves	Generally few blood vessels and nerves		
Function	• Supports microvasculature and nerves • Initial and primary site of inflammation	Withstands mechanical stress in multiple directions due to the irregular organization	Strong resistance to force in the direction of the parallel collagen fibers	Mechanical strength while allowing stretch and recoil
Location	Underlie epithelia, e.g., in lamina propria	For example, in dermis and organ capsules	For example, in tendons and ligaments	For example, in elastic ligaments and lamellae

Table 7.5 Structure of embryonic and reticular connective tissue

	Embryonic connective tissue		Reticular connective tissue
	Mesenchyme	Mucous connective tissue	
Extracellular matrix	Few, fine collagen fibers in a viscous ground substance	Few, fine collagen fibers in a gelatin-like ground substance called Wharton's jelly (stains like mucin)	Anastomosing meshwork of reticular fibers ensheathed by reticular cell extensions
Cells	Small spindle-shaped mesenchymal cells: • Contact each other through cell extensions → 3D cellular network	Small spindle-shaped mesenchymal cells: • Scattered and widely separated • With long thin cell extensions	Reticular cells in a 3D network
Blood vessels and nerves	Generally many blood vessels and nerves		
Function	Precursor of mature connective tissues	• Supports the blood vessels of the umbilical cord • Intermediate between mesenchyme and mature connective tissues	Stroma in bone marrow and lymphatic tissues (except in the thymus)
Location	Mesoderm of the early embryo	For example, in the umbilical cord	In bone marrow and lymphoid tissues (except in the thymus)

Inflammation

General
- Unspecific reaction to harmful stimuli, e.g., tissue damage or pathogens
  - Immune cells, e.g., resident macrophages, secrete cytokines → inflammation
- Commonly takes place locally in the loose connective tissue, the initial tissue that pathogens reach after penetrating epithelium
- Sometimes seen in combination with systemic reactions, e.g., fever and leukocytosis (increased concentration of leukocytes in blood)

Function
Most important human defense mechanism:
- Restricts tissue damage to limited area
- Weakens microorganisms
- Assists the removal of damaged/dead tissue
- Helps regenerate the tissue

Cytokines

General
- Paracrine and autocrine mediators, which regulate the immune system
- Secreted mainly by immune cells

Function
- Regulate the immune system
- Induce inflammation
  - Induce the expression of cell adhesion molecules on endothelial cells
  - Recruit leukocytes from the blood to connective tissue
  - Increase permeability of capillaries
  - Increase local blood flow

Cardinal signs of inflammation
General
- Increased permeability of capillaries → edema ⎤
- Increased local blood flow → heat and reddening ⎬ The five cardinal signs of inflammation
- Edema and cytokines → pain and loss of function ⎦

Leukocyte Extravasation

General
- Recruitment of leukocytes from the blood to the connective tissue
- Takes place in postcapillary venules

Steps of leukocyte extravasation:

1. Primary adhesion phase
   - Cytokines released at site of inflammation induce the endothelium to rapidly express selectins on the luminal surface.
   - Selectins bind loosely to receptors on leukocytes, which slow down and roll along the endothelium (like a tennis ball rolling on Velcro).
2. Secondary adhesion phase
   - Cytokines induce:
     - Expression of certain integrins on the rolling leukocyte
     - Expression of certain cell adhesion molecules, e.g., ICAM-1, on the luminal surface of endothelium
     - Loosening of cell junctions between endothelial cells
   - Cell adhesion molecules of endothelium bind integrins on leukocytes → leukocytes adhere tightly to endothelium.
3. Diapedesis
   - Leukocyte cell extension penetrates between endothelial cells (now with loosened cell junctions) → secretes proteases to break down the basal lamina.
   - Leukocyte migrates out of blood between endothelial cells and into the connective tissue.
4. Chemotaxis
   - Leukocyte migrates towards the site of inflammation, attracted by chemoattractant molecules released there.

Guide to Practical Histology: Connective Tissue

LOOSE CONNECTIVE TISSUE

General
Contains more cells than fibers

Loose (Areolar) Connective Tissue

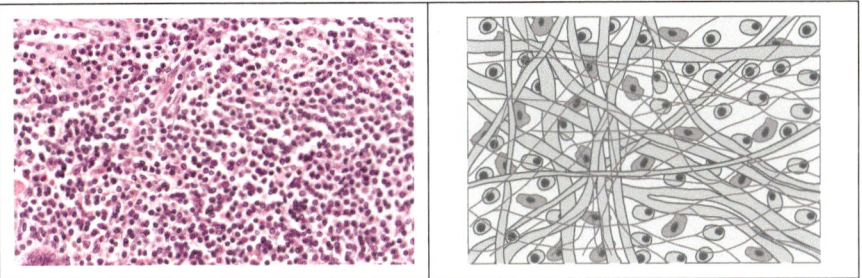

Left: photomicrograph of loose connective tissue. Magnification: high. Stain: PAS-hematoxylin (Courtesy of professor Jørgen Tranum-Jensen, University of Copenhagen). *Right*: simplified illustration of loose connective tissue

Characteristics
- Abundant cells of many different types
- Few, thin fibers
- Multiple blood vessels

Location
Found at many locations, e.g.:
- In dermis, as a thin layer underlying the epidermis of the skin
- In lamina propria, as a thicker layer underlying mucous membranes

Reticular Connective Tissue

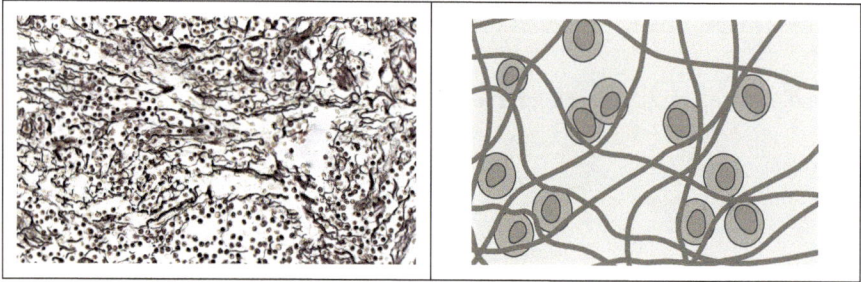

Left: photomicrograph of reticular connective tissue. Magnification: high. Stain: silver (Courtesy of professor Jørgen Tranum-Jensen, University of Copenhagen). *Right*: simplified illustration of reticular connective tissue

Characteristics
Resembles loose connective tissue in HE stain (reticular fibers are not visible)

Location
Constitutes the stroma in bone marrow and lymphatic tissues (except the thymus)

Special staining
Fibers are seen forming a network in close relation to the cells of the tissue, if stained with, e.g.:
- Silver: stains the reticular fibers black/brown
- Reticulin: stains the reticular fibers blue/black
- PAS: stains reticular fibers pink

Mesenchyme

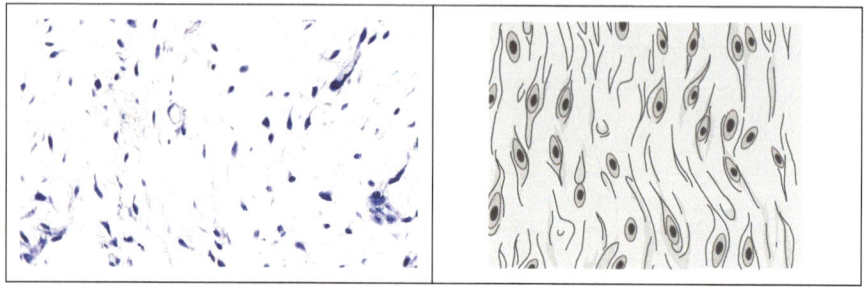

Left: photomicrograph of mesenchyme. Magnification: high. Stain: toluidine blue (Courtesy of professor Jørgen Tranum-Jensen, University of Copenhagen). *Right*: simplified illustration of mesenchyme

Characteristics
- Small spindle-shaped cells
- Few, fine fibers

Location
For example, in the mesoderm of the early embryo

Can be mistaken for
Mucous connective tissue
- Cells are more widely distributed.

Mucous Connective Tissue

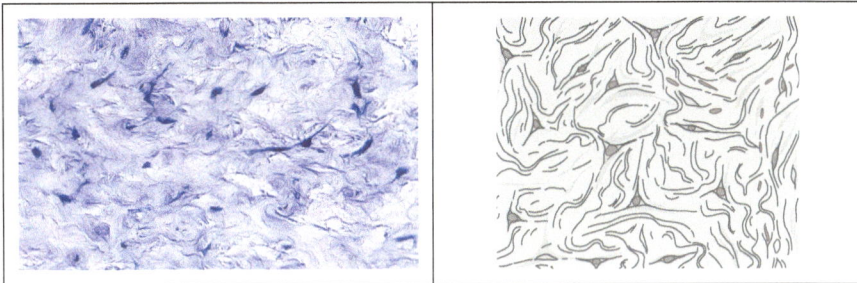

Left: photomicrograph of mucous connective tissue. Magnification: high. Stain: toluidine blue and Alcian blue (Courtesy of professor Jørgen Tranum-Jensen, University of Copenhagen). *Right*: simplified illustration of mucous connective tissue

Characteristics
- Scattered and widely separated spindle-shaped cells with long thin cell extensions
- Few, fine wavy fibers
- Ground substance stains similar to mucin (must be fixed first, as it leaches out during routine preparation)

Location
For example, found in the umbilical cord

Special staining
- Alcian blue: stains the ground substance blue
- PAS: stains the ground substance pink

Can be mistaken for
Mesenchyme
- Cells are less widely distributed.

DENSE CONNECTIVE TISSUE

General
Contains more fibers than cells

Dense Irregular Connective Tissue

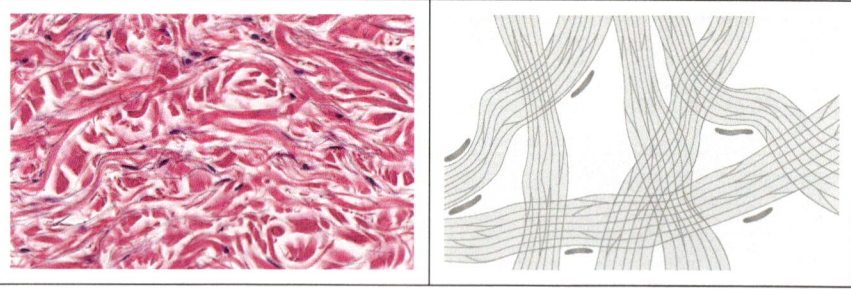

Left: photomicrograph of dense irregular connective tissue. Magnification: high. Stain: HE (Courtesy of associate professor Steen Seier Poulsen, University of Copenhagen). *Right*: simplified illustration of dense irregular connective tissue

Characteristics
- Thick bundles of weakly eosinophilic collagen fibers in an irregular pattern
- Small white spaces and few scattered nuclei between the fibers

Location
For example, found in:
- The dermis of the skin
- Organ capsules

Can be mistaken for
Smooth muscle tissue
- Smooth muscle fibers
   - Are densely packed, with no spaces in between
   - Are arranged in parallel in the individual layers of smooth muscle tissue
   - Are more eosinophilic
- The nuclei are located within the smooth muscle fibers.

Dense Regular Connective Tissue

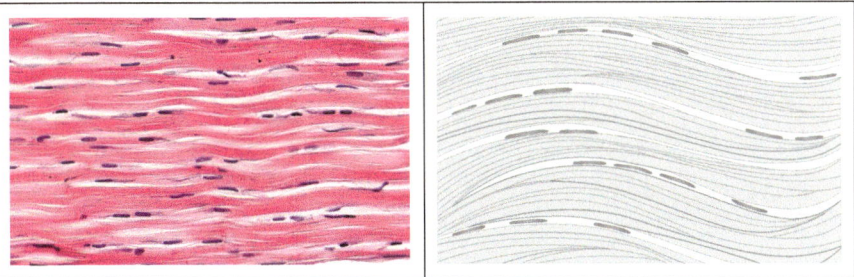

Left: photomicrograph of dense regular connective tissue. Magnification: high. Stain: HE (Courtesy of professor Jørgen Tranum-Jensen, University of Copenhagen). *Right*: Simplified illustration of dense regular connective tissue

Characteristics
- Longitudinal section:
  - Thick bundles of dense, parallel, often wavy, weakly eosinophilic collagen fibers.
  - Dark flattened nuclei are aligned in rows between the fiber bundles (as the stripes between the lanes of a highway).
- Cross section:
  - Weakly eosinophilic collagen fibers
  - Indistinct borders between the fibers
  - Small dark nuclei located between the fibers

Location
For example, in tendons and ligaments

Can be mistaken for
- Longitudinal section
  - Skeletal muscle tissue
    - Skeletal muscle fibers
      - Are more eosinophilic
      - Have cross striations
    - Nuclei are located within the muscle fibers.
  - Smooth muscle tissue
    - Smooth muscle fibers are
      - More eosinophilic
      - Thinner
    - Nuclei are located within the muscle fibers.
- Cross section
  - Skeletal muscle tissue
    - Skeletal muscle fibers are more eosinophilic.
    - White spaces are seen between the muscle fibers.
    - Nuclei are located within the muscle fibers.

Dense Elastic Connective Tissue

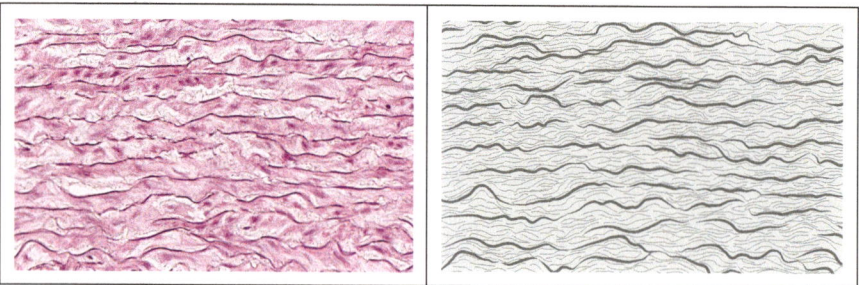

Left: photomicrograph of dense elastic connective tissue. Magnification: high. Stain: HE (Courtesy of professor Jørgen Tranum-Jensen, University of Copenhagen). *Right*: simplified illustration of dense elastic connective tissue

Characteristics
- Parallel bundles of thick, wavy, elastic fibers.
- The elastic fibers are strongly refractive and "flash" when focusing in and out of the focal plane.

Location
For example, found in the wall of elastic arteries

Special staining
- Orcein: elastic fibers stain red/brown and lose their refractive properties.
- Weigert's (resorcin-fuchsin): elastic fibers stain blue/black and lose their refractive properties.

References

5, 25, 33, 34, 45.

Chapter 8
Cartilage

Contents

General
- Specialized connective tissue
- Avascular
  - Cells are nourished from the surrounding tissues via diffusion through the ground substance.
- A sheath of dense irregular connective tissue (perichondrium) surrounds all cartilage, except:
  - Articular cartilage (Chap. 15)
  - Epiphyseal plates (Chap. 9)
  - Fibrocartilage

Function
- Mechanical support
  - Fibers:
    - Resist tensile strength
  - Ground substance (viscous gel):
    - Firm, yet pliable and resilient (like a wet sponge) → resists compression and adapted to bear weight
- Specific functions of the different types of cartilage are listed in Table 8.1.

© Springer International Publishing Switzerland 2017
A. Rehfeld et al., *Compendium of Histology*, DOI 10.1007/978-3-319-41873-5_8

Table 8.1 Types of cartilage

	Hyaline cartilage	Elastic cartilage	Fibrocartilage
Macroscopically	Glassy/bluish	Yellowish	Whitish
Light microscopy	Homogenous, amorphous extracellular matrix	Non-homogenous, filamentous extracellular matrix	Dense connective tissue with clumps of hyaline cartilage
Composition	• Chondrocytes/-blasts in lacunae, solitary or in clusters (isogenous groups) • Extracellular matrix with thin collagen fibrils	As hyaline cartilage plus a network of elastic fibers	Mixture of dense connective tissue and hyaline cartilage
Collagen type	Type II	Type II	Type I and II
Perichondrium	+, Except in articular cartilage and epiphyseal plates	+	−

Function	• Form articular cartilage
	  ○ Smooth, low-friction surface
	  ○ Resists compression
	• Form fetal skeleton → precursor for most bones via endochondral ossification (Chap. 9)
	• Able to grow fast → lengthwise bone growth via epiphyseal plates (Chap. 9)
	• Fracture-resistant skeleton in respiratory tract
		• Provides flexible support
		• Fracture-resistant skeleton in ear
			• Resistance to compression via hyaline cartilage clumps
			• Resistance to shearing forces via dense connective tissue

Staining of extracellular matrix	• HE:
	  ○ Weakly basophilic
	  ○ More strongly basophilic in deep regions and around lacunae
	• Toluidine blue: metachromatic (blue/ red)
		• HE: Elastic fibers are weakly stained but highly refractile
		• Orcein: elastic fibers stain brown
		• Resorcin-fuchsin: elastic fibers stain blue
			HE: small basophilic hyaline cartilage clumps between dense eosinophilic collagen fiber bundles

Location	Most common type, e.g. in rings of trachea	For example, in external ear	For example, in intervertebral discs

Divided into (Table 8.1)
- Hyaline cartilage
- Elastic cartilage
- Fibrocartilage

Consist of
- Cells
- Extracellular matrix

CELLS OF CARTILAGE

Divided into (Table 8.2)
- Chondroblasts
- Chondrocytes
- Fibroblasts (only in fibrocartilage)

EXTRACELLULAR MATRIX OF CARTILAGE

General
The extracellular matrix is especially abundant in cartilage and makes up >95 % of the volume.

Divided into
- Ground substance
- Fibers
- Multiadhesive glycoproteins

Consists of
- Ground substance
  - Proteoglycan aggregates with abundant negative charges.
  - Negative charges bind cations and $H_2O \rightarrow$ formation of a highly hydrated gel:
    - H_2O makes up $\approx 70 \%$ of cartilages weight.
    - The high H_2O content permits diffusion to deep regions of the cartilage.

- Fibers
  - Thin, ⊘ 20 nm, collagen fibrils of type II collagen → 3D meshwork
  - Only in elastic cartilage: elastic fibers
  - Only in fibrocartilage: thicker collagen fibers of type I collagen
- Multiadhesive glycoproteins, e.g., fibronectin

Table 8.2 Cells of cartilage

	Location	Light microscopy	Function
Chondroblasts	• In all types of cartilage • Located just beneath the perichondrium in lacunae (spaces) in the extracellular matrix	• Flattened cells • Ovoid nucleus • Basophilic cytoplasm due to abundant rER	Production of extracellular matrix of cartilage

Chondrocytes	• In all types of cartilage
	• Located deep in the cartilage in lacunae in the extracellular matrix
		• Rounded cells
		• Round/ovoid nucleus
		• Contain lipid droplets and glycogen granules (nutritional storage)
		• Appearance vary with activity
		  ○ Active production of extracellular matrix
		    ■ Basophilic cytoplasm due to abundant rER
		    ■ Pale area in cytoplasm corresponds to the Golgi apparatus (negative Golgi stain)
		  ○ No active production of extracellular matrix
		    ■ Acidophilic cytoplasm due to low amounts of rER
			Active/inactive production of extracellular matrix of cartilage

Fibroblasts	Only in fibrocartilage	• Large flattened cell • Elongated dark (heterochromatic) nucleus • Pale cytoplasm with low amount of rER → only nucleus is visible in the light microscope	Production of extracellular matrix of the dense connective tissue component in fibrocartilage

Light microscopy
- Unlike the other types of connective tissue, the ground substance in cartilage is retained during routine preparation.
- Ground substance stains basophilic/metachromatic.

MEMO-BOX
- **Hyaline cartilage: H**omogenous extracellular matrix
- **ELASTIC** cartilage: contains **ELASTIC** fibers
- **FIB**rous cartilage: contains **FIB**roblasts and dense **FIB**ers of collagen type I.

Formation and Modulation of Cartilage

FORMATION OF CARTILAGE (CHONDROGENESIS)

General
Begins at 5th week of gestation

Formation
- Cartilage:
  1. Mesenchymal cells aggregate into a mass of closely apposed cells (chondrogenic nodule).
  2. Cells in the chondrogenic nodule differentiate into chondroblasts.
  3. Chondroblasts produce extracellular matrix, which surrounds the individual cells.
  4. Cells are now chondrocytes in lacunae.
- Perichondrium:
  1. Mesenchymal cells surrounding the chondrogenic nodule differentiate into fibroblasts.
  2. Fibroblasts produce a sheath of dense irregular connective tissue (perichondrium).

GROWTH OF CARTILAGE

General
Cartilage grows until the end of puberty.

Divided into
- Interstitial growth
  - Formation of new cartilage within existing cartilage.
  - Chondrocytes located deep in cartilage divide → additional chondrocytes which produce extracellular matrix.
- Appositional growth
  - Formation of new cartilage on the surface of existing cartilage.
  - Cells from the innermost layer of the perichondrium differentiate into chondroblasts, which produce extracellular matrix.

CALCIFICATION OF CARTILAGE

General
- A naturally occurring process
- Takes place in:
  - Hyaline cartilage
    - During endochondral ossification (Chap. 9)
    - In innermost part of articular cartilage (near the surface of the bone)
    - During aging, e.g., in tracheal rings
  - Fibrocartilage
    - During repair of bone fractures

Formation
1. Embedding of calcium phosphate crystals in extracellular matrix
   ↓
2. Diminished diffusion
   ↓
3. Chondrocytes die
   ↓
4. Cartilage removal and bone tissue formation

REPAIR OF CARTILAGE

General
Limited due to lack of blood vessels:
- Most commonly defects are replaced by dense connective tissue.
- If defects involve the perichondrium, a slow and often incomplete, repair takes place.
  - ○ Cells from inner layer of the perichondrium differentiate into chondroblasts, which form new cartilage.

Guide to Practical Histology: Cartilage

Hyaline Cartilage

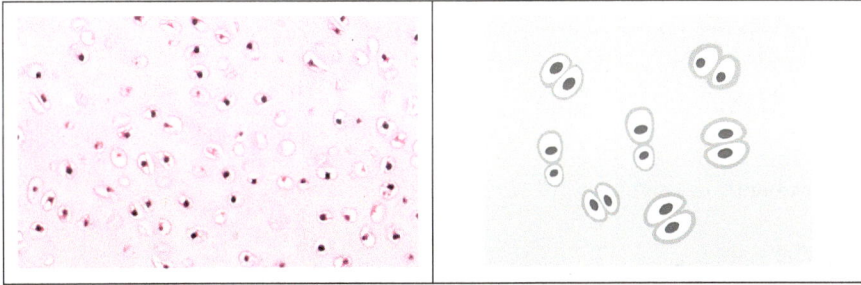

Left: photomicrograph of hyaline cartilage. Magnification: high. Stain: HE (Courtesy of professor Jørgen Tranum-Jensen, University of Copenhagen). *Right*: simplified illustration of hyaline cartilage

Characteristics
Homogenous mass with cells in small spaces (lacunae):
- The mass is weakly basophilic near the surface.
- The mass is more intensely basophilic in the deeper areas, especially near the lacunae.

Location
- Adult skeletal parts, e.g., in the rings of trachea
- Fetal skeletal parts
  - ○ Macroscopically resemble miniature models of adult skeletal parts
  - ○ Often contain areas of endochondral ossification

Special staining
Toluidine blue: stains the cartilage mass metachromatic (blue/red).

Elastic Cartilage

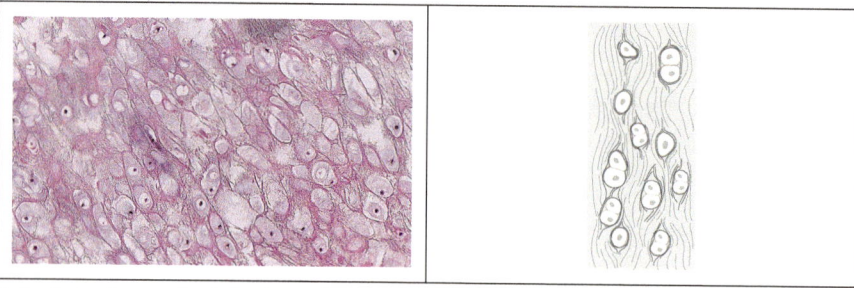

Left: photomicrograph of elastic cartilage. Magnification: high. Stain: HE.(Courtesy of professor Jørgen Tranum-Jensen, University of Copenhagen). *Right*: simplified illustration of elastic cartilage

Characteristics
- Non-homogenous mass with:
    - ○ Elastic fibers
    - ○ Cells in large, densely packed spaces (lacunae), resembling "eyes"
- The elastic fibers of the mass are strongly refractive and "flash" when focusing in and out of the focal plane.

Location
For example, in epiglottis

Special staining
- Orcein: elastic fibers stain red/brown and lose their refractive properties.
- Weigert's (resorcin-fuchsin): elastic fibers stain blue/black and lose their refractive properties.

Fibrocartilage

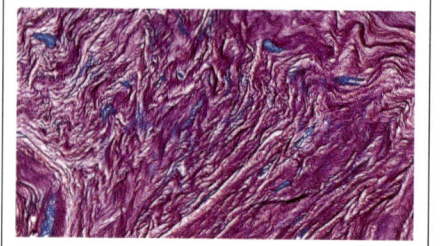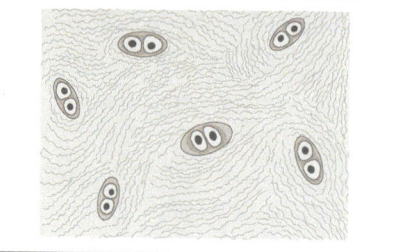

Left: photomicrograph of fibrocartilage. Magnification: low. Stain: Van Gieson and Alcian blue (Courtesy of professor Jørgen Tranum-Jensen, University of Copenhagen). *Right*: simplified illustration of fibrocartilage

Characteristics
- Small basophilic masses (hyaline cartilage)
- Surrounded by thick bundles of eosinophilic collagen fibers (dense irregular connective tissue)

Location
For example, in intervertebral discs

References

5, 25, 33, 34.

Chapter 9
Bone Tissue

Contents

General
- A specialized form of connective tissue with a mineralized extracellular matrix.
- The major component of bones (Chap. 15).
- The surface of bone tissue is covered with:
  - Endosteum: on internal surfaces of bones
  - Periosteum: on external surfaces of bones, except areas with articular cartilage

© Springer International Publishing Switzerland 2017

A. Rehfeld et al., *Compendium of Histology*, DOI 10.1007/978-3-319-41873-5_9

Function
- Very hard and strong tissue, which provides mechanical support in bones
  - The functions of bones are listed in Chap. 15.
- Take part in calcium and phosphate homeostasis, through Ca^{2+} and PO_4^{3-} storage

Divided into
- Lamellar (mature) bone tissue:
  - Compact (cortical) bone tissue
  - Spongy (cancellous, trabecular) bone tissue
- Immature (nonlamellar, woven) bone tissue

Consist of
- Cells (Fig. 9.4)
  - Osteoprogenitor cells
  - Osteoblasts
  - Osteocytes
  - Bone lining cells
  - Osteoclasts
- Extracellular matrix
  - Osteoid
    - Fibers
    - Ground substance
    - Multiadhesive glycoproteins
  - Mineral
    - Hydroxyapatite crystals

MEMO-BOX
OS is Latin for bone → most words concerning bone tissue contain "**OS**," e.g., peri**OS**teum and **OS**teocyte

---

BONE CELLS

Osteoprogenitor Cells

Function
- Stem cells, derived from mesenchymal stem cells
- Differentiate into the other bone cell types, except osteoclasts:

○ Osteoprogenitor cells

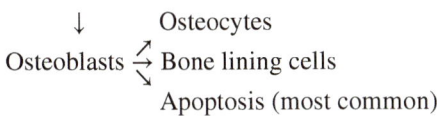

Light microscopy
- Osteoprogenitor cells resemble bone lining cells:
  - ○ Flattened cell body
  - ○ Elongated, light (euchromatic) nucleus
  - ○ Acidophilic/weak basophilic cytoplasm
- Found in inner layer of periosteum and in endosteum.

Osteoblasts

General
- Bone tissue forming cells
- Turn into osteocytes and bone lining cells:
  - ○ During bone tissue formation:
    - ▪ 10–20 % of osteoblasts turn into osteocytes as the osteoblasts embed themselves within lacunae in the extracellular matrix.
  - ○ When bone tissue formation is completed:
    - ▪ Remaining 80–90 % of osteoblasts either:
      - • Undergo apoptosis (most commonly)
      - • Turn into bone lining cells, which line the surface of the newly formed bone
- Osteoblasts are connected by cell extensions that form gap junctions:
  - ○ The osteoblast-derived osteocytes and bone lining cells remain connected after bone tissue is formed.

Function
Production of the extracellular matrix of bone tissue:
- Secrete unmineralized extracellular matrix (osteoid)
- Initiate mineralization in the osteoid via:
  - ○ Secretion of factors that locally elevate the concentration of Ca^{2+}, e.g., osteocalcin
  - ○ Budding off small matrix vesicles into the osteoid, which:
    - ▪ Contain factors that locally elevate the concentration of PO_4^{3-}, e.g., alkaline phosphatase
    - ▪ Serve as foci for the initial hydroxyapatite crystal formation

Light microscopy
- Single layer of cuboidal/polygonal cells, resting on a thin layer of weak acidophilic osteoid.
- Light (euchromatic) nucleus, located in the cell pole facing away from the osteoid.
- Basophilic cytoplasm, due to abundant rER.
- Pale area in cytoplasm corresponding to the Golgi apparatus (negative Golgi stain).
- Thin cell extensions can be seen between neighboring osteoblasts.

Osteocytes

General
- Major cell type in bone tissue (95 % of bone cells)
- Life span: 10–20 years
- Osteocytes are connected to adjacent osteocytes and bone lining cells via numerous thin cell extensions forming gap junctions.

Function
- Take part in calcium and phosphate homeostasis:
  - Through local remodeling of surrounding extracellular matrix (lacuna and canaliculi)
- Maintenance of bone tissue via:
  - Mechanosensitivity:
    - Osteocytes respond to mechanical stress in the extracellular matrix:
      - Decreased mechanical stimuli, e.g., during immobilization:
        - Osteocytes induce bone tissue loss by transmitting signals to other bone cells
      - Increased mechanical stimuli:
        - Osteocytes induce bone tissue formation by transmitting signals to other bone cells
  - Signal transmission to other cells:
    - Osteocytes transmit signals to other bone cells in response to changes, e.g., mechanical stimuli, in the surrounding bone extracellular matrix:
      - Direct signaling:
        - To neighboring osteocytes and bone lining cells, through gap junctions
      - Indirect signaling:
        - To other cells, e.g., distant osteoblasts, through secretion of signaling molecules

Light microscopy
- Located in lacunae between the lamellae of the bone extracellular matrix.
- Dark (heterochromatic), ovoid nucleus.
- Cytoplasm is pale/weak basophilic.
- Numerous narrow tunnels (canaliculi), containing thin cell extensions, spread out from lacunae:
  - Routine preparation: canaliculi are not seen.
  - Ground section: canaliculi are black/brown

Bone Lining Cells

General
- Cover all inner and outer surfaces of bones, except:
  - Where remodeling (bone formation/resorption) is taking place
  - Areas covered with articular cartilage
- Communicate directly with adjacent bone lining cells and osteocytes through numerous thin cell extensions with gap junctions

Function
Role in bone resorption:
- Osteoclasts cannot resorb bone tissue covered with osteoid.
- Bone lining cells produce collagenases, which break down osteoid, allowing osteoclasts to start bone resorption directly on the mineralized bone extracellular matrix.

Light microscopy
- Resemble osteoprogenitor cells:
  - One layer of flattened cells
  - Elongated light (euchromatic) nucleus
  - Acidophilic/weak basophilic cytoplasm
- Bone lining cells rest on a thin layer of osteoid, which cover the underlying mineralized bone tissue.

Osteoclasts

General
- Bone tissue resorbing cells
- Part of the mononuclear phagocyte system (Chap. 7), derived from monocyte progenitor cells:
  - The only bone cell not derived from osteoprogenitor cells:
    - Granulocyte/monocyte progenitor cells
      ↓ Fusion of multiple cells

- ▪ Osteoclast precursor
  ↓ Differentiation
- ▪ Osteoclast
- Motile cells, which move to areas where bone resorption is needed
- Undergo apoptosis after finishing bone resorption:
  - ○ Have a life span of a few days

Function

Bone resorption:

- Dissolve crystals of mineralized bone extracellular matrix
- Phagocytize osteocytes and degraded extracellular matrix products

Light microscopy

- Often located in a resorption lacuna (Howship's lacuna) on the surface of the bone tissue.
- ◯ up to 100 μm.
- 5–10 nuclei.
- Cytoplasm is weakly basophilic in young osteoclasts → acidophilic in older osteoclasts.
- Contain multiple copies of organelles, including numerous lysosomes.

The bone resorption process of osteoclasts

General

Bone resorption is regulated by, e.g.:

- Parathyroid hormone:
  - ○ Enhances bone resorption by indirectly increasing the osteoclast activity
- Calcitonin:
  - ○ Inhibits bone resorption by directly inhibiting the osteoclast activity

Structure (Fig. 9.4)

Three important zones are seen in the osteoclast during bone resorption:

- Ruffled border:
  - ○ Plasma membrane of the osteoclast in direct contact with bone tissue:
    - ○ Forms multiple deep infoldings
    - ○ Infoldings → increased surface area for secretion/phagocytosis
- Clear zone (sealing zone):
  - ○ Boundary of ruffled border
  - ○ Contains multiple cell–extracellular matrix junctions between the osteoclast and the bone extracellular matrix → tight seal of resorption lacuna

- Resorption lacuna:
  - The area between the ruffled border and the bone tissue, bounded by the clear zone
  - Site of the bone resorption process:
    1. Exocytosis of lysosomal enzymes
    2. Secretion of H^+:
       - Decrease pH → activation of lysosomal enzymes
       - Dissolves hydroxyapatite crystals into free Ca^{2+} and PO_4^{3-}
    3. Phagocytosis of remaining material, e.g., osteocytes, degraded extracellular matrix components and mineral

MEMO-BOX
OsteoBlasts: Build up bone tissue
OsteoClasts: Crush (resorb) bone tissue

EXTRACELLULAR MATRIX OF BONE TISSUE

General
- The extracellular matrix of bone tissue is mineralized, in contrast to other connective tissues.
- The hard, mineralized extracellular matrix forms the structural basis of the functions of bone tissue.

Function
- Fibers:
  - Provide tensile strength and some elasticity
- Minerals:
  - Provide great hardness to the extracellular matrix

Consists of
- Osteoid (unmineralized bone extracellular matrix):
  - Fibers:
    - Collagen fibers of type I collagen (90 % of protein in osteoid)
  - Ground substance
  - Multiadhesive glycoproteins
    - For example, osteonectin, which connects collagen to hydroxyapatite crystals
- Minerals ($\approx$75 % of weight):
  - $Ca^{2+} + PO_4^{3-} \rightarrow$ hydroxyapatite crystals, $Ca_{10}(PO_4)_6(OH)_2$
  - The crystals both precipitate within:
    - Small gaps in the collagen fibers
    - The ground substance

Light microscopy
- Osteoid is weakly acidophilic.
- Mineralized bone extracellular matrix is acidophilic.

Mineralization of Osteoid

General
Begins 10–20 days after the deposition of osteoid by osteoblasts

Divided into
- Primary mineralization
- Secondary mineralization

Primary mineralization
General
- Duration 3–4 days.
- 80 % of minerals are deposited during this period.

Formation
Osteoblasts initiate mineralization of the osteoid:
1. Release factors that locally elevate the concentration of Ca^{2+}, e.g., osteocalcin.
2. Bud off small matrix vesicles into osteoid. Matrix vesicles contain factors that locally elevate the concentration of PO_4^{3-}, e.g., alkaline phosphatase.
3. Solubility equilibrium for $CaPO_4$ is reached $\rightarrow$ hydroxyapatite crystals, $Ca_{10}(PO_4)_6(OH)_2$, precipitate using matrix vesicles as initial foci.
4. Further mineralization of osteoid due to expansion of the formed crystals.

Secondary mineralization

General
- Duration 3–4 months.
- Remaining 20 % of minerals are deposited during this period, by substituting crystal-bound H_2O with mineral.

Lamellar (Mature) Bone Tissue

COMPACT BONE TISSUE

General (Fig. 9.1)
- Compact mass
- Without macroscopically visible spaces
- Extracellular matrix is arranged in lamellae
- Forms:
  - The outer layer of all bones
  - The major part of the diaphysis (shaft) of long bones

Consists of
- Osteons (Haversian systems)
  - Concentric lamellae surrounding a central canal
  - Structural units of compact bone
- Interstitial lamellae
  - Found between osteons
  - Remnant lamellae of former osteons, which have been incompletely removed during remodeling
- Circumferential lamellae
  - Few parallel lamellae, just beneath the periosteum and the endosteum.
  - The lamellae follow the entire circumference of outer bone surface and medullary cavity.

Light microscopy
A homogenous mass of eosinophilic lamellae:
- Indistinct borders between the lamellae.
- Osteocytes are located in small white spaces between the lamellae.

Staining
Ground bone (not a staining, but a special preparation technique for bone tissue):
- Bone tissue is brownish with dark spaces (lacunae).
- Dark lines (canaliculi) are seen radiating out from lacunae.

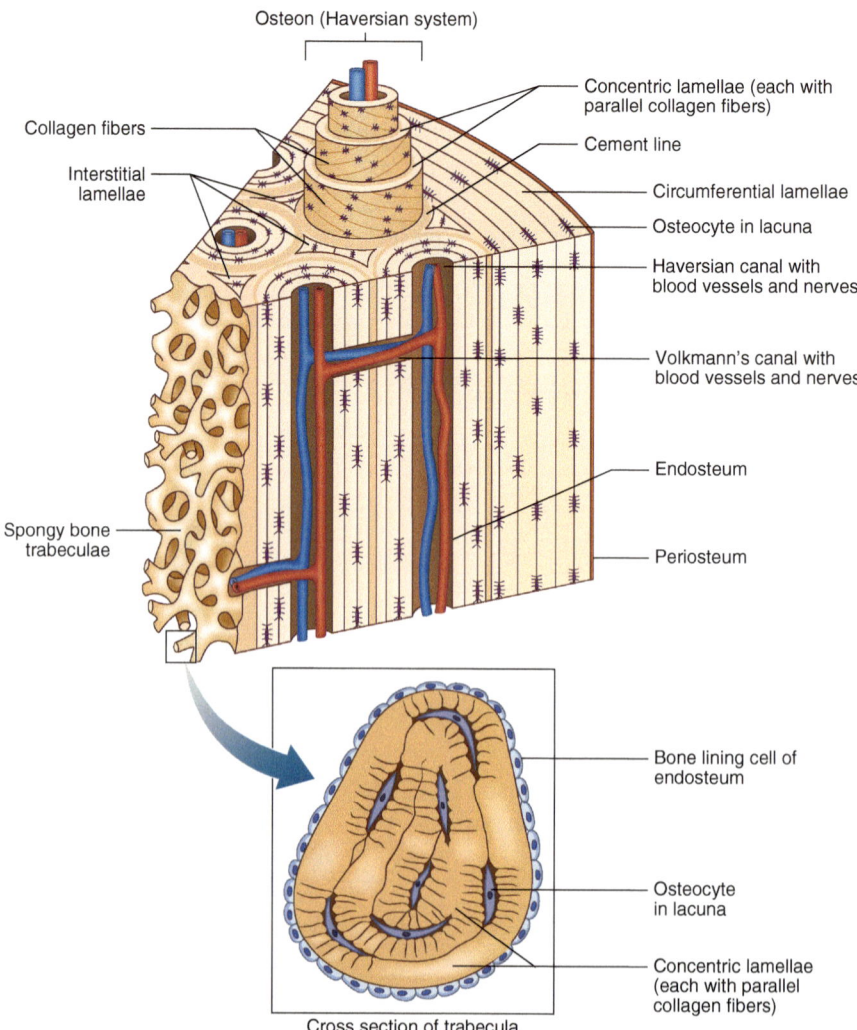

Fig. 9.1 Bone tissue structure: the structure of compact and spongy bone tissue

Osteon (Haversian System)

General
The structural units of compact bone tissue

Structure (Fig. 9.1)
- 3 mm long, $\oslash \approx 200$ µm
- A hollow cylinder, with the long axis parallel to the long axis of the bone
- A cement line, an outer layer rich in collagen, forms the boundary of the osteon and attaches it to adjacent osteons
- Haversian canal (osteonal canal):
  - The canal central in the "hollow cylinder," surrounded by the concentric lamellae
  - $\oslash$ 50 µm
  - Contain loose connective tissue, blood vessels, and nerves

Consists of
- Extracellular matrix:
  - Organized in lamellae:
    - Multiple concentric 3–7 µm thick rings, encircling the central osteonal canal.
    - Lamellae have parallel collagen fibers, organized in different directions in adjacent lamellae → osteon has high tensile strength in multiple directions.
- Osteocytes:
  - Located in lacunae between the lamellae.
  - Thin cell extensions run in narrow tunnels (canaliculi) and form contact with adjacent osteocytes and bone lining cells through gap junctions.
  - Canaliculi anastomose with:
    - Each other
    - Haversian canals
    - Volkmann's canals
    - Medullary spaces
    - The outer bone surface
  - Osteocytes are nourished by diffusion through the fluid surrounding the cell extensions in the canaliculi.

Light microscopy
Round unit of concentric eosinophilic lamellae, surrounding a central large round white space

Perforating canals (Volkmann's canals)

Structure (Fig. 9.1)
- Transverse canals, connecting Haversian canals to:
  - Other Haversian canals
  - Medullary spaces
  - The outer bone surface
- Contain loose connective tissue, blood vessels, and nerves
- Not surrounded by concentric lamellae

SPONGY BONE TISSUE

General
- Thin anastomosing trabeculae forming a spongelike 3D meshwork:
  - Organized to provide maximal strength in the directions of the mechanical load
- Spaces between trabeculae are macroscopically visible.
- Extracellular matrix is arranged in lamellae.
- Forms:
  - The inner layer of all bones
  - The major part of the epiphyses (ends) of long bones

Structure (Fig. 9.1)
- Fine bone trabeculae forming a spongelike 3D meshwork:
  - Trabeculae thickness: 50–500 μm.
  - The pattern and thickness vary with mechanical stress acting on the bone.
- Trabeculae are formed from lamellar bone tissue similar to compact bone tissue, but with some differences:
  - Spongy bone tissue is composed mainly of trabecular osteons.
  - Most trabeculae contain no blood vessels and nerves.
    - Bone cells are nourished from blood vessels in the bone marrow.
  - The thickest trabeculae are too thick to nourish the deep-seated osteocytes by diffusion from the bone marrow:
    - These trabeculae contain Haversian systems and Volkmann's canals with blood vessels to nourish these deep-seated osteocytes.

Light microscopy
Eosinophilic homogenous masses, with irregular shapes (trabeculae):
- Composed of eosinophilic lamellae.
- Indistinct borders between lamellae.
- Osteocytes are located in small white spaces between the lamellae.

Trabecular Osteon (Trabecular Packet)

Structure
- ≈ 1 mm long, $\oslash \approx 50$ µm.
- Half-moon shaped.
- A cement line, an outer layer rich in collagen, forms the boundary of the trabecular osteon and attaches it to adjacent osteons.

Consist of
- Extracellular matrix:
  - Organized in lamellae:
    - Multiple concentric 3–7 µm thick rings, which do not surround a central canal as in Haversian systems.
    - Lamellae have parallel collagen fibers, organized in different directions in adjacent lamellae → osteon has high tensile strength in multiple directions.
- Osteocytes:
  - Located in lacunae between the lamellae.
  - Thin cell extensions run in narrow tunnels (canaliculi) and form contact with adjacent osteocytes and bone lining cells through gap junctions.
  - Osteocytes are nourished through the canaliculi via diffusion from blood vessels in the bone marrow.

Immature (Nonlamellar, Wowen) Bone Tissue

General
- Initial bone tissue formed during:
  - Bone formation
  - Bone repair
- Extracellular matrix is not arranged in lamellae.
- Replaced with mature (lamellar) compact or spongy bone tissue during remodeling.

Structure
- Extracellular matrix:
  - Irregularly arranged collagen fibers → no lamellae and osteons.
  - Ground substance is more abundant.
  - No secondary mineralization occur.
- Cells:
  - Randomly arranged, within lacunae in the extracellular matrix

Endosteum and Periosteum

General
The surface of bone tissue is covered with:
- Endosteum: on internal surfaces of bones
- Periosteum: on external surfaces of bones, except areas with articular cartilage

Endosteum

General
Covers all inner surfaces of bone, including Haversian and perforating canals

Consist of
Single layer of:
- Bone lining cells
- Scattered osteoprogenitor cells

Periosteum

General
Covers outer surface of bone, except areas with articular cartilage

Function
- Appositional bone growth ⎤
- Bone repair   ⎦ via osteoprogenitor cells in inner periosteum.

Divided into
- Inner part:
  - Single layer of:
    - Bone lining cells
    - Scattered osteoprogenitor cells
- Outer part:
  - Dense connective tissue, containing larger blood vessels and lymph vessels
  - Sharpey's fibers:
    - Bundles of collagen fibers extending from periosteum into the extracellular matrix of the underlying bone tissue:
      - Anchors periosteum to the bone tissue
      - Numerous where tendons and ligaments attach to periosteum → attach tendons and ligaments to bone tissue

Bone Formation (Ossification)

General
Ossification begins early in fetal life:
1. Osteoblasts produce osteoid.
2. Osteoid is mineralized forming immature bone tissue.
3. Immature bone tissue is exchanged with mature (lamellar) bone tissue through bone remodeling.

Divided into
- Intramembranous ossification
  - Bone formation directly in mesenchyme
  - Formation of:
    - Cranial bones
    - Facial skeleton
    - Main part of the mandible
    - Main part of the clavicle
- Endochondral ossification
  - Bone formation within a preformed cartilage model
  - Formation of all bones not mentioned above.

INTRAMEMBRANOUS OSSIFICATION

General
- Bone formation directly in mesenchyme
- Takes place from 8th week of gestation

Formation (Fig. 9.2)

1. Ossification center forms:
   I. Mesenchymal stem cells condensate into a membranous aggregation.
   II. Mesenchymal stem cells within membranous aggregation differentiate into osteoblasts.
   III. Osteoblasts secrete osteoid.
   IV. Osteoid mass grows, mineralizes, and fuses with adjacent ossification centers within the membranous aggregation trabeculae of immature spongy bone tissue.
2. Periosteum forms:
   V. The membranous aggregation that sorrounds the multiple ossification centers forms the periosteum.

Light microscopy

- Initial ossification center:
  - Weak acidophilic osteoid mass
  - Surrounded by a single layer of basophilic osteoblasts
- Later ossification center:
  - Larger osteoid mass connected with adjacent osteoid masses.
  - Osteoid turns more acidophilic as it mineralizes.
  - Surrounded by a single layer of basophilic osteoblasts.

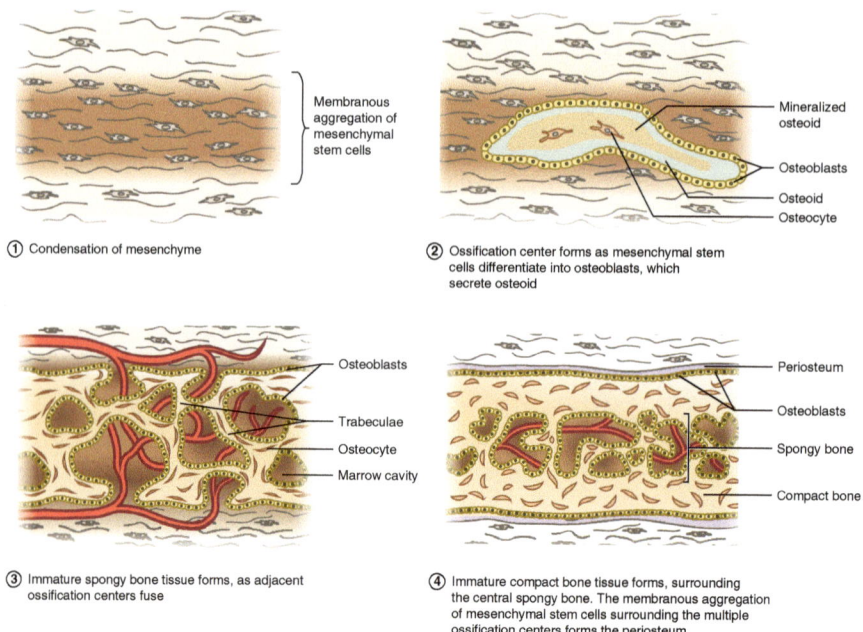

Fig. 9.2 Intramembranous ossification: the events of intramembranous ossification

ENDOCHONDRAL OSSIFICATION

General (Fig. 9.3)
- Bone formation within a preformed cartilage model:
  - Cartilage model with general shape of the bone is formed in the mesenchyme by chondrogenesis (Chap. 8).
- Takes place from the 8th week of gestation.
- Endochondral ossification of long bones is well studied and used as an example here.

Consists of
- Primary ossification center
- Lengthwise growth
- Secondary ossification centers

Primary Ossification Center

General
- Forms from 12th week of gestation.
- Located in the mid-diaphysis of the cartilage model of a long bone

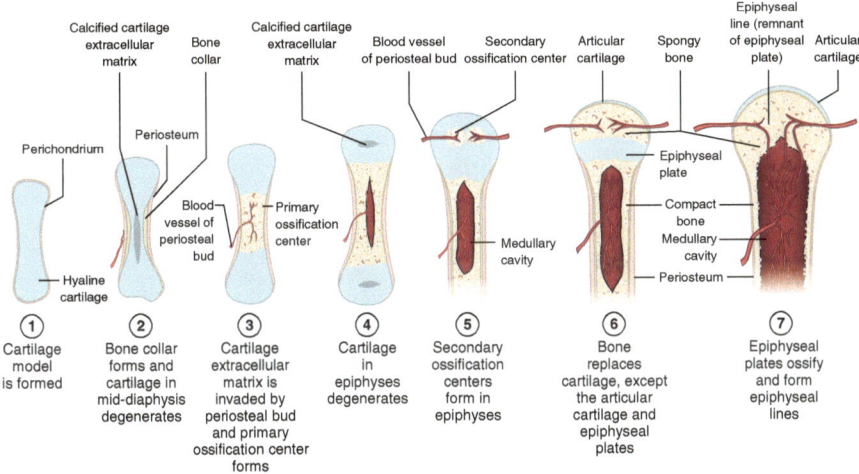

Fig. 9.3 Endochondral ossification: the events of endochondral ossification of a long bone

Formation
1. Bone collar forms:
   I. Perichondrium of cartilage model acquires ability to form osteoblasts and is now called periosteum.
   II. Osteoblasts form a thin bone collar around the mid-diaphysis by intramembranous ossification.
2. Cartilage in mid-diaphysis degenerates:
   I. Bone collar impedes diffusion in underlying cartilage.
   II. Chondrocytes enlarge → larger lacunae and less extracellular matrix.
   III. Chondrocytes secrete alkaline phosphatase → calcification of extracellular matrix → diffusion is further reduced → death of chondrocytes.
   IV. "Scaffold" of calcified cartilage extracellular matrix remains.
3. Cartilage extracellular matrix is invaded by vascularized connective tissue (periosteal bud):
   I. Osteoclasts resorb a tunnel in the bone collar at mid-diaphysis.
   II. Vascularized connective tissue from periosteum (the periosteal bud) penetrates tunnel in bone collar and fills empty spaces of calcified cartilage extracellular matrix.
4. Primary ossification center forms:
   I. Mesenchymal stem cells of the periosteal bud differentiate into osteoblasts.
   II. Osteoblasts use the calcified cartilage extracellular matrix as a "scaffold" and form osteoid on its surface (the true endochondral ossification).
   III. Osteoid mineralizes and form "mixed" trabeculae of immature bone tissue covering a core of calcified cartilage extracellular matrix.

Light microscopy
- Early signs of primary ossification center:
  - Degeneration of cartilage in mid-diaphysis:
    - Chondrocytes enlarge → many large spaces (lacunae).
    - Cartilage extracellular matrix calcifies → turns basophilic
  - Bony collar:
    - Acidophilic layer around the mid-diaphysis
- Later signs of primary ossification center:
  - "Mixed" trabeculae are seen within cartilage:
    - A core of basophilic calcified cartilage extracellular matrix.
    - Acidophilic bone tissue layer surrounds the core.
    - Basophilic osteoblasts cover bone layer.

MEMO-BOX
- Intramembranous ossification: "Intra" is Latin for inside. Bone formation inside a membranous aggregation of cells in the mesenchyme.
- Endochondral ossification: "Endo" is Greek for within and "chondro" is Greek for cartilage. Bone formation within a model of cartilage.

Lengthwise Growth

General
- Occurs in long bones after formation of a primary ossification center
- Lasts until the end of puberty
- Takes place in:
  1. Epiphyseal cartilage
     ↓ Formation of secondary ossification centers
  2. Epiphyseal growth plate: the remaining part of the epiphyseal cartilage

Formation (Table 9.1)
Growth takes place in five distinct zones found within the cartilage (from epiphysis → diaphysis):
1. Zone of reserve cartilage
2. Zone of proliferation
3. Zone of hypertrophy
4. Zone of calcified cartilage
5. Zone of bone formation and resorption

Epiphyseal growth plate

General
- The persistent disc of epiphyseal cartilage between the primary ossification center of the diaphysis and the secondary ossification center of an epiphysis.
- After the end of puberty, proliferation of chondrocytes ceases in the zone of reserve cartilage (zone 1):
  ○ The activity in the other zones persists until the epiphyseal growth plate disappears and medullary cavities of diaphysis and epiphysis join.

Memo-Box
The five zones of the epiphyseal growth plate can be remembered with the sentence "**R**eal **P**eople **H**ave **C**ollar **B**ones," referring to the zones of **R**eserve cartilage, **P**roliferation, **H**ypertrophy, **C**alcified cartilage, **B**one formation and resorption.

Table 9.1 Lengthwise growth

Zone	Name	Characteristics	Light microscopy	Function
1	Zone of reserve cartilage	Slow cartilage growth in all directions	Normal hyaline cartilage	Cartilage reserve, which makes further lengthwise growth possible
2	Zone of proliferation	• Chondrocytes arrange into columns parallel to the length axis of the bone • Chondrocytes proliferate → increasing height of columns → lengthwise growth	Columns of multiple small chondrocytes	Induce lengthwise growth
3	Zone of hypertrophy	Hypertrophy of chondrocytes → • Increasing height of columns → lengthwise growth • Larger lacunae and less extracellular matrix	Columns of multiple large chondrocytes	Induce lengthwise growth
4	Zone of calcified cartilage	• Extracellular matrix undergo calcification → Turns more basophilic • Chondrocytes die → leave behind "scaffold" of calcified extracellular matrix	Basophilic calcified cartilage extracellular matrix	Scaffold for bone tissue formation
5	Zone of bone formation and resorption	1. Empty lacunae are invaded by vascularized connective tissue from the medullary cavity 2. Mesenchymal stem cells differentiate into osteoblasts 3. Osteoblasts produce osteoid on the "scaffold" of calcified extracellular matrix 4. Osteoid mineralizes and forms trabeculae of immature bone tissue 5. Osteoclasts resorb the diaphyseal ends of the trabeculae, at the same rate as they are formed: • Keeps epiphyseal growth plate width constant • Increase medullary cavity towards epiphyseal ends	"Mixed" trabeculae: • Basophilic calcified cartilage extracellular matrix form a core • Acidophilic bone tissue layer surrounds the core • Basophilic osteoblasts rest on bone layer	• Bone tissue formation • Cartilage removal

Growth of the bone collar

General
- The bone collar is extended towards the epiphyseal ends, during the lengthwise growth.
- ⊘ of bone is increased by simultaneous:
  ○ Formation of new bone tissue on the outer surface of the bone
  ○ Resorption of bone tissue from the medullary cavity
- Bone collar thickness increases as the formation exceeds resorption.

Secondary Ossification Center

General
- Forms shortly after birth.
- Located in the epiphyses of the long bone.
- No bone collar is formed → cartilage at articulating surface persists as articular cartilage.

Formation
1. Cartilage in epiphysis degenerates:
   I. Chondrocytes enlarge → larger lacunae and less extracellular matrix.
   II. Chondrocytes secrete alkaline phosphatase → calcification of extracellular matrix → diffusion is further reduced → death of chondrocytes.
   III. "Scaffold" of calcified cartilage extracellular matrix remains.
2. Cartilage extracellular matrix is invaded by vascularized connective tissue (periosteal bud):
   I. Enters epiphysis from the perichondrium (now called periosteum).
   II. Fills empty spaces in calcified cartilage extracellular matrix.
3. Secondary ossification center forms:
   I. Mesenchymal stem cells in the periosteal bud differentiate into osteoblasts.
   II. Osteoblasts form osteoid on calcified cartilage extracellular matrix "scaffold."
   III. Osteoid mineralizes and forms "mixed" trabeculae of immature bone tissue covering a core of calcified cartilage extracellular matrix.

Light microscopy
- Early signs of secondary ossification center:
  ○ Degeneration of epiphyseal cartilage:
    ▪ Chondrocytes enlarge → many large spaces (lacunae).
    ▪ Cartilage extracellular matrix calcifies → turns basophilic.
- Later signs of secondary ossification center:
  ○ "Mixed" trabeculae are seen within cartilage:
    ▪ A core of basophilic calcified cartilage extracellular matrix.
    ▪ Acidophilic bone tissue layer surrounds the core.
    ▪ Basophilic osteoblasts cover bone layer.

Bone Modeling, Remodeling, and Repair

Bone Modeling

General
- Takes place during the growth period, i.e., until the end of puberty
- For example, seen during the lengthwise growth in long bones

Function
Displacement of inner and outer bone surfaces → alters the shape of the young bone towards its final adult shape.

Consist of
Two processes that are uncoupled and independent, with an excess of bone formation:
- Bone formation by osteoblasts
- Bone resorption by osteoclasts

> **MEMO-BOX**
> Modeling: as in "shaping" → process shaping the young bone towards its final adult shape.

Bone Remodeling

General
- Occurs during the entire life.
- Bone formation and resorption processes are under normal conditions in equilibrium:
  - Peak bone mass is reached around 30 years of age.
  - Bone loss:
    - Reversible bone loss:
      - After the peak bone mass is reached, bone tissue is slowly lost.
      - A result of slightly more bone resorption than bone formation.
    - Irreversible bone loss:
      - Takes place, e.g., when a trabeculae of spongy bone is perforated.
      - Osteoblasts can only form new osteoid on an existing surface, e.g., a "scaffold" of cartilage or bone extracellular matrix and can thus not repair the perforated trabecule.

Function
- Replacement of existing bone tissue with new bone tissue:
  - Initially, mature (lamellar) bone tissue replaces immature bone tissue → lamellae and osteons are formed.
  - Later on old mature bone tissue, containing dead osteocytes and microfractures, is replaced by new mature bone tissue.
- Reorganizing the 3D structure of bone tissue in relation to changes in mechanical stress on the bone
- Takes part in the calcium and phosphate homeostasis

Consist of
Two processes that are coupled and form bone remodeling units:
- Bone resorption by osteoclasts
- Bone formation by osteoblasts

Regulation of bone remodeling

General
Bone remodeling is regulated by, e.g.:
- Mechanical stress, sensed by the osteocytes
- Hormones, e.g., parathyroid hormone, thyroid hormones, and estrogen/ testosterone
- Signaling molecules, e.g., cytokines and growth factors

Bone remodeling units

General (Fig. 9.4)
Differs between the two bone tissue types:
- In compact bone tissue:
  - Cutting cone:
    1. Osteoclasts form a cutting cone, which resorbs bone and forms a tunnel with $\varnothing \approx 200$ μm, corresponding to the $\varnothing$ of an osteon.
    2. Vascularized connective tissue containing mesenchymal stem cells grows into the tunnel.
  - Reversal phase:
    3. Mesenchymal stem cells differentiate into osteoblasts.
  - Closing cone:
    4. Osteoblasts form successive lamellae of a new osteon.
- In spongy bone tissue:
  - Similar process as in compact bone.
  - Osteoclasts only resorb a ≈ 50 μm deep furrow, corresponding to the thickness of a trabecular osteon.

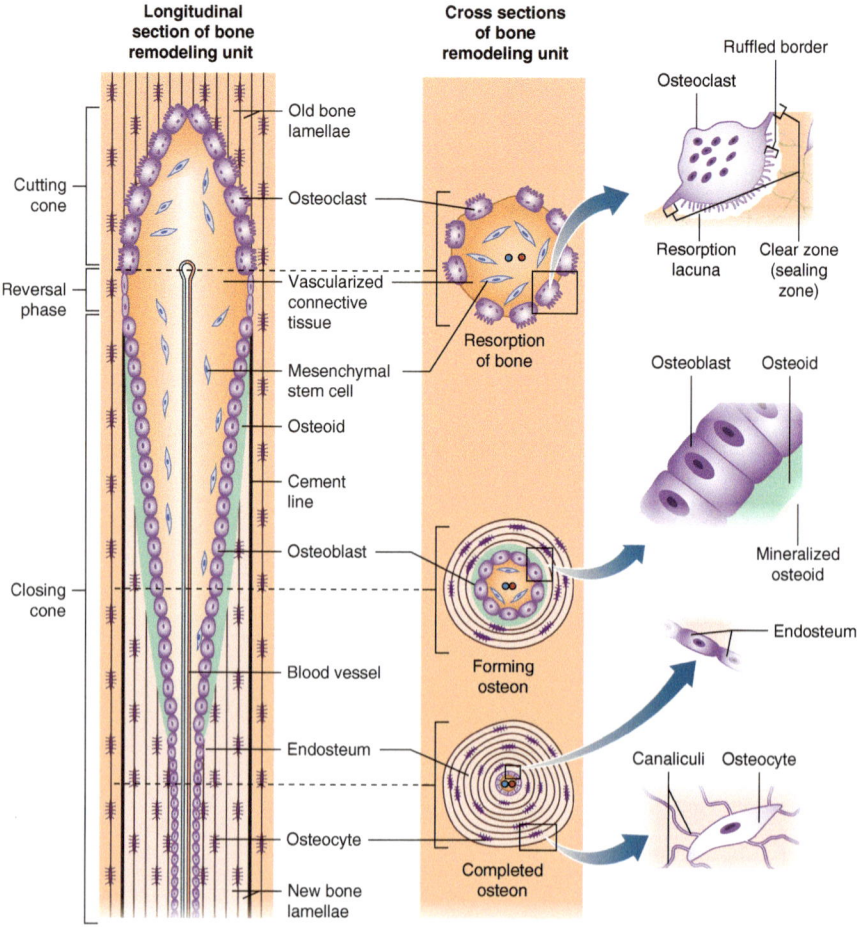

Fig. 9.4 Bone remodeling unit of compact bone tissue and the cells of bone tissue

Local remodeling

General

Local remodeling by osteocytes also takes place:
- Remodeling of extracellular matrix surrounding the osteocytes (lacunae and canaliculi)
- Does not involve the bone remodeling units

Function

Takes part in the calcium and phosphate homeostasis:
- The single osteocytes only remodel a small part of the bone extracellular matrix.
- As osteocytes make up 95 % of bone cells, the combined effect of local remodeling on the calcium and phosphate homeostasis can be large.

Bone Repair

General
- Bone tissue can repair itself after fractures.
- Duration: 6–14 weeks until a hard callus is formed.

Function

Restores bone structure and shape after a fracture

Bone repair process

1. Granulation tissue forms:
    I. A large hematoma forms from ruptured blood vessels at the fracture site → induces inflammation.
    II. Ingrowth of fibroblasts from periosteum.
    III. Fibroblasts produce loose connective tissue (granulation tissue), which replace the hematoma.
2. Soft callus forms:
    I. Fibrocartilage forms within the granulation tissue forming a soft callus, which stabilizes the fracture.
    II. Cells from the inner periosteum differentiate into osteoblasts.
    III. Osteoblasts form a bony sheath, by intramembranous ossification, on the surface of the soft callus.
3. Hard callus forms:
    I. Osteoblasts from the bony sheath invade the soft callus.
    II. Osteoblasts form bone tissue within the soft callus by endochondral ossification forming a hard callus of immature bone tissue.
4. Original bone shape and structure is restored through remodeling:
    I. Mature (lamellar) bone tissue replaces the immature bone tissue.
    II. Original bone shape is restored.

Guide to Practical Histology: Bone

Compact Bone

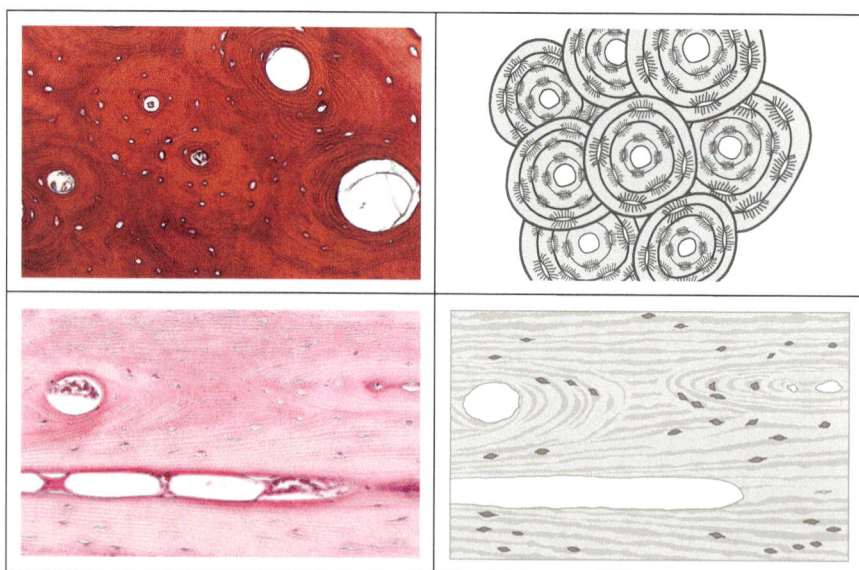

Top left: photomicrograph of cross sectioned compact bone tissue. Magnification low. Stain Mallory-Azan (Courtesy of professor Jørgen Tranum-Jensen, University of Copenhagen). *Top right*: simplified illustration of cross sectioned compact bone tissue. *Bottom left*: photomicrograph of longitudinal sectioned compact bone tissue. Magnification low. Stain HE (Courtesy of professor Jørgen Tranum-Jensen, University of Copenhagen). *Bottom right*: simplified illustration of longitudinal sectioned compact bone tissue

Characteristics
- Homogenous mass of eosinophilic lamellae:
  - Indistinct borders between the lamellae.
  - Cells are located in small white spaces between the lamellae (lacunae).
- Cross section:
  - Multiple round units (osteons) of concentric eosinophilic lamellae, surrounding a large round white space (osteonal canal)
- Longitudinal section:
  - Long parallel eosinophilic lamellae, with two types of scattered larger white spaces:
    - Round spaces (perforating canals)
    - Elongated spaces (osteonal canals)

Location
For example, the diaphysis of long bones

Special staining
Ground bone (not a staining, but a special preparation technique for bone tissue):
- Bone tissue is brownish with dark spaces (lacunae).
- Dark lines (canaliculi) are seen radiating out from lacunae.

Spongy Bone Tissue

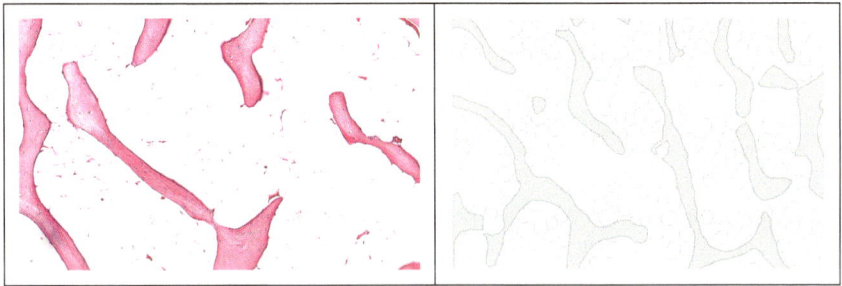

Left: photomicrograph of spongy bone tissue. Magnification low. Stain HE (Courtesy of professor Jørgen Tranum-Jensen, University of Copenhagen). *Right*: simplified illustration of spongy bone tissue

Characteristics
- Eosinophilic homogenous masses, with irregular shapes (trabeculae):
  - Composed of eosinophilic lamellae.
  - Indistinct borders between lamellae.
  - Cells are located in small white spaces between the lamellae.
- Bone marrow is seen between the trabeculae.

Location
For example, the epiphyses of long bones

Intramembranous Ossification

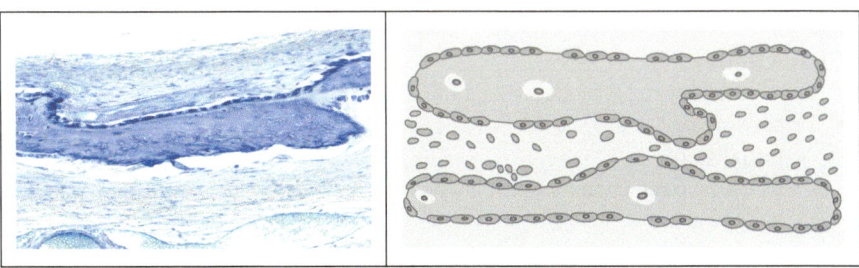

Left: photomicrograph of a trabecula formed by intramembranous ossification. Magnification: high. Stain: Toluidine blue (Courtesy of professor Jørgen Tranum-Jensen, University of Copenhagen). *Right*: simplified illustration of a trabecula formed by intramembranous ossification

Characteristics

At low magnification:

- A membranous aggregation of cells in loose connective tissue (mesenchyme):
  - Within the membranous aggregation, eosinophilic homogenous masses of irregular shapes (trabeculae) are seen.
- A single layer of basophilic cells (osteoblasts) covers the trabeculae.

Location

Commonly found in specimens of:

- Ossification of cranial bones:
  - Flat specimen.
  - Large, round basophilic hair follicles are seen at the surface opposite to the trabeculae.
- Ossification of mandible:
  - Specimen often contains a large basophilic "bell-like" structure (developing tooth), which is seen near the trabeculae.

Endochondral Ossification

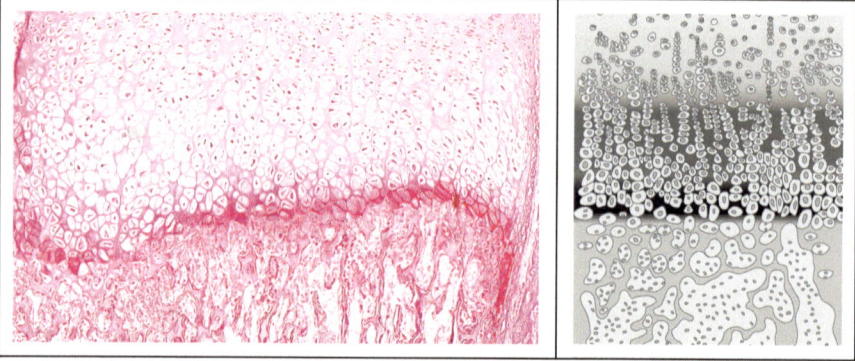

Left: photomicrograph of endochondral ossification. Magnification: high. Stain: HE (Courtesy of professor Jørgen Tranum-Jensen, University of Copenhagen). *Right*: simplified illustration of endochondral ossification

Characteristics

- Seen within skeletal models made of hyaline cartilage.
- Depending on the stage of the ossification process, different changes are seen:
  - Initial stage:
    - Cells in the center of the cartilage are larger than in remaining parts of the cartilage.
  - Later stage:
    - Bone trabeculae are seen within the cartilage.
    - A distinct straight border between bone formation and cartilage is visible.

Location

For example, seen in fetal skeletal parts:

• Macroscopically resemble miniature models of adult skeletal parts.

References

5, 7, 23, 25, 33, 34.

Chapter 10
Bone Marrow

General
- Specialized connective tissue of two types:
  - Red bone marrow
  - Yellow bone marrow
- Found within the spaces of bone:
  - Newborns solely have red bone marrow.
  - Adults have a 50/50 ratio between red and yellow bone marrow.
    - Red bone marrow is primarily located within the bones of the axial skeleton, corresponding to the area covered by a one-piece swimsuit.
    - Yellow bone marrow occupies the remaining spaces in the bone.
- Formed during the formation of bone (ossification).

Divided into
Two types, which may transform into each other:
- Red bone marrow
- Yellow bone marrow

© Springer International Publishing Switzerland 2017   187
A. Rehfeld et al., *Compendium of Histology*, DOI 10.1007/978-3-319-41873-5_10

Red Bone Marrow

General
- Red color is due to:
  - Abundant blood vessels
  - High content of erythrocyte stem cells containing hemoglobin
- May transform into yellow bone marrow

Function
The site of blood cell formation (hemopoiesis)

Consists of
- Vascular space
  - Sinusoids (discontinuous capillaries)
- Hemopoietic space
  - Parenchyma
    - Hemopoietic cells in cords/islets
  - Stroma
    - Reticular connective tissue

Vascular Space

Sinusoids

General
- Special capillary with large, varying $\oslash$ (Chap. 17)
- Supplied by the blood vessels of the bone (Chap. 15)

Function
- Sinusoid wall forms the barrier between the hemopoietic space and vascular system.
- Newly formed blood cells reach the bloodstream by transcellular passage through temporary pores in endothelial cells.

Consist of
- Endothelium
  - Thin simple squamous epithelium without tight junctions
- Basal lamina
  - Discontinuous
- Reticular cells (adventitial cells)
  - Cover outer vessel surface partially

Hemopoietic Space

Consists of
- Parenchyma
  - Hematopoietic cells in cords/islets
- Stroma
  - Reticular connective tissue
    - Reticular cells
      - Produce reticular fibers
      - Ensheath the reticular fibers completely with their cell extensions → form an anastomosing 3D cellular meshwork
      - Can differentiate into adipocytes → yellow bone marrow
    - Extracellular matrix
      - Reticular fibers → forming an anastomosing meshwork
      - Ground substance
      - Multiadhesive glycoproteins
  - Other cells in stroma
    - Macrophages
    - Mast cells
    - Adipocytes

Hemopoiesis

General
- The formation of new blood cells.
- Main location of hemopoiesis changes during embryonic life (Table 10.1).

Table 10.1 Main site of hemopoiesis during embryonic and postnatal life

Time line	Main location	Major type of erythrocyte	
		Nucleus	Hemoglobin type
First trimester, from third week of gestation	Yolk sac	+	Fetal type
Second trimester	Liver and spleen	−	Fetal type
Third trimester	Red bone marrow	−	Fetal type
Postnatally	Red bone marrow	−	Adult type

Function
- Formation of new blood cells
  - Erythrocyte development (erythropoiesis)
  - Thrombocyte development (thrombopoiesis)
  - Leukocyte development (leukopoiesis)
- Maintain steady levels of blood cells, which all have limited life spans

EARLY STEPS IN HEMOPOIESIS

General
Development of unipotent progenitor cells from a common pluripotent progenitor cell

Formation
See Fig. 10.1.

LATE STEPS IN HEMOPOIESIS

General
- Development of mature blood cells from unipotent progenitor cells.
- Unlike the stem cells going through the earlier steps in hemopoiesis, many cells going through the later steps have a distinct morphology in the light microscope (Table 10.2).

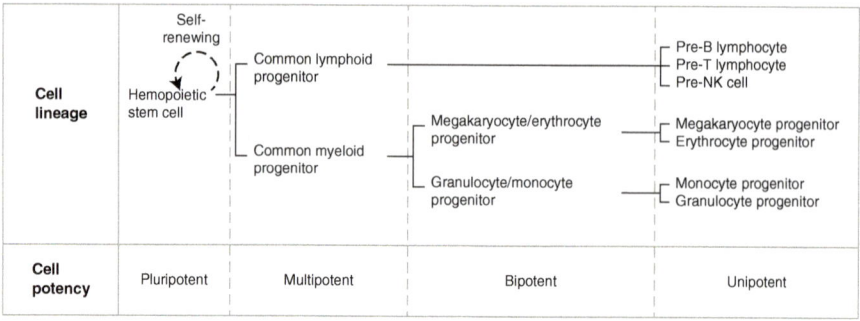

Cell lineage	Self-renewing Hemopoietic stem cell	Common lymphoid progenitor Common myeloid progenitor		Pre-B lymphocyte Pre-T lymphocyte Pre-NK cell
			Megakaryocyte/erythrocyte progenitor	Megakaryocyte progenitor Erythrocyte progenitor
			Granulocyte/monocyte progenitor	Monocyte progenitor Granulocyte progenitor
Cell potency	Pluripotent	Multipotent	Bipotent	Unipotent

Fig. 10.1   Early steps in hemopoiesis and the cell potency of the cells

Table 10.2 Simplified later steps in hemopoiesis

Cell	⊘	Nucleus	Cytoplasm
Stem cell (−blast) Mitoses and ↓differentiation	Large	• Large • Light (euchromatic)	• Basophilic • Without specific contents
Differentiated cell (−cyte)	Small	• Small • Dark (heterochromatic)	• Less basophilic • With specific contents

Divided into
- Erythropoiesis, erythrocyte development
- Leukopoiesis, leukocyte development:
  - Granulopoiesis, granulocyte development
  - Monopoiesis, monocyte development
  - Lymphopoiesis, lymphocyte development
- Thrombopoiesis, thrombocyte development

Erythropoiesis

General
- Duration 7 days
- Stimulated by erythropoietin

Structure
- Erythroblasts form erythroblastic islets around macrophages, which phagocytize extruded nuclei.
- Erythroblastic islets are formed in the hemopoietic space adjacent to the sinusoid wall.
- Mature erythrocytes are pushed through temporary pores in the endothelium and into the bloodstream.

Light microscopy (Table 10.3 and Fig. 10.2)
Overview of changes during erythropoiesis:
- Cell size decreases
- Nucleus
  - Decreases in size
  - Turns dark (heterochromatic)
  - Is lost at the end of development
- Cytoplasm goes from basophilic to acidophilic staining, as:
  - It fills up with the acidophilic hemoglobin.
  - Organelles are lost, including the basophilic ribosomes.

Table 10.3 Erythropoiesis

Cell	⦰	Nucleus	Cytoplasm	Free ribosomes (basophilic)	Hemoglobin (acidophilic)
Proerythroblast ↓ Mitoses	12–20 μm	• Large • Spherical	Mild basophilic due to free ribosomes	+++	−
Basophilic erythroblast ↓ Mitoses	10–16 μm	• Smaller • Darker (more hetero-chromatic)	Strongly basophilic due to many free ribosomes	++++	−
Polychro-matophilic erythroblast ↓ Mitoses	10–15 μm	• Smaller • Hetero-chromatin in checkerboard pattern	• Basophilic with acido-philic areas due to hemoglobin • Seen as distinct regions or a blend gray color	+++	+
Orthochro-matophilic erythroblast (normoblast) ↓ Nucleus extruded	8–10 μm	• Small • Dark (hetero-chromatic)	Acidophilic due to large amounts of hemoglobin, with slight basophilia due to remaining ribosomes	++	++
Reticulocyte (polychro-matophilic erythrocyte) ↓ Ribosomes lost	≈7.5 μm	No nucleus	Acidophilic with trace basophilia due to remaining ribosomes	+	+++
Mature erythrocyte	≈7.5 μm	No nucleus	Acidophilic	−	+++

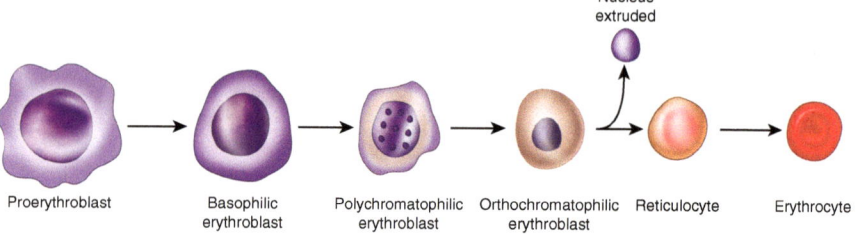

Fig. 10.2 Erythropoiesis: stages of erythrocyte development

> **MEMO-BOX**
> Use the names from erythropoiesis to remember events:
> - **BASOPHILIC** erythroblast: has a strongly **BASOPHILIC** cytoplasm due to large amounts of free ribosomes, which are needed to synthesize hemoglobin.
> - Polychromatophilic erythroblast: "polychrom" is Greek for multicolored, as it has acidophilic areas of hemoglobin in the basophilic cytoplasm.
> - Orthochromatophilic erythroblast: "orthochrom" is Greek for correct colored, as it is now purely acidophilic similar to a mature erythrocyte, as its cytoplasm is filled up with hemoglobin.

Granulopoiesis

General
- Duration 14 days
- Stimulated by colony-stimulating factors

Structure
- Myeloblasts form clusters within the hemopoietic space some distance from the sinusoid wall.
- Mature granulocytes are motile and migrate into the lumen of sinusoids.

Light microscopy (Table 10.4 and Fig. 10.3)
Overview of changes during granulopoiesis:
- Cell size decreases slightly
- Nucleus:
  1. Decreases in size and turns dark (heterochromatic)
  2. Elongates
  3. Forms lobes at the end of development
- Cytoplasm fills with granules:
  1. Primary granules (lysosomes)
  2. Secondary (specific) granules

Monopoiesis

General
- Duration ≈ 2 days
- Stimulated by colony-stimulating factors

Light microscopy
See Table 10.5.

Table 10.4 Granulopoiesis

Cell	⊘	Nucleus	Cytoplasm	Primary granules (lysosomes)	Secondary (specific) granules
Myeloblast Mitoses ↓	14–20 µm	• Large • Spherical • Light (euchromatic)	• Intensely basophilic • Without granules	–	–
Promyelocyte Mitoses ↓	18–24 µm	• Large • Spherical • Light (euchromatic)	• Basophilic • Primary granules (lysosomes), which are only produced at this stage	+++	–
Myelocyte Mitoses ↓	≈15 µm	• Smaller • Indented/elliptical • Darker (more heterochromatic)	• Weakly basophilic • Few secondary (specific) granules	++	+
Metamyelocyte Formation of nuclear lobes ↓	≈15 µm	Elongated/kidney shaped	Many secondary (specific) granules → cells are clearly identified as • Neutrophilic • Eosinophilic • Basophilic	+	+++
Mature granulocyte	12–15 µm	Lobulated	Many secondary (specific) granules	+	+++

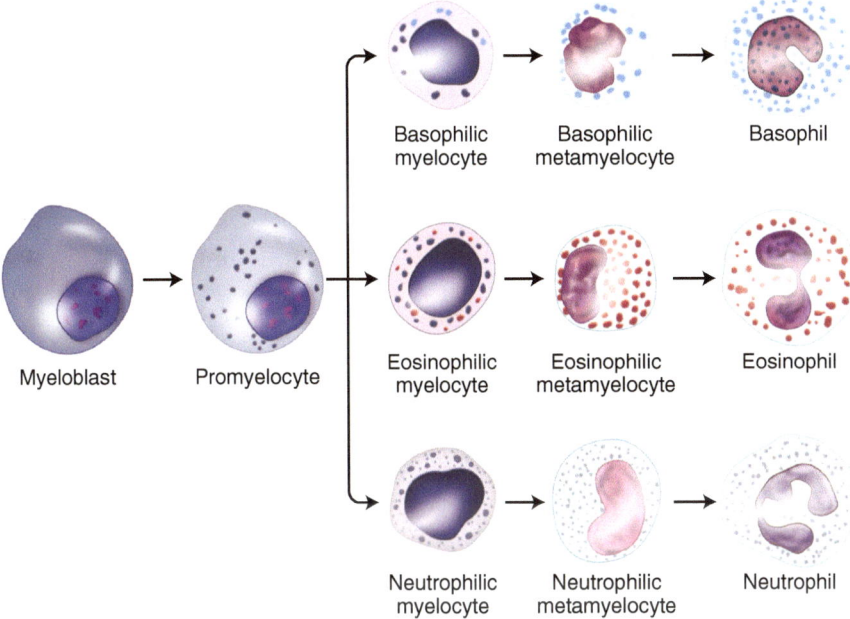

Fig. 10.3 Granulopoiesis: stages of granulocyte development

Table 10.5 Monopoiesis

Cell	⊘	Nucleus	Cytoplasm
Monoblast ↓ Mitoses	14–18 μm	• Large • Ovoid	• Basophilic • Without granules
Promonocyte ↓ Mitoses	14–18 μm	• Large • Slightly indented	• Mild basophilic • Without granules
Mature monocyte	12–18 μm	Indented/kidney shaped	• Pale basophilic • Many granules (lysosomes)

MEMO-BOX
Remember events of granulopoiesis:
- **PR**omyelocyte: **PR**imary granules in cytoplasm, which are only **PR**oduced at this stage.
- First the primary granules are formed, later the secondary granules.
- **META**myelocyte: as is "**META**morphosis" the Greek word for a change in physical form → first cell in granulopoiesis, which is clearly seen as becoming a neutrophil, eosinophil, or basophil in the light microscope, because of the many secondary granules.
- The nucleus must first be elongated, before nuclear lobes can be formed, analogous to when you need an elongated balloon to make balloon animals.

Lymphopoiesis

General
- Pre-B lymphocytes and pre-NK cells stay in bone marrow during further development (Chap. 19).
- Pre-T lymphocytes migrate to the thymus for further development (Chap. 19).

Light microscopy
See Table 10.6.

Table 10.6 Lymphopoiesis

Cell	⊘	Nucleus	Cytoplasm
Lymphoblast Mitoses ↓	10–20 µm	• Large • Light (euchromatic)	• Sparse • Basophilic • Without granules

Mature lymphocyte	≈7 µm	• Smaller
		• Dark
		  (heterochromatic)
			• Thin rim
			• Basophilic due to
			  many free ribosomes
			• Without granules

> **MEMO-BOX**
> Pre-B lymphocyte: stays in Bone marrow for further development
> Pre-T lymphocyte: migrates to Thymus for further development

Thrombopoiesis

General
- Duration 10 days
- Stimulated by thrombopoietin

Structure
Megakaryocytes:
- Reside in the hemopoietic space adjacent to the sinusoid wall
- Send long cell extensions through endothelial pores and into the bloodstream, where small fragments are broken off as thrombocytes

Light microscopy
See Table 10.7.

Table 10.7 Thrombopoiesis

Cell	⊘	Nucleus	Cytoplasm
Megakaryoblast Endomitoses (chromosomes replicate without nuclear- and cell ↓ division)	≈30 μm	• Large • Ovoid	Basophilic
Megakaryocyte Breaks off small fragments as ↓ thrombocytes	50–70 μm	• Multilobed • Polyploid, i.e., contains multiple sets of chromosomes	• Weakly acidophilic • Basophilic granules
Mature thrombocytes	≈3 μm	No nucleus	• Central darker-stained zone with basophilic granules • Peripheral weakly stained zone

Yellow Bone Marrow

General
- White adipose tissue (Chap. 11) found within the spaces of bone
- Yellow color due to the abundant adipocytes
- Has no active hemopoiesis
  - Retains hemopoietic potential, i.e., can transform into red bone marrow if necessary

Function
As white adipose tissue of other locations, e.g., storage of lipids

Guide to Practical Histology: Bone Marrow

Red Bone Marrow Smear

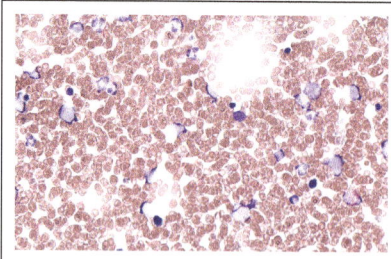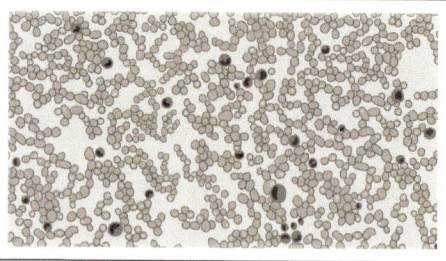

Left: photomicrograph of red bone marrow smear. Magnification: high. Stain: Giemsa (Courtesy of professor Jørgen Tranum-Jensen, University of Copenhagen). *Right*: simplified illustration of red bone marrow smear

Characteristics
- Numerous eosinophilic erythrocytes.
  - Erythrocytes are often seen in clumps or rows.
- Numerous hemopoietic cells with nuclei.
- Large round white (empty) spaces, (lipid droplets formed from rupturing of adipocytes during aspiration of the bone marrow specimen).

Special staining
Giemsa or Wright's stain:
- Methylene blue (basic dye): stains basophilic
- Azure dyes (basic dyes): stain azurophilic (dark blue/purple), e.g., lysosomes
- Eosin (acidic dye): stains eosinophilic

Can be mistaken for
Blood smear:
- Contains no hemopoietic stem cells → Few cells with nuclei.
- No large round white (empty) spaces.
- At large magnification, it is easy to find fields of view lacking cells with nuclei, unlike in the red bone marrow smear.

Bone Marrow

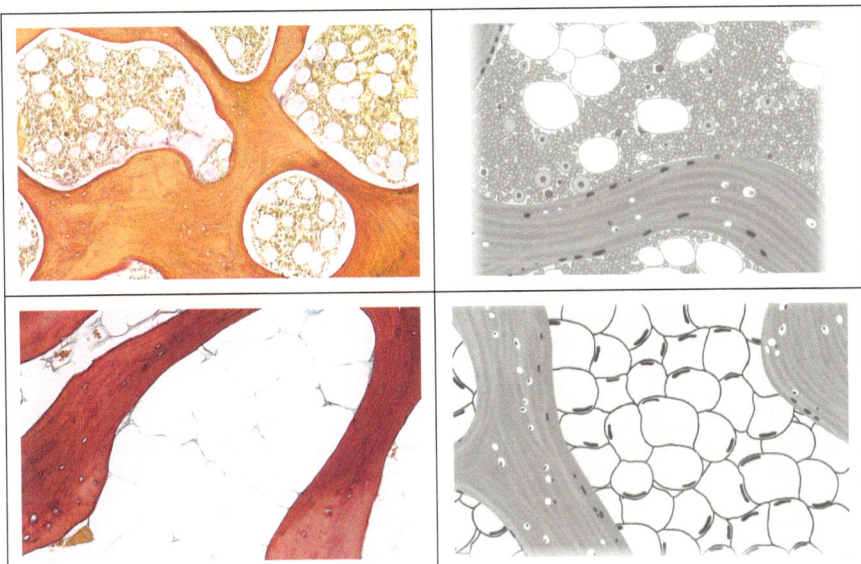

Top left: photomicrograph of red bone marrow. Magnification: low. Stain: Van Gieson and Alcian blue (Courtesy of professor Jørgen Tranum-Jensen, University of Copenhagen). *Top right*: simplified illustration of red bone marrow. *Bottom left*: photomicrograph of white bone marrow. Magnification: low. Stain: Mallory-Azan. (Courtesy of professor Jørgen Tranum-Jensen, University of Copenhagen). *Bottom right*: simplified illustration of white bone marrow

Characteristics

- Surrounded by bone tissue
- Two types of bone marrow:
  - Red bone marrow
    - Multiple tightly packed hemopoietic stem cells
    - Multiple white spaces:
      - Sinusoids containing erythrocytes
      - Adipocytes, seen as large white (empty) polyhedral cells
  - White bone marrow
    - Multiple adipocytes
      - Large white (empty) polyhedral cells.
      - Cells form a polygonal meshwork (resembles chicken wire).

Location

- Red bone marrow
  - ○ Primarily located within the bones of the axial skeleton, corresponding to the area covered by a one-piece swimsuit
  - ○ For example, within the vertebrae
- White bone marrow
  - ○ Occupies the remaining spaces in bone
  - ○ For example, in the bones of the fingers

References

5, 25, 33, 34, 36.

Chapter 11
Adipose Tissue

Contents

General
- Specialized loose connective tissue
- Consist of large groups of adipocytes (fat cells)

Divided into (Table 11.1)
- White (unilocular) adipose tissue
- Brown (multilocular) adipose tissue

Formation
- Both white and brown adipocytes are derived from mesenchymal stem cells but via different cell lineages.
- White and brown adipocytes can transdifferentiate into each other if stimulated, e.g.:
  - White → brown during long-term exposure to cold
  - Brown → white during longer periods where caloric intake exceeds energy expenditure

© Springer International Publishing Switzerland 2017   201
A. Rehfeld et al., *Compendium of Histology*, DOI 10.1007/978-3-319-41873-5_11

Table 11.1 White and brown adipose tissues

	White adipose tissue	Brown adipose tissue
Macroscopically	White/yellow	Brown
Cells of tissue:		
• Type	White adipocytes	Brown adipocytes
• Shape	Rounded/polyhedral	Polygonal
• Size	⊘ 15–150 μm	⊘ 10–25 μm
• Nucleus	Peripheral and flattened	Round
• Cytoplasm	• A single large lipid droplet, which fills up almost all of the cytoplasm • Abundant sER	• Multiple small lipid droplets • Abundant spherical mitochondria
• External lamina (similar to a basal lamina)	Surrounds cell	Surrounds cell
Main function	Energy homeostasis via storage of lipids	Heat production (thermogenesis)
Location	Found in multiple locations, e.g., as subcutaneous fat	Present in small amounts in adults, primarily around internal organs

Growth

Divided into
- Hypercellular growth:
  ○ Increased number of adipocytes
  ○ Through differentiation of new adipocytes from mesenchymal stem cells
- Hypertrophic growth:
  ○ Increased size of lipid droplets within the adipocytes

White (Unilocular) Adipose Tissue

General
- Macroscopically white/yellow
- Found in multiple locations, e.g., as subcutaneous fat
- Make up ≈ 20 % of body weight in healthy adults.

Structure
- Well vascularized
- Contain scattered sympathetic nerve fibers

Function
- Energy homeostasis:
  - When caloric intake exceeds energy expenditure, excess energy is stored in lipid droplets as triglycerides (three fatty acids bound to glycerol).
  - When energy expenditure exceeds caloric intake, triglycerides are broken down → fatty acids are released to the blood and used in cells as a source of energy through β-oxidation.
- Water homeostasis:
  - β-oxidation of fatty acids generates H_2O in addition to ATP.
- Insulation:
  - White adipose tissue has a low thermal conductivity, due to the high lipid content.
  - For example, seen for subcutaneous fat, which reduce heat loss from body surface.
- Endocrine function:
  - Adipocytes secrete, e.g.:
    - Hormones, e.g., leptin, which regulates the appetite
    - Growth factors
    - Cytokines

Consist of
- Parenchyma:
  - White adipocytes in groups
- Stroma:
  - Connective tissue septa, which divides the tissue into lobes and lobules
  - Reticular fibers underlying the external laminae of the adipocytes

Divided into
- Storage depot type:
  - Most white adipose tissue is of this type.
  - Degraded and used as energy source during reduced caloric intake.
- Essential depot type:
  - White adipose tissue found at specific locations, e.g.:
    - In orbital cavities
    - Under the soles and palms
    - Around kidneys
    - In bone marrow
  - Essential function in supporting and cushioning organs and structures
  - Remains intact during reduced caloric intake

MEMO-BOX
TriGLYCERides: "Tri" means three → Three fatty acids bound to GLYCERol

White (Unilocular) Adipocytes

General
- Found in loose connective tissue both as:
  - Solitary cells
  - Groups of cells
- Large groups are called white adipose tissue.

Function
- Lipid storage
- Secretion of, e.g.:
  - Hormones
  - Growth factors
  - Cytokines

Light microscopy
See Table 11.1

Staining
- Lipid leaches out during routine preparation:
  - Only the nucleus and a thin rim of cytoplasm remain:
    - A single adipocyte looks like a signet ring.
    - Groups of adipocytes form a polygonal meshwork (resembles chicken wire).
- Lipid can be preserved using frozen sections or fixed and stained, e.g., with osmium tetroxide which stains the cell black/brown.

Regulation of energy homeostasis in white adipose tissue

Divided into
- Regulation via sympathetic nervous system:
  - Norepinephrine (noradrenaline) stimulates breakdown of triglycerides.
- Regulation via endocrine system:
  - Insulin stimulates increased storage of triglycerides.
  - Glucagon stimulates breakdown of triglycerides.
  - Catecholamines stimulate breakdown of triglycerides.

Brown (Multilocular) Adipose Tissue

General
- Macroscopically brown, due to the abundant mitochondria of the multilocular adipocytes
- Found abundantly in the fetus
- Make up 5 % of body mass in newborns
- Present in small amounts in adults, primarily around internal organs

Structure
- Very well vascularized
- Contain numerous sympathetic nerve fibers

Function
Heat production (thermogenesis):
- Heat is generated through β-oxidation of fatty acids within the abundant spherical mitochondria:
  - Specific proteins uncouple the β-oxidation from ATP production → energy from β-oxidation is released as heat and not used to produce ATP.
- Heat is distributed to the rest of the body with the blood flowing through the tissue.
- The heat production is regulated by the sympathetic nerve system:
  - Norepinephrine (noradrenaline) stimulates heat production.

Consists of
- Parenchyma:
  - Brown adipocytes in closely packed groups
- Stroma:
  - Connective tissue septa, which divide the tissue into lobes and lobules

Brown (Multilocular) Adipocytes

Light microscopy
See Table 11.1

MEMO-BOX
- White (unilocular) adipocytes: "Uni" means one. Cells only contain a single lipid droplet.
- Brown (**MULTI**locular) adipocytes: Cells have **MULTI**ple lipid droplets.

Guide to Practical Histology: Adipose Tissue

White Adipose Tissue

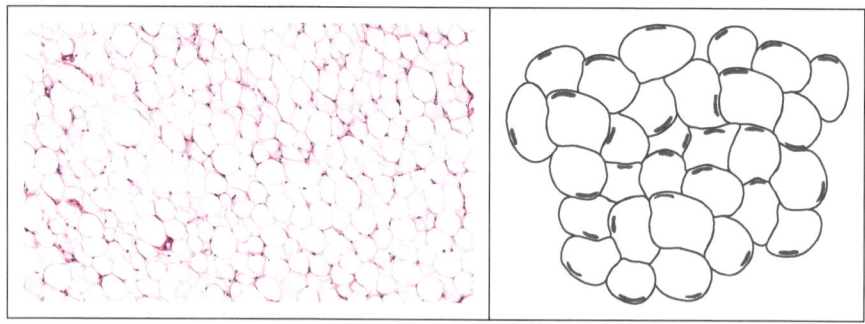

Left: photomicrograph of white adipose tissue. Magnification: high. Stain: HE (Courtesy of professor Jørgen Tranum-Jensen, University of Copenhagen). *Right*: simplified illustration of white adipose tissue

Characteristics
Aggregations of large white (empty) polyhedral cells:
- A peripheral nucleus seen in some of the cells.
- A single cell resembles a signet ring.
- Groups of cells form a polygonal meshwork (resembles chicken wire).

Location
Found in multiple locations in the human body, e.g., as subcutaneous fat

Special Staining
- Osmium tetroxide: Stains cells black/brown
- Sudan black: Stains cells black

Brown Adipose Tissue

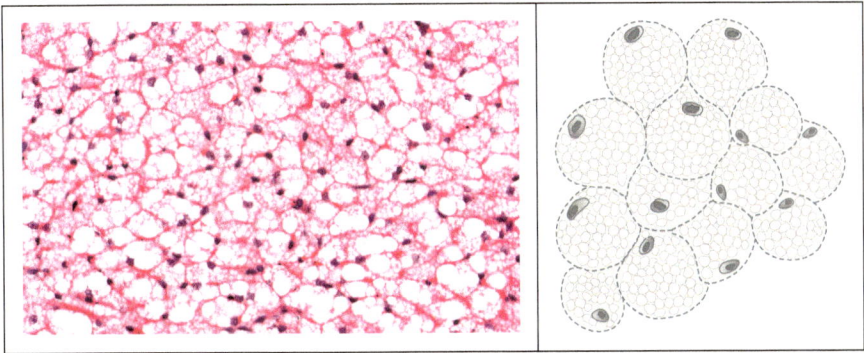

Left: photomicrograph of brown adipose tissue. Magnification: high. Stain: HE (Courtesy of professor Jørgen Tranum-Jensen, University of Copenhagen). *Right*: simplified illustration of brown adipose tissue

Characteristics
- Aggregations of cells with:
  - Eosinophilic cytoplasm
  - Many small lipid droplets, seen as white (empty) vacuoles
  - Ovoid nucleus
  - Indistinct cell borders
- Contains multiple capillaries:
  - Seen as narrow white spaces with multiple eosinophilic erythrocytes

Location
Only present in small amounts in adults, e.g., around the internal organs

Can be mistaken for
Trabecular endocrine tissue:
- Cells in strands, not in aggregations.
- Vacuoles are indistinct or smaller.
- Often divided into morphologically different areas.

References
5, 25, 33, 34.

Chapter 12
Blood

Contents

General
- Specialized type of connective tissue.
- Extracellular matrix (plasma) is fluid, unlike in other types of connective tissue.
- ≈5 L in adults, but depends on body size.
- Blood circulate through the cardiovascular system (Chap. 17).

Function
- Transport media:
  - Delivers nutrients and O_2 to cells
  - Removes wastes and CO_2 from cells
  - Distributes hormones and other regulatory substances
  - Transports immune cells and antibodies
- Maintain homeostasis, e.g., by acting as a pH buffer and participating in thermoregulation.

Consists of
- Cells (formed elements) (Table 12.1):
  - Erythrocytes (red blood cells) ≈ 5.000.000/µL
  - Thrombocytes (platelets) ≈ 300.000/µL
  - Leukocytes (white blood cells) ≈ 7.000/µL
- Extracellular matrix (plasma)

© Springer International Publishing Switzerland 2017
A. Rehfeld et al., *Compendium of Histology*, DOI 10.1007/978-3-319-41873-5_12

Table 12.1 Overview of blood cells

	Erythrocytes	Thrombocytes	Leukocytes					
			Agranulocytes		Granulocytes			
			Monocyte	B/T lymphocyte	Neutrophil	Eosinophil	Basophil
⊘	≈7.5 μm	≈3 μm	12–18 μm	≈7 μm	10–15 μm	10–15 μm	10–15 μm
Cell shape	Biconcave disc	Discus shaped	Round	Round	Round	Round	Round
Nucleus	No nucleus	No nucleus	Indented/ C-shaped	Large, round, and dark (heterochromatic)	2–4 lobes	Two lobes	2–3 lobes
Cytoplasm	Acidophilic	Central dark and peripheral pale zone	Weakly stained with lysosomes	Thin basophilic rim	Many weakly stained granules	Many eosinophilic granules	Many basophilic granules
Function	Transport of O_2 and CO_2	Hemostasis	Differentiates into, e.g., macrophages	Important roles in both innate and adaptive immune response	Phagocytosis	Fight parasitic infections	Role in innate immune response

Staining

Special mixtures of dyes are often used for staining blood smears, e.g., Giemsa or Wright's stain:

- Methylene blue (basic dye): Stains basophilic
- Azure dyes (basic dyes): Stain azurophilic (dark blue/purple), e.g., lysosomes
- Eosin (acidic dye): Stains acidophilic

Blood Cells

ERYTHROCYTES (RED BLOOD CELLS)

General

- Life span of ≈ 120 days
- ≈1 % of all erythrocytes are removed every day:
  - 90 % are phagocytized by macrophages in the liver, spleen, and bone marrow
  - 10 % are broken down intravascularly, as they get fragile with age
- Continuously produced in the bone marrow (Chap. 10)

Structure

- Biconcave disc
- ⊘ ≈ 7.5 μm
- Anucleate, i.e., without a nucleus.
- Cytoplasm is fully packed with hemoglobin (stain acidophilic).

- Contain no organelles except:
  - Plasma membrane
  - Cytoskeleton with unique composition:
    - Integral membrane proteins:
      - Attach plasma membrane to cytoskeleton.
      - Extracellular domains are glycosylated and form blood group antigens
    - Peripheral membrane proteins, spectrins:
      - Cover inner surface of plasma membrane as a 2D lattice network.
      - Stabilize plasma membrane and maintain biconcave cell shape.
      - Makes erythrocytes elastic, flexible, and able to withstand shearing and deformation as they pass through narrow blood vessels.

Function

Transport of O_2 and CO_2 bound to hemoglobin

Light microscopy
- Small, $\oslash \approx 7.5$ μm, biconcave acidophilic discs
- Anucleate, i.e., without a nucleus

Erythrocytes as a histological ruler

General
- Erythrocytes can be used as a "histological ruler" of $\oslash \approx 7.5$ μm to measure the sizes of other cells and structures in specimens.
- The sizes of leukocytes in blood are easily remembered in relation to erythrocytes:
  - B and T lymphocytes are ≈ 1x erythrocyte size.
  - Granulocytes and monocytes are ≈ 2x erythrocyte size.

THROMBOCYTES (PLATELETS)

General

Life span ≈ 10 days

Structure
- Discus shaped
- $\oslash \approx 3$ μm
- Anucleate (without a nucleus)
- Cytoplasm:
  - Central zone:
    - Darker staining with basophilic granules
  - Peripheral zone:
    - Weakly stained rim of cytoplasm containing:
      - Microtubules → maintain discoid shape.
      - Actin filaments and myosin → responsible for thrombocyte contraction during clot retraction.

Function

Play an important part in hemostasis (control of bleeding)

Light microscopy

- Very small, $\oslash \approx 3$ µm, discus-shaped structures:
  - Darker staining centrally
  - Weakly stained peripherally
- Anucleate (without a nucleus)
- Are often seen in aggregates

Hemostasis

Divided into

- Primary hemostasis (platelet plug formation)
- Secondary hemostasis (blood coagulation)
- Clot retraction

Formation (Fig. 12.1)
1. Damage to endothelium of blood vessel
2. Platelet plug formation (primary hemostasis):
   (a) Primary aggregation:
     - Damaged endothelium → exposed connective tissue → platelets adhere to collagen → form a platelet plug
   (b) Secondary aggregation:
     - Platelets in plug release mediators, e.g.:
       - Adenosine diphosphate (ADP) → further aggregation of platelets → increase plug size.
       - Serotonin → vasoconstriction → limits blood loss.
       - Coagulation factors → promote coagulation.
3. Blood coagulation (secondary hemostasis):
   - The damaged endothelium and aggregated platelets release coagulation factors → initiation of coagulation cascade:
     (a) Fibrinogen is cleaved to fibrin → fibrins cross-link to form an impermeable mesh over platelet plug.
     (b) Fibrin mesh traps blood cells → blood clot (thrombus).
4. Clot retraction:
   - Contraction of platelets in blood clot:
     - Clot shrinks and bulges less into lumen → permit normal blood flow in vessel
     - Pulls the edges of the lesion together → aids the regeneration of vessel wall.

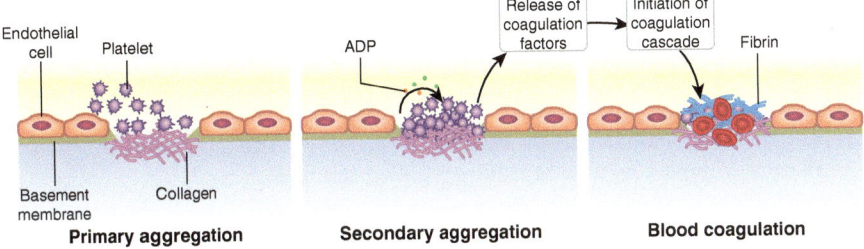

Fig. 12.1 The steps of hemostasis

LEUKOCYTES (WHITE BLOOD CELLS)

General

- Motile cells
- Spend most of their lifetime outside the blood circulation, e.g., in connective tissues, where they perform their major functions (Chaps. 7 and 19).
- For a detailed description of leukocytes, see Chap. 7.

Divided into (Table 12.2)

- Granulocytes: Contain many specific granules
- Agranulocytes: Contain no specific granules (only the nonspecific lysosomes)

Table 12.2 Leukocytes in blood circulation

	Granulocytes			Agranulocytes	
	Neutrophils	Eosinophils	Basophils	Monocytes	Lymphocytes
Specific granules	Yes	Yes	Yes	No	No
% of leukocytes in blood	≈60%	≈3%	≈0.5%	≈5%	≈30%
Time in blood circulation	Circulate for ≈10h before migrating into connective tissue: • 50%: In a freely circulating pool • 50%: In a marginated (slowly transiting) pool ○ Adhesion of granulocytes to the endothelium of capillaries and postcapillary venules → slows transit			Circulate for ≈1h before migrating into connective tissue	• Variable • Commonly in transit from one lymphatic tissue to another • Are able to recirculate between blood and tissues

Plasma

General
- The fluid extracellular matrix of blood.
- Plasma without coagulation factors is called serum.

Structure
Opaque yellow liquid

Consist of
- H_2O, >90 % of volume
- Solutes, e.g.:
  - Proteins, e.g.:
    - Albumin: ≈50 % of blood proteins:
      - Major contributor of colloid osmotic pressure
      - Carrier protein for, e.g., hormones and metabolites
    - Globulins:
      - Immunoglobulins (antibodies)
      - Nonimmune globulins, e.g., coagulation factors
  - Electrolytes
  - Nutrients

Guide to Practical Histology: Blood

Blood Smear

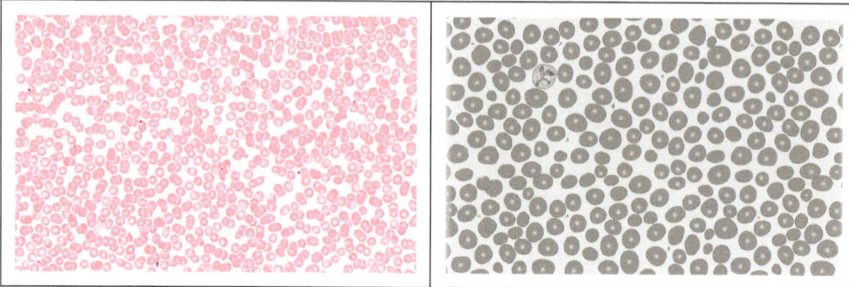

Left: photomicrograph of blood smear. Magnification: high. Stain: Giemsa. (Courtesy of professor Jørgen Tranum-Jensen, University of Copenhagen). *Right*: simplified illustration of blood smear

Characteristics
- Many eosinophilic erythrocytes
- Few cells with nuclei
- At large magnification: Easy to find fields of view without any cells with nuclei

Special staining
Giemsa or Wright's stain:
- Methylene blue (basic dye): Stains basophilic
- Azure dyes (basic dyes): Stain azurophilic (dark blue/purple), e.g., lysosomes
- Eosin (acidic dye): Stains eosinophilic

Can be mistaken for
Red bone marrow smear:
- Contains hemopoietic stem cells.
- Large round white (empty) spaces in the specimen (lipid droplets formed from rupturing of adipocytes during aspiration of bone marrow).
- At large magnification, it is difficult to find fields of view lacking cells with nuclei.

References
5, 25, 33, 34.

Chapter 13
Muscle Tissue

Contents

General
- One of the four basic tissue types.
- A special nomenclature exists for muscle tissue (Table 13.1).

Structure
An aggregation of elongated, contractile cells

© Springer International Publishing Switzerland 2017   217
A. Rehfeld et al., *Compendium of Histology*, DOI 10.1007/978-3-319-41873-5_13

Table 13.1 Muscle tissue nomenclature

Standard nomenclature	Nomenclature in muscle tissue
Cytoplasm	Sarcoplasm
Smooth endoplasmic reticulum (sER)	Sarcoplasmic reticulum
Plasma membrane (plasmalemma)	Sarcolemma

Function

Contraction → movement:
- "External" movement, e.g., of the limbs
- "Internal" movement → changes in shape of internal organs, e.g., the peristaltic movements in the intestines

Consists of

Muscle fibers:
- Skeletal muscle tissue: Fibers = the individual skeletal muscle cells
- Cardiac muscle tissue: Fibers = chains of multiple, connected cardiac muscle cells
- Smooth muscle tissue: Fibers = the individual smooth muscle cells

Divided into (Table 13.5)
- Striated muscle tissue, with microscopically visible cross striations:
  - Skeletal muscle tissue
  - Cardiac muscle tissue
- Smooth muscle tissue, without cross striations

Skeletal Muscle Tissue

General (Fig. 13.1)
Found in the skeletal muscles (Chap. 15)

Consists of
Skeletal muscle cells, also called skeletal muscle fibers.

Skeletal Muscle Cell

General
- Multinucleated cell
- Formed from fusion of multiple progenitor cells (myoblasts)

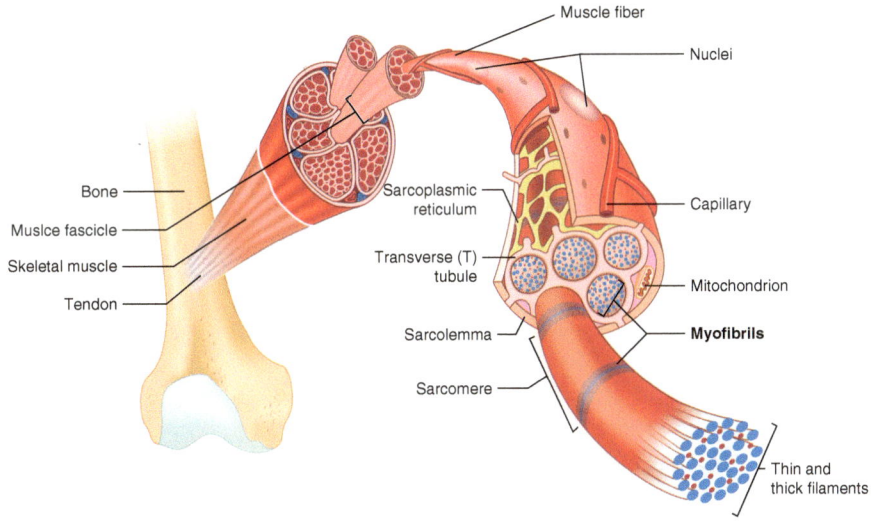

Fig. 13.1 The structure of a skeletal muscle, attached to bone via a tendon

Structure
- Long cylindrical cell:
  - ○ Length up to 100 cm
  - ○ ⊘ 10–100 μm
- Multiple peripherally located nuclei
- Cytoplasm:
  - ○ Myofibrils:
    - ▪ Multiple, parallel, and densely packed rod-like units
    - ▪ Gives rise to the cross striations seen in the light microscope
  - ○ Sarcoplasmic reticulum surrounding the myofibrils
  - ○ Multiple mitochondria
  - ○ Tubular invaginations of the plasma membrane (T tubules)
  - ○ Glycogen granules and lipid droplets
- Surrounded by an external lamina (similar to a basal lamina)

Function
Contraction (commonly voluntary)

Light microscopy
- Long acidophilic cells, with cross striations
- Multiple peripherally located nuclei

Skeletal muscle cell types

General
- Several types of skeletal muscle cells exist, e.g., types I, IIa, and IIb (Table 13.2).
- Most skeletal muscles contain a mixture of the different types.
- The ratio between the types within a muscle can be changed, e.g., through physical exercise.

Table 13.2   Skeletal muscle cell types

	Type I (red)	Type IIa (intermediate)	Type IIb (white)
Physiological properties:			
Function:			
• Main function	High endurance	Intermediate	High force generation
• Contraction speed	+	++	+++
• Force generated	+	++	+++
• Resistance to fatigue	+++	++	+
Sequence of recruitment in muscle	First (by small exertion)	Second (by medium exertion)	Third (by large exertion)
Major type of muscle cell in:	For example, postural muscles of back	For example, leg muscles	For example, extraocular muscles
Structure:			
In vivo color	Red (due to high myoglobin content)	Intermediate	White (light pink)
Muscle cell ⊘	Small	Medium	Large
Mitochondria	+++	++	+
Capillaries surrounding muscle cell	+++	++	+
Metabolic aspects:			
Source of ATP	Oxidative phosphorylation	• Oxidative phosphorylation • Anaerobic glycolysis	Anaerobic glycolysis
Myoglobin content	+++	++	+
Glycogen content	+	++	+++
Myosin ATPase activity	+	++	+++

MYOFIBRILS

General
- Contractile rod-like units of striated muscle tissue.
- Fill up cytoplasm.

Structure
- $\oslash$ 1–2 μm
- Extend the entire length of the cell.
- Formed from chains of sarcomeres, connected through Z discs.

Consist of
- Z discs
- Sarcomeres

Z Disc (Z Line)

Structure (Fig. 13.2)
- Zigzag structure
- Contain α-actinin, which attach to actin filaments on each side of the Z disc at the angles of the zigzag
- Z discs are, via intermediate filaments, connected to:
  - Each other } Keep sarcomeres in
  - Plaques in the plasma membrane } register → cross striations.

Sarcomere

General
- The myofibril segment between two adjacent Z discs
- The basic contractile unit in striated muscle

Structure (Fig. 13.2)
- 2.5 μm long (in relaxed muscle cells)
- Divided into A, I, and H bands:
  - A band: corresponds to the full length of the thick filaments
  - I band: corresponds to the part of the sarcomere without thick filaments
  - H band: corresponds to the part of the sarcomere without thin filaments
- The sarcomere, I band, and H band shortens with contraction

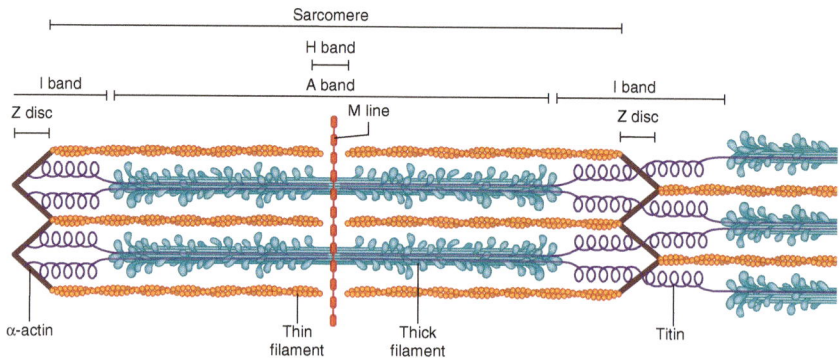

Fig. 13.2 Sarcomere: a longitudinally sectioned part of a sarcomere

Consist of
- Thick filaments
- Thin filaments
- Accessory proteins, e.g.:
  ○ Titin: Connects the Z disc to the M line
  ○ M line proteins: Connect adjacent thick filaments

Thick filaments

Structure
- 1.6 μm long
- ⌀ 15 nm
- Located corresponding to the A band
- Attached to the M line by M line proteins

Consist of
200–300 myosin II molecules, each containing:
- Two heavy chains, which form:
  ○ A long tail
  ○ Two heads, each with an:
    ▪ Actin-binding site
    ▪ ATP-binding site
- Two accessory light chains per myosin head, i.e., four light chains

Formation (Fig. 13.3)
- Tails of myosin II molecules:
  ○ Aggregate in an alternating parallel array
  ○ Arrange "tail to tail" around the M line → bipolar filament
- Heads of myosin II molecules:
  ○ No heads are found adjacent to M line (called the bare zone), which correspond to the H band in relaxed sarcomeres.
  ○ In remaining part, heads spiral out from the filament.

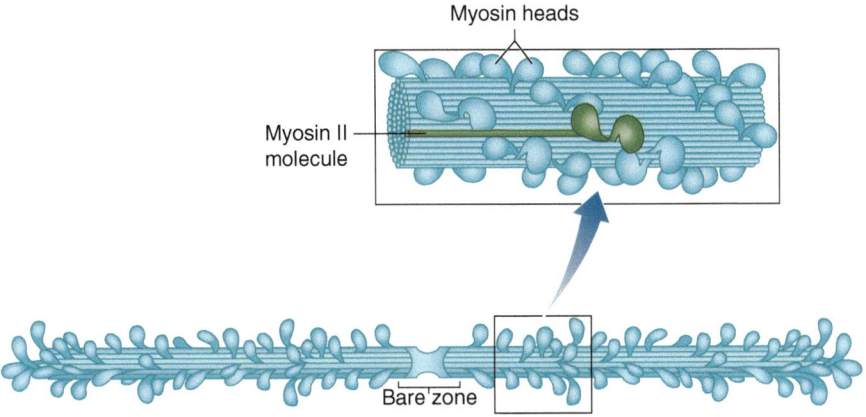

Fig. 13.3 Thick filament: a bipolar thick filament of a sarcomere

MEMO-BOX
- **Myosin II** molecules: Attach to the **M** line
- **H** band (in relaxed sarcomeres): Contains no myosin **Heads**

Thin filaments

Structure
- 1 μm long
- ⊘ 7 nm
- Located corresponding to the whole sarcomere, except the H band.
- Plus end is attached to a Z disc by α-actinin.

Consist of
- Actin filament
  - Double spiral of two F-actin strands, made from G-actin monomers.
  - Each G-actin monomer contains a myosin-binding site.
- Associated proteins:
  - Tropomyosin:
    - 40 nm long
    - Located in rows within the groove between the two F-actin strands
    - Covers the myosin-binding sites
  - Troponin complex:
    - Troponin C: Binds to Ca^{2+}
    - Troponin T: Binds to tropomyosin
    - Troponin I: Binds to the actin filament → keeps tropomyosin in place and thus inhibits binding of myosin heads

MEMO-BOX
- **I** band: Only contains actIn filaments
- Troponin **C**: Binds to Ca^{2+}
- Troponin **T**: Binds to **T**ropomyosin
- Troponin **I**: Binds to the actIn filament, keeping tropomyosin in place → **I**nhibits binding of myosin heads

Titin

Structure
- Large protein with springlike domains
- Spans half the sarcomere from the Z disc, through the thick filament, to the M line.

Function
- Keeps thick filaments in place
- Connects the Z disc to the M line → Resists overstretching of the sarcomere

T TUBULES

Structure (Fig. 13.1)
- Long tubular invaginations of the plasma membrane.
- Transverse the cytoplasm and encircle the myofibrils.
- Two T tubules per sarcomere at A–I band junctions.

Function
Distribute depolarization from the cell surface into the center of the cell → synchronized contraction in all myofibrils

MEMO-BOX
T tubules: **T**ransverse the cytoplasm

SARCOPLASMIC RETICULUM

General (Fig. 13.1)
- Network of sER tubules surrounding the myofibrils
- Broken into segments, which run between A and I band junctions:
  - At each A–I band junction, the sER forms a terminal cistern in contact with a T tubule.

Function
Ca^{2+} store

Triad

General
Surrounds the myofibril at A–I band junctions.

Consists of
- Terminal cistern of one sER segment
- T tubule
- Terminal cistern of the adjacent sER segment

INNERVATION OF SKELETAL MUSCLE CELLS

General
- Contraction of skeletal muscle cells is controlled via:
  - The central nervous system (mostly voluntary)
  - Reflex arches (involuntary), e.g.:
    - Stretch reflex, via muscle spindles (Chap. 15)
    - Golgi tendon reflex, via Golgi tendon organs (Chap. 15)
- Skeletal muscle cells are directly innervated by motor neurons of the spinal cord:
  - The axon of a motor neuron divides into multiple branches, each forming a neuromuscular junction (synapse) with a skeletal muscle cell.
  - A motor neuron and the muscle cells it innervates form a motor unit.

Motor unit

General
- Formed by a motor neuron and the muscle cells it innervates.
- A motor unit only contains one type of skeletal muscle cells.
- The number of muscle cells per motor unit varies from several to hundreds, according to how delicate movements the muscle performs, e.g.:
  - The muscles of the eye: Few muscle cells per motor unit
  - The postural muscles of the back: Multiple muscle cells per motor unit

Neuromuscular Junction (Motor End Plate)

Structure
- The synapse between a motor neuron and a skeletal muscle cell.
- Located near midpoint of the skeletal muscle cell.
- Only one neuromuscular junction per muscle cell.

Consists of
- Axon terminal
  - Contains vesicles with acetylcholine
- Synaptic cleft, 30–50 nm wide
  - Contains acetylcholine esterase, which breaks down acetylcholine
- Plasma membrane of skeletal muscle cell
  - Forms multiple deep folds → increase surface area
  - Contains acetylcholine-gated Na^+-channels

Mechanism of contraction in skeletal muscle cells
- Neuromuscular signal transmission:
  1. An action potential reaches the axon terminal.
  2. Acetylcholine is released to the synaptic cleft.
  3. Acetylcholine binds acetylcholine-gated Na^+-channels in the plasma membrane of the skeletal muscle cell.
  4. Na^+-channels open → Local Na^+ influx in the skeletal muscle cell.
  5. Na^+ influx triggers an action potential in the skeletal muscle cell.

- Excitation–contraction coupling:
  6. The action potential spreads to the T tubules.
  7. Voltage-sensitive proteins in the T tubules change conformation →
     mechanical opening of underlying Ca^{2+}-channels in sER terminal cisterns
     of triads (called excitation–contraction coupling).
  8. Ca^{2+} flows from the sER into the cytoplasm.
  9. Troponin C binds Ca^{2+} → conformational change in troponin
     complex → repositioning of tropomyosin away from myosin-binding sites
     on actin filament → myosin heads can now bind to the actin filaments.
- Actomyosin crossbridge cycle (see below):
  10. Myosin heads attach to the actin filaments → actomyosin crossbridge cycle,
      using ATP as energy source.
  11. Actin filaments slide parallel with the myosin filaments towards the
      M line → shorten the muscle cell.
- End of contraction:
  12. The contraction ends with a fall in Ca^{2+} concentration, through reuptake in
      sER, and by pumping Ca^{2+} out across plasma membrane → resting Ca^{2+}
      concentration is reached in less than 30 milliseconds.

Actomyosin crossbridge cycle

Consists of (Fig. 13.4)
1. Attachment: Myosin heads are bound to actin filaments in unbent confirmation.
2. Release: Myosin heads bind ATP and detach from actin filament.
3. Bending: Myosin heads use the energy from ATP to bend into "pre-power
   stroke" position.
4. Force generation: Myosin heads bind to actin filaments again and return
   to unbent confirmation (called a power stroke), which pulls in actin
   filaments → back to 1.

Enhancement of the contractive force

- A skeletal muscle cell always contract fully (shorten 30%) in an "all-or-none"
  fashion with each action potential.
- Enhancement of the contractive force in skeletal muscles takes place by
  recruiting more motor units → contraction of more muscle cells within the
  muscle.

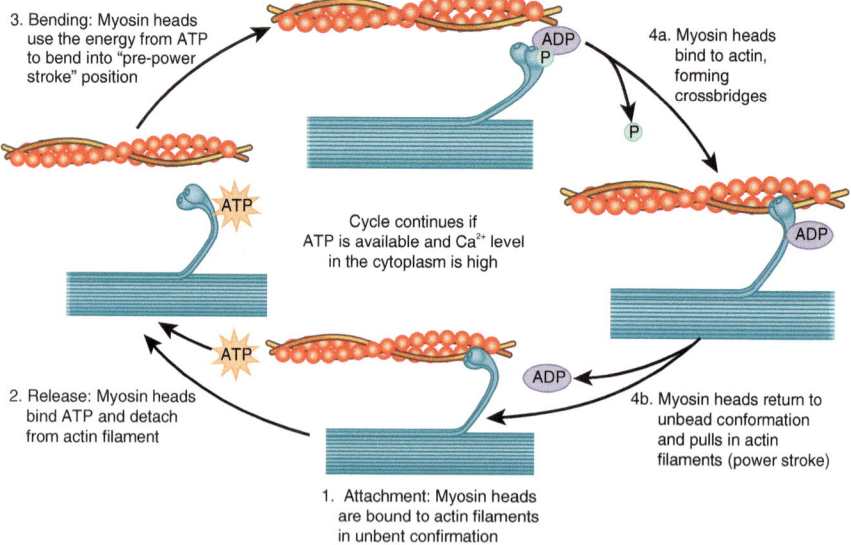

Fig. 13.4 The actomyosin crossbridge cycle

GROWTH AND REGENERATION OF SKELETAL MUSCLE TISSUE

Growth

General

Skeletal muscle tissue grows by hypertrophy:
- More myofibrils within the single skeletal muscle cells.
- Triggered by, e.g., strenuous exercise.

Regeneration

General

Skeletal muscle tissue has limited regeneration, only after smaller injuries:
- Intact external lamina:
  - Regeneration of muscle cells through satellite cells
- Damaged external lamina:
  - Muscle tissue is replaced with connective tissue.

Satellite cells

Structure
- Small flattened cells found between the skeletal muscle cell and its external lamina.
- Have smaller and darker nuclei, than those of the skeletal muscle cell.
  - 5% of the nuclei associated with a skeletal muscle cell are from the satellite cells.

Function
Stem cells:
- Responsible for the limited regenerative ability of skeletal muscle tissue
- Differentiate into myoblasts, which fuse into new skeletal muscle cells

Cardiac Muscle Tissue

General
- Constitutes the myocardium of the heart (Chap. 17).
- Cardiac muscle cells connect to each other end to end through intercalated discs → branching network of cardiac muscle fibers:
  - Each cardiac muscle fiber consists of chains of multiple, connected cardiac muscle cells.

Consists of
Cardiac muscle cells.

Cardiac Muscle Cell

Structure
- Branching "Y-shaped" cells
  - 80–100 μm long
  - $\oslash$ 10–20 μm
- 1–2 central, large, ovoid light (euchromatic) nuclei
- Cytoplasm:
  - Similar to in the skeletal muscle cell, with some differences (Table 13.3).
- Intercalated discs where cells connect to each other end to end
- Surrounded by an external lamina (similar to a basal lamina)

Table 13.3 Differences between skeletal and cardiac muscle cell cytoplasm

	Skeletal muscle cell	Cardiac muscle cell
Myofibrils	Densely packed	Less densely packed → weaker cross striations
Mitochondria	Multiple	• More numerous • Densely packed in rows between myofibrils → length striations
Glycogen granules	Small	Large
T tubules	Two per sarcomere at A–I band junctions	• Larger tubules • Only one per sarcomere at Z discs
Sarcoplasmic reticulum (sER)	• Well-developed network surrounding myofibrils • In segments between A–I band junctions • Forms terminal cisterns in contact with T tubules	• More simple network surrounding myofibrils • In segments between Z discs • Form noncontinuous, small terminal cisterns in contact with T tubules

Triads or diads	Triads are formed from:
	• Terminal cistern of one sER segment
	• T tubule
	• Terminal cistern of the adjacent sER segment
		• No triads, since there are no regular terminal cisterns
		• Diads are formed from:
		  ○ One T tubule
		  ○ Small terminal cistern of a single sER segment

Function
- Contraction (involuntary)
- Pacemaker   ⎤ Modified cardiac muscle cells are
- Impulse propagation ⎦ specialized for these functions (Chap. 17)

Light microscopy
- Short, Y-shaped acidophilic cells
- 1–2 central, large, ovoid light (euchromatic) nuclei
- Striations:
  ○ Weak cross striations   ⎤ Checkered appearance
  ○ Distinct length striations ⎦
- Intercalated discs:
  ○ Transverse/steplike dark lines
  ○ Seen where cells connect to each other end to end

Intercalated Discs

General
Steplike junction between cardiac muscle cells (Fig. 13.5)

Structure
- Cardiac muscle cells contact each other end to end
- The plasma membranes of the two cells interdigitate and form:
  ○ Transverse surfaces:
    ▪ Located corresponding to a Z disc relative to the sarcomeres of the cell
    ▪ Contain cell–cell junctions:
      • Fascia adherens
      • Desmosomes
  ○ Longitudinal surfaces:
    ▪ Contain cell–cell junctions:
      • Desmosomes
      • Gap junctions

Function
- Adhesion, mediated by the desmosomes and fascia adherens:
  ○ Adhere cardiac muscle cells to each other.
  ○ Conduct contractile forces.
- Electrical synapse, mediated by the gap junctions:
  ○ Allow direct flow of electrical impulses between cardiac muscle cells → heart contracts as a syncytium

Mechanism of contraction in cardiac muscle cells
Similar to that of skeletal muscle cells, with some differences (Table 13.4)

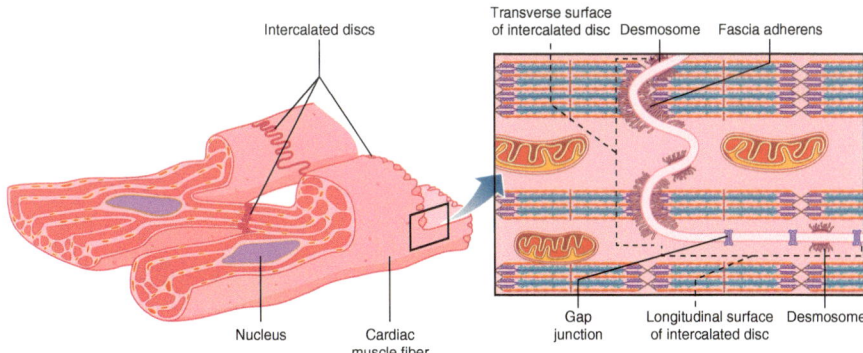

Fig. 13.5 The structure of an intercalated disc

Table 13.4 Differences in contraction mechanism between skeletal and cardiac muscle cells

	Skeletal muscle cell	Cardiac muscle cell
Initiation of contraction via	Action potential in muscle cell: • Triggered by an action potential in the motor neuron	Action potential in muscle cell: • Initiated in pacemaker cells in the sinus node • Spreads to the other cardiac muscle cells through an impulse propagating system (Chap. 17)
Effect of action potential reaching T tubules	1. Voltage-sensitive proteins in the T tubule change conformation 2. Mechanical opening of underlying Ca^{2+}-channels in sER terminal cisterns 3. Ca^{2+} enter cytoplasm from sER	1. Voltage-sensitive proteins in T tubule change conformation into open Ca^{2+}-channels 2. Influx of extracellular Ca^{2+} 3. Ca^{2+}-triggered opening of Ca^{2+} channels in sER → additional rise in cytoplasmic Ca^{2+} concentration
Source of cytoplasmic rise in Ca^{2+} concentration	Ca^{2+} stored in sER	• Extracellular Ca^{2+} from T tubule lumen (primary source) • Ca^{2+} stored in sER
Contraction in muscle cell with each action potential	Full	Submaximal, since too few Ca^{2+} ions enter cytoplasm to bind all troponin-C molecules
Enhancement of contraction	Recruitment of more motor units in muscle	Increasing intracellular Ca^{2+} concentration
Innervation	Somatic nervous system, which initiate contraction	Autonomic nervous system, which modulate: • Frequency (heart rate) • Contractile force

GROWTH AND REGENERATION OF CARDIAC MUSCLE TISSUE

Growth

General

Cardiac muscle tissue grows by hypertrophy:
- Additional myofibrils within the single cardiac muscle cells
- Triggered by increased workload, e.g., from strenuous exercise, or increased resistance in cardiovascular system

Regeneration

General
- Very limited in cardiac muscle tissue, as cardiac muscle cells lack satellite cells.
- Dead cardiac muscle cells are replaced by connective tissue.

Smooth Muscle Tissue

General

Primarily found in:
- The wall of internal organs
- The wall of blood vessels

Consists of

Smooth muscle cells

Divided into
- Unitary type (tonic smooth muscle tissue)
- Multiunit type (phasic smooth muscle tissue)

Smooth Muscle Cell

Structure
- Elongated, fusiform (spindle-shaped) cells:
  - 20–200 µm long (up to 500 µm in pregnant uterus)
  - $\oslash$ 2–10 µm
- A single central flattened nucleus.
- Cytoplasm:
  - Multiple, long fiber units (correspond to the myofibrils of striated muscle tissue)
  - Sarcoplasmic reticulum (sER) forms longitudinal tubules between the fiber units
  - No T tubules
  - Numerous mitochondria
  - Well-developed rER and Golgi apparatus
- Surrounded by an external lamina (similar to a basal lamina).
- Cells are kept together by a network of reticular fibers, on the outer surface of the external lamina.

Function
- Contraction (involuntary)
- Production of extracellular matrix components, e.g., in the tunica media of blood vessels

Light microscopy
- Elongated, thin fusiform (spindle-shaped) acidophilic cells
- A single central flattened nucleus, often twisted (corkscrew shape)
- Lack striations

FIBER UNITS (CONTRACTILE APPARATUS)

General (Fig. 13.6)
- Contractile rod-like units of smooth muscle tissue (correspond to myofibrils)
- The contractile units of the fiber units are called filament bundles (correspond to sarcomeres).
- Contraction is regulated through thick filaments of the filament bundles, in contrast to in sarcomeres, where it is regulated through thin filaments (via troponin complex).

Structure
- Transverse the cytoplasm obliquely
- Formed from chains of filament bundles, connected through dense bodies
- Connect to the cell membrane via plaques, and hereby distribute contractile force to the cell membrane

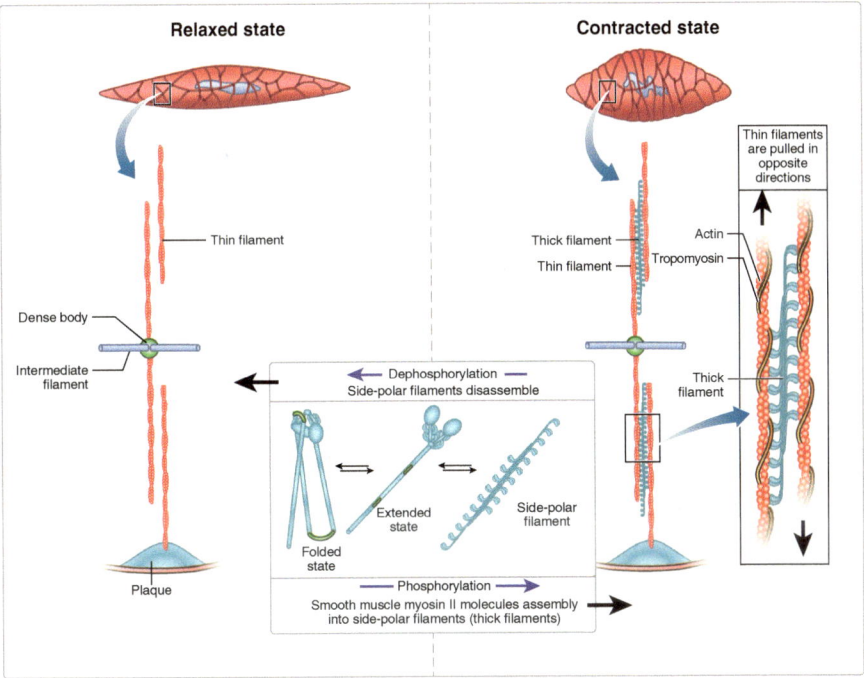

Fig. 13.6 Contractile apparatus of smooth muscle cells: Left, myosin II molecules are in the folded state and do form side-polar myosin filaments. No contraction takes place. Right, myosin II molecules aggregate into side-polar myosin filaments and contraction can take place

Consists of
- Dense bodies (correspond to Z discs)
- Filament bundles (correspond to sarcomeres)

Dense bodies

Structure
- Contain multiple proteins, e.g., α-actinin, which binds to both actin and intermediate filaments.
- Connect the filament bundles end to end, forming long fiber units.
- Intermediate filaments connect dense bodies to each other and with plaques → keep the contractile apparatus in place.

Filament Bundles

Structure
- Run obliquely in cell between dense bodies
- The dense bodies connect the filaments end to end, forming long fiber units.

Function
The contractile unit of smooth muscle tissue

Consist of (Fig. 13.6)
- Thick filaments
  - Only formed during contraction
  - One thick filament
  - Located centrally within a "cylinder" of thin filaments
- Thin filaments
  - Several thin filaments form a "cylinder" around the central thick filament
  - Attach to a dense body (or plaque) with the plus end:
    - Thin filaments on one side of the thick filament attach to a dense body in one end.
    - Thin filaments on the other side of the thick filament attach to a dense body in the opposite end.

Thick filaments

Consist of
Multiple smooth muscle myosin II molecules

Formation (Fig. 13.6)
- Tails of smooth muscle myosin II molecules:
  - Aggregate aligned in one direction on one side of the filament and in the opposite direction on the other.
- Heads of smooth muscle myosin II molecules:
  - Heads are polarized towards opposite ends on the upper side and lower side of filament (side-polar filament) (Fig. 13.6).
  - Found along almost the full length of the filament, except at opposite "bare ends" on each side of the filament.

Thin filaments

Consist of
- Actin filaments
  - Double spiral of two F-actin strands, made from G-actin monomers.
  - Each G-actin monomer contains a myosin-binding site.
- Associated proteins:
  - Tropomyosin and caldesmon:
    - Regulate myosin ATPase activity.

Initiation of contraction in smooth muscle cells

Contraction is initiated by a rise in cytoplasmic Ca^{2+} that can be triggered by:

- Action potential in smooth muscle cell:
  - Leads to influx of extracellular Ca^{2+} though voltage gated Ca^{2+}-channels.
    - This alone is insufficient to induce contraction and needs to be supplemented by release of Ca^{2+} from sER.
  - Action potential is initiated by:
    - Ligand-gated ion channels, responsive to, e.g., acetylcholine, or norepinephrine (noradrenaline).
    - Mechanosensitive ion channels, responsive to, e.g., stretch of the cell.
- Second messengers:
  - Second messengers can induce a rise in cytoplasmic Ca^{2+} via:
    - Second messenger-gated Ca^{2+}-channels in sER → release of Ca^{2+} from sER.
    - Second messenger-gated Ca^{2+}-channels in cell membrane → influx of extracellular Ca^{2+}.
  - Second messenger formation is triggered by the binding of ligands to various receptors of the cell membrane, e.g., G protein-coupled receptors.
    - The ligands that trigger second messenger are, e.g., hormones:
      - Epinephrine (adrenaline) and norepinephrine (noradrenaline)
      - Angiotensin II
      - Oxytocin

Mechanism of contraction in smooth muscle cells

1. Cytoplasmic rise in Ca^{2+} concentration.
2. Ca^{2+} binds and activates calmodulin.
3. Calmodulin activates the myosin light chain kinase.
4. Myosin light chain kinase phosphorylates myosin heads.
5. Smooth muscle myosin II molecules assemble into side-polar filaments.
6. Myosin heads attach to the actin filaments → actomyosin crossbridge cycle (using ATP at 10 % the rate of in striated muscle) → slow contraction.
7. Actin filaments on each side of the myosin filament are pulled in opposite directions, which shortens the smooth muscle cell (up to 80 %).
8. Contraction ends because of:
   a. A fall in Ca^{2+} concentration, through reuptake in sER and by pumping Ca^{2+} out across plasma membrane → inactivation of myosin light chain kinase
   b. Dephosphorylation of:
      - Myosin heads which are detached from actin filaments → disassembly of myosin filaments → contraction ends fully
      - Myosin heads still attached to actin filaments → remain attached, but now unable to use ATP (called latch state) → sustained contractive state, without further shortening

TYPES OF SMOOTH MUSCLE TISSUE

Divided into
- Unitary type (tonic smooth muscle tissue):
  - Dense bundles or layers of smooth muscle cells
  - A syncytium of cells, which contracts as a single unit
- Multiunit type (phasic smooth muscle tissue):
  - Solitary smooth muscle cells
  - Cells contract independently

Unitary Type (Tonic Smooth Muscle Tissue)

General
- Most abundant type, e.g., in the wall of internal organs and blood vessels.
- Smooth muscle fibers in dense bundles or layers
- Cells are connected through gap junctions → syncytium, which contracts as a single unit.
- Innervated loosely by autonomic nerve endings:
  - Enlargements (bouton en passant) of nerve endings release autonomic neurotransmitters.
  - The enlargements are located 10–20 μm from the smooth muscle cells.
  - No synapses (motor end plates) are formed.

Function
Tonic contraction:
- Slow contraction
- Often sustained contraction through long periods of time (myosin heads in latch state).
- Contraction is regulated by:
  - Spontaneous contractile activity:
    - Modulated by acetylcholine and norepinephrine (noradrenaline) from autonomic nerves
  - Activation of mechanosensitive ion channels, through stretching of smooth muscle cells
  - Hormones, which can trigger either contraction or relaxation

Multiunit Type (Phasic Smooth Muscle Tissue)

General
- Solitary smooth muscle cells
- Rare, e.g., found in the iris of the eye and ductus deferens.
- Cells act independently of each other.

- Innervated closely by autonomic nerve endings:
  - Enlargements of nerve endings release autonomic neurotransmitters.
  - The enlargements are in direct contact with the smooth muscle cell.
  - No synapses (motor end plates) are formed.

Function
Phasic contraction:
- Fast contraction followed by full relaxation.
- Contraction is initiated by action potential in the smooth muscle cell.
- Exhibit no spontaneous activity.
- Contraction is regulated by autonomic neurotransmitters.
  - Acetylcholine
  - Norepinephrine (noradrenaline)

> **MEMO-BOX**
> UNITary type: Multiple smooth muscle cells contract simultaneously as a single **UNIT**.

GROWTH AND REGENERATION OF SMOOTH MUSCLE TISSUE

Growth

General
Smooth muscle tissue grows by:
- Hypertrophy: Additional filament bundles in the single smooth muscle cells
- Hyperplasi: Proliferation of smooth muscle cells

Regeneration

General
Smooth muscle tissue regenerates well:
- Smooth muscle cells are able to divide and continuously replace old and damaged cells.
- Mesenchymal stem cells can form new smooth muscle cells.

Table 13.5 Overview of muscle cells

	Skeletal muscle cells	Cardiac muscle cells	Smooth muscle cells
Function	Voluntary contraction	Involuntary contraction	Involuntary contraction
Location, e.g.:	Muscles of skeleton	Heart	Wall of internal organs
Cross striation	++	+	−
Length striation	−	+	−
Nucleus:			
• Number per cell	Multiple	1–2	1
• Location	Peripheral	Central	Central
• Morphology	Flattened	Ovoid, light (euchromatic)	Flattened, sometimes twisted (corkscrew shape)
Shape	Cylindrical	Branching "Y-shaped"	Spindle shaped
Length	Up to 100 cm	80–100 μm	20–200 μm
⌀	10–100 μm	10–20 μm	0.2–10 μm
Contractile unit	Sarcomere	Sarcomere	Filament bundle
Contraction	Shortens cell 30 %	Shortens cell 30 %	Shortens cell up to 80 %
T tubules	• Two per sarcomere • At A–I band junctions	• One per sarcomere • At Z discs	None
Sarcoplasmic reticulum (sER)	• Well-developed network of tubules surrounding myofibrils • With terminal cisterns, forming triads with T tubules	• Simple network of tubules surrounding myofibrils • With small, noncontinuous terminal cisterns, forming diads with T tubules	Longitudinal tubules between filament bundles
Regulation of contraction	Through thin filaments, via troponin complex	Through thin filaments, via troponin complex	Through thick filament, via phosphorylation of myosin heads
Intracellular activator of contraction	Rise in cytoplasmic Ca^{2+} concentration	Rise in cytoplasmic Ca^{2+} concentration	Rise in cytoplasmic Ca^{2+} concentration
Innervation	Somatic nervous system	Autonomic nervous system	Autonomic nervous system
End of contraction	Fall in cytoplasmic Ca^{2+} concentration	Fall in cytoplasmic Ca^{2+} concentration	• Fall in cytoplasmic Ca^{2+} concentration • Dephosphorylation of myosin heads

Guide to Practical Histology: Muscle Tissue

Skeletal Muscle Tissue

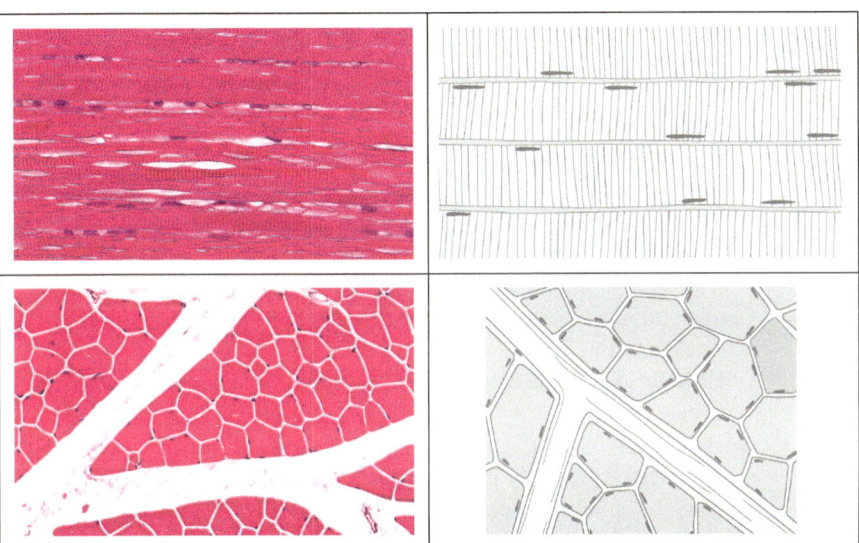

Top left: photomicrograph of longitudinal sectioned skeletal muscle tissue. Magnification: high. Stain: HE (Courtesy of professor Jørgen Tranum-Jensen, University of Copenhagen). *Top right*: simplified illustration of longitudinal sectioned skeletal muscle tissue. *Bottom left*: photomicrograph of cross sectioned skeletal muscle tissue. Magnification: high. Stain: HE (Courtesy of professor Jørgen Tranum-Jensen, University of Copenhagen). *Bottom right*: simplified illustration of cross sectioned skeletal muscle tissue

Characteristics
- Skeletal muscle cells (fibers) are eosinophilic.
- Longitudinal section:
  - Long, straight, parallel, and non-branched fibers
  - Distinct cross striations
  - Multiple peripheral nuclei
- Cross section:
  - Polyhedral cross sections of fibers of relatively uniform size.
  - Multiple peripheral nuclei.
  - Small white gaps are seen between the fibers.
  - Dense connective tissue organizes fibers into bundles → resembles marbled meat at low magnification.

Location
In skeletal muscles

Special staining
Van Gieson:
- Stains muscle cells yellow
- Stains collagen fibers red

Can be mistaken for
- Longitudinal section:
  - Dense regular connective tissue:
    - Collagen fibers:
      - Are less eosinophilic
      - Lack cross striations
      - Are often slightly wavy
    - The nuclei are located outside the collagen fibers.
  - Cardiac muscle tissue:
    - Cardiac muscle fibers:
      - Are branching
      - Have weaker cross striations and distinct length striations → checkered appearance
    - Nuclei:
      - Are located centrally in the cardiac muscle cells.
      - Only 1–2 nuclei per cell.
- Cross section:
  - Dense regular connective tissue:
    - Collagen fibers:
      - Are less eosinophilic
      - Have indistinct borders and no white spaces separating them
    - Nuclei are located outside the collagen fibers.
  - Cardiac muscle tissue:
    - Contains larger white spaces between the muscle fibers.
    - Nuclei are located centrally in the cardiac muscle cells.

Cardiac Muscle Tissue

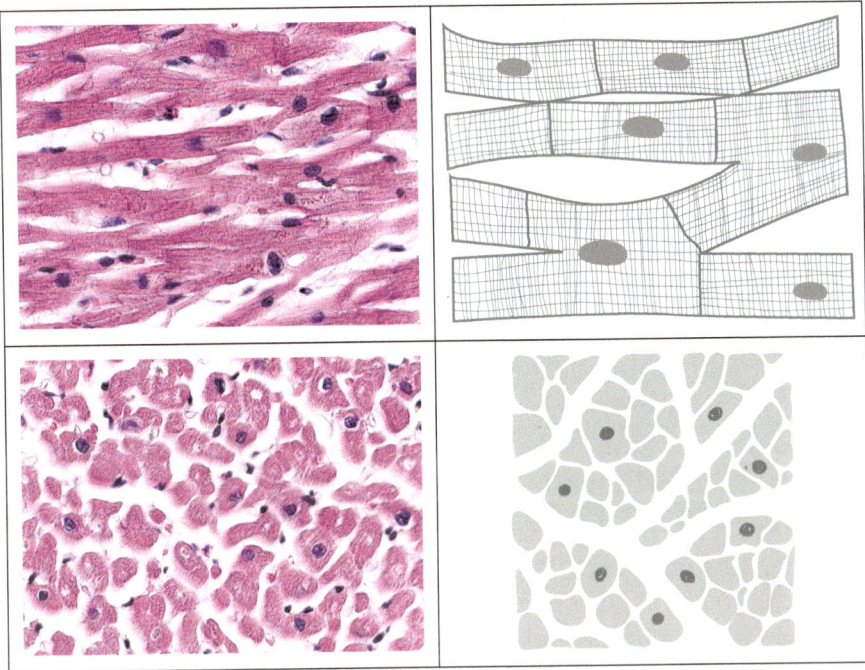

Top left: photomicrograph of longitudinal sectioned cardiac muscle tissue. Magnification: high. Stain: HE (Courtesy of professor Jørgen Tranum-Jensen, University of Copenhagen). *Top right*: simplified illustration of longitudinal sectioned cardiac muscle tissue. *Bottom left*: photomicrograph of cross sectioned cardiac muscle tissue. Magnification: high. Stain: HE (Courtesy of professor Jørgen Tranum-Jensen, University of Copenhagen). *Bottom right*: simplified illustration of cross sectioned cardiac muscle tissue

Characteristics
- Cardiac muscle cells (fibers) are eosinophilic.
- Multiple capillaries are seen between the muscle fibers:
  - Narrow white spaces with multiple eosinophilic erythrocytes
- Both cross, oblique and longitudinal sections of muscle fibers are seen in the same specimen:
  - Longitudinal section:
    - Short, branching "Y-shaped" cells:
      - Form an irregular network
      - Have 1–2 central light nuclei
      - Have weak cross striations and distinct length striations → checkered appearance
    - Intercalated discs (often indistinct) are seen where two cardiac muscle cells contact each other.
  - Cross section:
    - Rounded cross sections of fibers of varying sizes.
    - White spaces are seen between fibers.
    - Central nuclei are seen in some of the cross sectioned fibers.

Location

Only found in the myocardium of the heart.

Can be mistaken for
- Longitudinal section:
  - ○ Skeletal muscle tissue:
    - ▪ Skeletal muscle fibers:
      - • Are longer, parallel and not branching
      - • Have more distinct cross striations and no length striations
      - • Contain multiple peripheral nuclei
- Cross section:
  - ○ Skeletal muscle tissue:
    - ▪ Contains smaller white spaces between the muscle fibers.
    - ▪ Nuclei are located peripherally in the cells.

Smooth Muscle Tissue

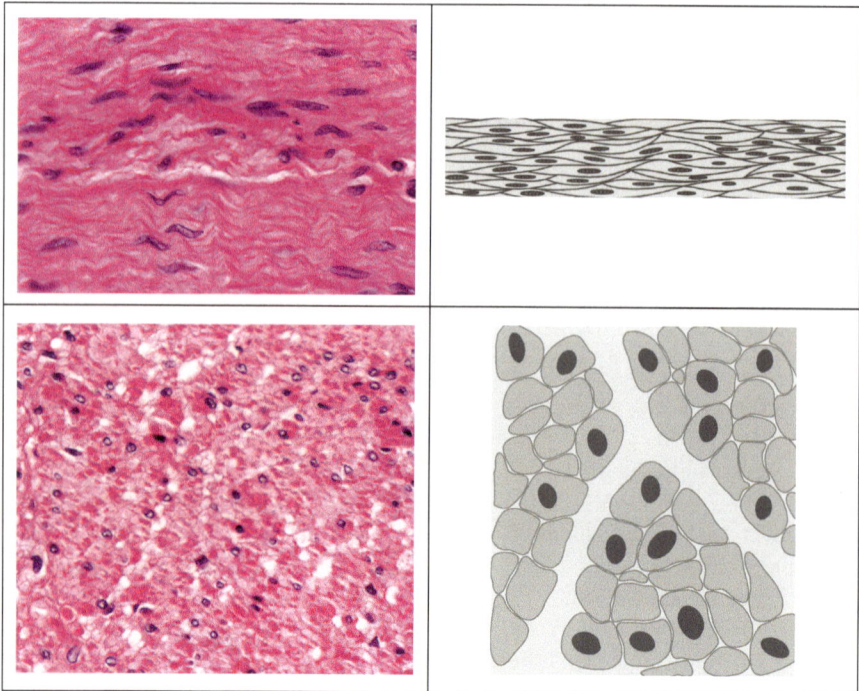

Top left: photomicrograph of longitudinal sectioned smooth muscle tissue. Magnification: high. Stain: HE (Courtesy of professor Jørgen Tranum-Jensen, University of Copenhagen). *Top right*: simplified illustration of longitudinal sectioned smooth muscle tissue. *Bottom left*: photomicrograph of cross sectioned smooth muscle tissue. Magnification: high. Stain: HE (Courtesy of professor Jørgen Tranum-Jensen, University of Copenhagen) *Bottom right*: simplified illustration of cross sectioned smooth muscle tissue

Characteristics
- Smooth muscle cells (fibers) are eosinophilic.
- Both cross and longitudinal sections of fibers are normally seen in the same specimen but in distinct, separate layers:
  - Longitudinal section:
    - Thin, often a bit wavy, densely packed parallel muscle fibers.
    - The borders between fibers are indistinct.
    - Each cell contains a single central elongated nucleus (sometimes corkscrew-shaped).
  - Cross section:
    - Thin, rounded cross sections of fibers of varying sizes:
      - The thickest of the cross sections contains a nucleus.
    - The fibers are densely packed, separated by thin white spaces.
    - Resembles a "salami slice" at low magnification.

Location
Seen in the wall of most internal hollow organs, e.g., the urinary bladder

Can be mistaken for
- Longitudinal section:
  - Peripheral nerve:
    - Nerve fibers are longer and more wavy.
    - White "cloudy" material is seen surrounding the axons.
    - Nuclei are of different sizes, in contrast to the smooth muscle nuclei, which are of similar size.
  - Dense regular connective tissue:
    - The collagen fibers are weaker eosinophilic.
    - Collagen fibers are commonly less wavy.
    - The nuclei are located in rows between the fibers.
  - Dense irregular connective tissue:
    - Collagen fibers:
      - Are weaker eosinophilic
      - Are separated by small white spaces
      - Are arranged in irregular directions
    - Nuclei are scarce and found between the fibers.

References
5, 13, 21, 25, 33, 34, 45.

Chapter 14
Nerve Tissue

Contents

General
- One of the four basic tissue types.
- Main component of the nervous system (Chap. 16):
  - Central nervous system (CNS):
    - Brain:
      - Cerebrum
      - Cerebellum
      - Brain stem
    - Spinal cord
  - Peripheral nervous system (PNS):
    - Peripheral nerves
      - Cranial nerves
      - Spinal nerves
    - Ganglia
      - Sensory ganglia
      - Autonomic ganglia

© Springer International Publishing Switzerland 2017
A. Rehfeld et al., *Compendium of Histology*, DOI 10.1007/978-3-319-41873-5_14

Function
Communication:
- Reaction to stimuli
- Processing of information
- Transmission of signals

Consists of
- Neurons (nerve cells)
- Glial cells (supporting cells)

Neuron (Nerve cell)

General (Fig. 14.1)
- A terminally differentiated cell, not capable of dividing
- The structural and functional unit of the nervous system

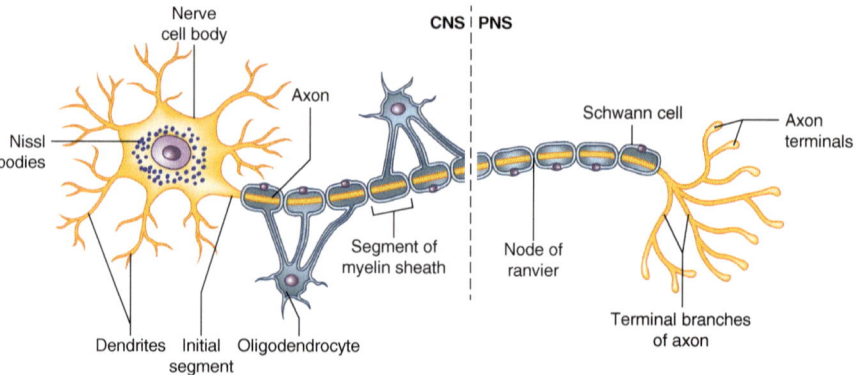

Fig. 14.1 A neuron, with a myelinated axon, traveling through both the central part (CNS) and peripheral part (PNS) of the nervous system

Function
- Excitable:
  - Neurons at rest keep a membrane potential of ≈ -70 mV.
  - Neurons can react to various stimuli through rapid changes in their membrane potential, i.e., depolarization (rise in membrane potential) or hyperpolarization (fall in membrane potential).

- Depolarization can trigger the initiation of an action potential
  (a depolarization wave) in the axon, followed by a rapid repolarization
  to resting membrane potential.
- Process signals:
  ○ Multiple stimuli, each leading to changes in membrane potential, are
    summarized and converted into a certain frequency of action potentials in
    the axon.
- Conduction of signals:
  ○ Action potentials propagate distally along the axon → Signals can be sent
    directly to remote cells.
- Transmission of signals:
  ○ Signals are transmitted to other cells through synapses.
  ○ At the synapsis, action potentials trigger the release of neurotransmitters,
    which induce effects in target cell.

Consists of
- Nerve cell body (soma, perikaryon)
- Cell extensions:
  ○ Dendrites
  ○ Axon

Divided into (Fig. 14.2)
- Anatomically:
  ○ Multipolar neurons
  ○ Bipolar neurons
  ○ Pseudounipolar (unipolar) neurons
- Functionally:
  ○ Sensory neurons
  ○ Motor neurons
  ○ Interneurons

NERVE CELL BODY (SOMA, PERIKARYON)

Structure
- Great variation in size and shape:
  ○ ⌀ 4–135 μm
  ○ Often polygonal, with cell extensions at the corners
- Nucleus:
  ○ Centrally located
  ○ Round, large, and light (euchromatic)
  ○ Contains a single prominent nucleolus

- Cytoplasm:
  - Nissl bodies (basophilic):
    - Well-developed rER
    - Abundant free ribosomes
  - Golgi apparatus
  - Numerous mitochondria
  - Cytoskeleton:
    - Intermediate filaments (neurofilaments)
    - Microtubules
    - Actin filaments
- Axon hillock
  - The part of nerve cell body where the axon originates
  - Lack large organelles, including the Nissl bodies → no basophilic staining.

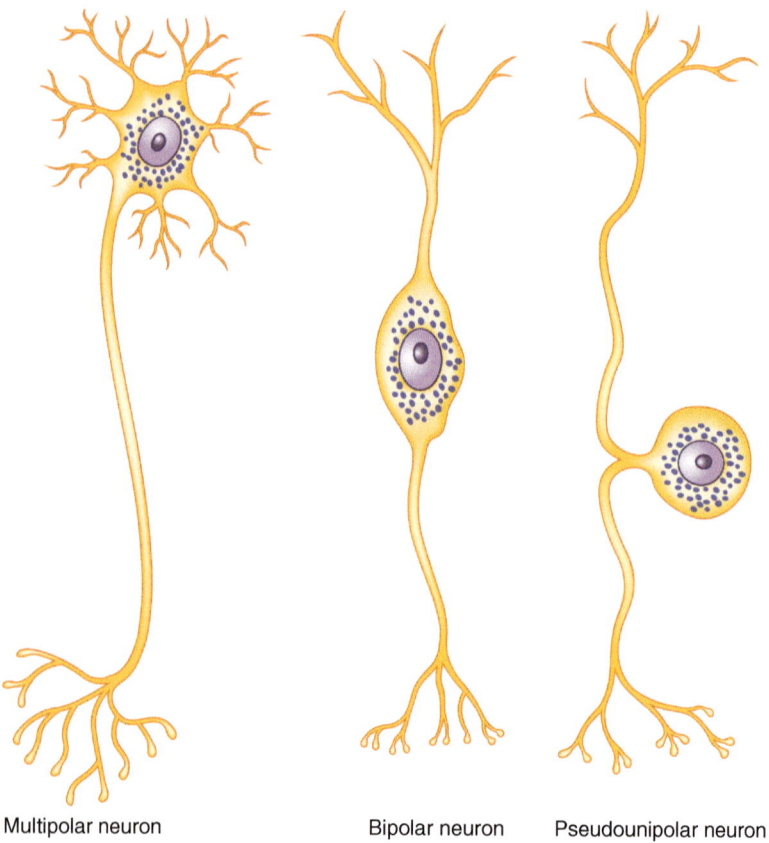

Multipolar neuron   Bipolar neuron   Pseudounipolar neuron

Fig. 14.2 The anatomical types of neurons

Light Microscopy
- A large, central, light (euchromatic) nucleus with a single central nucleolus (the nucleus resembles an eye).
- Basophilic clumps are seen in the cytoplasm surrounding the nucleus.

NERVE CELL EXTENSIONS

General
- Cytoskeletal components run parallel in the cell extensions and provide mechanical support.
- Microtubules form the basis of the transport systems within the cell extensions.

Divided into
- Dendrites
- Axon

Dendrites

General
- Most neurons have ≥1 dendrites
- Some neurons lack dendrites, e.g., rods and cones of the retina.

Structure
- Highly branched, forming a "dendritic tree."
- Base of the dendrite has a larger ⊘ than the axon.
- Dendrite narrows gradually as it branches.
- Most dendrites contain numerous small projections (spines), each forming a synapse with an axon:
  - Spines may emerge, disappear or change in size due to synaptic activity → implicated in learning and memory.

Function
- Increase the surface area of the neuron
- Receive stimuli from:
  - Synapses:
    - Axons of multiple other neurons form synapses with dendrite, usually on the dendritic spines.
  - External environment:
    - Dendrites can react to stimuli from the external environment through specific receptors.

MEMO-BOX
Dendron is Greek for "tree": Dendrites are highly branched "treelike" cell extensions.

Axon

General
- One axon per neuron:
  - Originates at the axon hillock of the nerve cell body.
  - Most proximal segment is called the initial segment.
  - Gives off perpendicular collaterals.
  - Forms terminal branches distally.
  - Ends as axon terminals.
- Lack in some neurons (anaxonic neurons), e.g., some interneurons
- Special nomenclature:
  - Axoplasm = cytoplasm
  - Axolemma = plasma membrane (plasmalemma)
- Axons with their sheaths are called nerve fibers

Structure
- Great variation in length: from less than 1 mm and up to 1 m or more
- ⌀ up to several μm and constant along the length of the axon
- Found with and without myelination, determined by the ⌀ of the axon:
  - ⌀ <1 μm → unmyelinated:
    - CNS: axons are bare, i.e., not ensheathed by glial cells
    - PNS: axons are ensheathed by Schwann cells
  - ⌀ ≥1 μm → myelinated: myelin sheath covers the axon from just distal to initial segment until the terminal branches.
    - CNS: axon is ensheathed by interfascicular oligodendrocytes
    - PNS: axon is ensheathed by Schwann cells

Function
- Generation of action potentials at the initial segment of the axon:
  - The initial segment contains numerous voltage-gated channels and therefore has the lowest threshold potential in the neuron:
    - Action potentials are always initiated at the initial segment as the membrane of the nerve cell body depolarizes.
  - The degree of depolarization in nerve cell body and dendrites is summarized at the initial segment and converted into a certain frequency of action potentials.
- Conduction of action potentials (like a flame along a fuse):
  - Unmyelinated axons: Conductive speed ≤1 m/s
  - Myelinated axons: Conductive speed up to 120 m/s

- Myelin sheath insulates the axon.
- Membrane depolarization can only occur at gaps, called nodes of Ranvier, located between the segments of the myelin sheath → saltatory "jumping" propagation of action potentials.
- Interaction with other cells:
  ○ Axonal enlargements form synapses with other neurons and effector cells.

Transport systems of nerve cell extensions

Function
- Transport intracellular contents along the parallel microtubules of dendrites and axon.
- Transport is driven by motor proteins:
  ○ Kinesins: wanders towards the plus end of microtubules
  ○ Dyneins: wanders towards the minus end of microtubules, which is embedded in the centrosome of the nerve cell body

Divided into (Table 14.1)
- Anterograde transport: away from nerve cell body
- Retrograde transport: towards the nerve cell body

Table 14.1 Transport systems of cell extensions

	Speed (mm/day)	Motor proteins	Transport of
Anterograde transport			
• Fast	50–400	Kinesins	For example, vesicles from the Golgi apparatus
• Slow	0.2–4	Unknown mechanism	For example, cytoskeletal components
Retrograde transport			
• Fast	50–400	Dyneins	For example: • Worn-out cellular components of nerve terminal • Endocytosed materials

---

MEMO-BOX
- Anterograde transport: **A**way from nerve cell body.
- "Retrograde" means moving backwards: Retrograde transport is transport back towards the nerve cell body.
- The **K**ing goes out to conquer: **K**inesins wanders out of nerve cell body.

TYPES OF NEURONS

Neurons are anatomically divided into

According to the number of cell extensions (Fig. 14.2, Table 14.2):
- Multipolar neurons
- Bipolar neurons
- Pseudounipolar (unipolar) neurons

Table 14.2 The anatomical types of neurons

	Multipolar neuron	Bipolar neuron	Pseudounipolar (unipolar) neuron
Cell extensions	Multiple: • One axon • ≥ 2 dendrites	Two: • One axon • One dendrite	A single T-shaped axon: • One end branches into a dendritic tree • The other end forms axon terminals
Location	Most common type, e.g., motor neurons	Rare, e.g., found in retina	For example, the sensory neurons of spinal ganglia

Neurons are functionally divided into

- Sensory neurons:
  - Convey signals from sensory receptors to the CNS via afferent nerves.
- Motor neurons:
  - Convey information from CNS or ganglia to effector cells via efferent nerves.
- Interneurons:
  - Form a communicating network between sensory and motor neurons.
  - Make up >99.9 % of all neurons.

REGENERATION OF NEURONS

Regeneration of nerve cell body

General

Regeneration of nerve cell bodies is highly limited as:
- Neurons are terminally differentiated and not capable of dividing.
- Neuronal stem cells, which can form new neurons, only are found in some areas of the CNS, e.g., hippocampus.

Regeneration of axons

General
Regeneration of axons depends on location:
- In the CNS: Injured axons do not regenerate.
- In the PNS: Injured axons can regenerate by growth from the proximal segment:
  1. Injury of axon.
  2. The part distal to the injury degenerates.
  3. The Schwann cells of the distal part dedifferentiate and arrange along their external lamina in long cellular cords, forming a "tube" of Schwann cells.
  4. Macrophages remove debris from degenerated part of axon and its surrounding myelin sheath within 2 weeks
  5. Axon regenerates with 3 mm/day by growth from proximal part guided by the "tube" of Schwann cells.
  6. Schwann cells redifferentiate and form a new myelin sheath.

SYNAPSES

General
- Specialized junction between neuron and other cells:
  - Neuron–neuron synapses:
    - In gray matter of CNS
    - In autonomic ganglia of PNS
  - Neuron–effector cell synapses:
    - For example, the neuromuscular junction with skeletal muscle cells
- Synapses occur at axonal enlargements, called boutons:
  - Along the axon (bouton en passant)
  - At axon terminals (bouton terminal)

Divided into
- Chemical synapses (most common type)
- Electrical synapses

Chemical Synapses

Function
- Transmission of signals (action potentials) via neurotransmitters.
- Transmission is unidirectional, i.e., from the presynaptic neuron to the postsynaptic cell.

Consist of (Fig. 14.3)
- Presynaptic axonal enlargement, e.g., an axon terminal:
  - Contains synaptic vesicles with neurotransmitters
- Synaptic cleft between the two cells:
  - ≈25 nm wide
- Postsynaptic cell membrane, e.g., a dendritic spine:
  - Contains membrane receptors for neurotransmitters

Divided into
According to location:
- Axodendritic synapse:
  - Between an axon and a dendrite
  - Most common type
- Axosomatic synapse:
  - Between an axon and a soma (nerve cell body)
- Axoaxonic synapse:
  - Between two axons

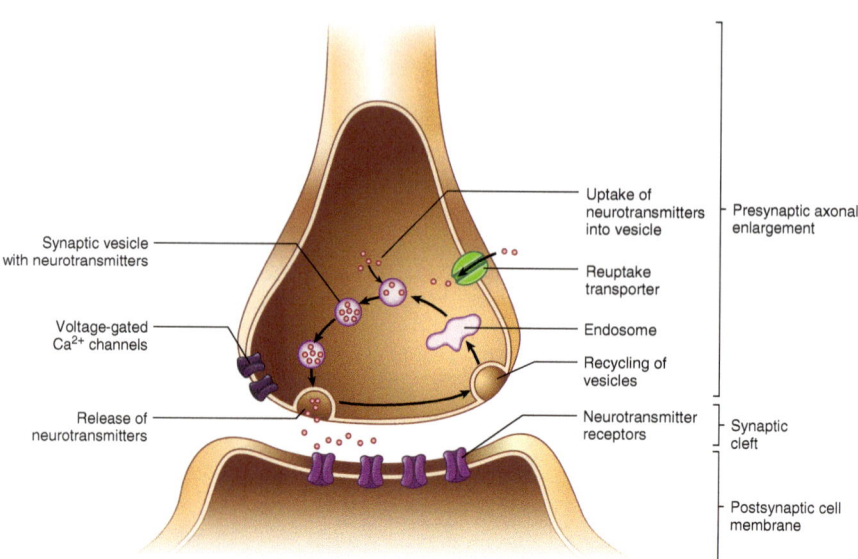

Fig. 14.3 Structure of a chemical synapse

Synaptic transmission in chemical synapses

1. An action potential reaches the axonal enlargement causing voltage-gated Ca^{2+} channels to open $\rightarrow Ca^{2+}$ influx
2. Local intracellular rise in Ca^{2+} concentration $\rightarrow$ synaptic vesicles release a fixed amount of neurotransmitters to the synaptic cleft
3. Neurotransmitters bind to specific receptors in the postsynaptic cell membrane $\rightarrow$ response, e.g., depolarization or hyperpolarization of the membrane potential in postsynaptic cell
4. Neurotransmitters are removed from the synaptic cleft by:
   ○ Reuptake into neurons or astrocytes (major part)
   ○ Enzymatic breakdown in the synaptic cleft

Membrane receptors on postsynaptic cell membrane

Function

Transduce neurotransmitter signal in synaptic cleft into response in postsynaptic cell.

Divided into (Table 14.3)

- Ionotropic receptors
- Metabotropic receptors

Neurotransmitters

General

- Molecules released by neurons to the synaptic cleft.
- Act as ligands for membrane receptors of the postsynaptic cell membrane.

Table 14.3 Membrane receptors on postsynaptic cell membrane

Receptor	Type	Transmission speed
Ionotropic receptor	Ligand-gated ion channel	Fast response: • Transmission via ions, e.g., Na^+ or Cl^- • Response within milliseconds
Metabotropic receptor	Ligand-gated receptor, coupled to G proteins	Commonly slower response: • Transmission via G proteins • Response occurs after milliseconds to minutes

Divided into
- In central nervous system:
  - Excitatory neurotransmitters
    - For example, glutamate and serotonin
  - Inhibitory neurotransmitters
    - For example, GABA and glycine
- In peripheral nervous system:
  - Neurotransmitters of somatic nervous system
    - Acetylcholine
  - Neurotransmitters of autonomic nervous system
    - Norepinephrine (noradrenaline)
    - Acetylcholine

Vesicle recycling in chemical synapses (Fig. 14.3)

1. Vesicles bud off from the trans-Golgi network and are transported to the axon terminal through fast anterograde transport.
2. Neurotransmitters are synthesized at the axon terminal and taken up into the vesicles.
3. Vesicles are docked adjacent to the cell membrane ready for fast release of neurotransmitters.
4. Vesicle fuse with cell membrane and release neurotransmitters to synaptic cleft.
5. After release, the vesicle is endocytosed and fuses with an endosome.
6. Vesicles bud off from the endosome and are again ready to be filled with neurotransmitter ($\rightarrow$ #2).

Electrical Synapses

General
- Rare in nerve tissue, e.g., found in the retina.
- Mediated by gap junctions.

Function
Direct transmission of electrical impulses between two cells

Glial Cells (Supporting Cells)

General
In contrast to neurons, glial cells are:
- Not forming synapses
- Not excitable
- Able to divide

Divided into
- Glial cells of CNS (central neuroglia) (Table 14.4):
  ○ Astrocytes
  ○ Oligodendrocytes
  ○ Microglia
  ○ Ependymal cells
- Glial cells of PNS (peripheral neuroglia):
  ○ Schwann cells
  ○ Satellite cells
  ○ Various other cells, e.g.:
    ▪ Enteric glial cells: Structurally and functionally similar to astrocytes
    ▪ Müller cells of retina (Chap. 28)

Table 14.4 Glial cells of the central nervous system

	Astrocyte	Oligodendrocyte	Microglia	Ependymal cells
Structure	• Large cell • Star shaped	Small cell	Smallest cell	Simple cuboidal/columnar epithelium
Cell extensions	• Many • Highly branched	• Few • Less branched	Short and thin	• Cilia • Microvilli
Nucleus	• Large • Light (euchromatic)	• Small • Dark (heterochromatic)	• Small, elongated • Dark (heterochromatic)	• Large • Round
Parts visible in routine preparations	Nucleus	Nucleus	Nucleus	Whole cell
Function	Multiple, e.g., mechanical support	Forms myelin sheaths in CNS	• Phagocytosis • Antigen presentation	• Produce cerebrospinal fluid • Aid movement of cerebrospinal fluid

GLIAL CELLS OF THE CENTRAL NERVOUS SYSTEM

Astrocytes

General
- The largest glial cell of the CNS
- Many highly branched cell extensions with end feet, covering:
  ○ Neuronal surfaces
  ○ Basal domain of ependymal cells
  ○ Basal lamina of blood vessels
  ○ Basal lamina of pia mater
- The end feet form barriers (glia limitans), which separate nerve tissue from other tissues and act as functional barriers, e.g., against immune cells.

Structure
- Large, star-shaped cell
- Many highly branched cell extensions with end feet
- Large, light (euchromatic) nucleus

Function
- Mechanical support:
  ○ The cell extensions prevent contact between neurons and:
    ▪ Other neurons
    ▪ Ependymal cells
    ▪ Blood vessels
    ▪ Pia mater
- Metabolic functions:
  ○ Reuptake of neurotransmitters
  ○ Synthesis of precursor molecules for neurotransmitters
  ○ Removal of waste products from neurons
- Form scar tissue within the CNS
- Ion buffer:
  ○ Astrocytes are connected through gap junctions and thereby form a syncytium able to act as a large ion buffer, e.g., for K^+ in the extracellular fluid
- Regulates and maintains the blood–brain barrier

Divided into
- Fibrous astrocytes:
  ○ Most abundant in white matter
  ○ Few cell extensions
  ○ Contain numerous intermediate filaments, made from GFAP (glial fibrillary acid protein) subunits, specific for astrocytes

- Protoplasmic astrocytes:
  - Most abundant in gray matter
  - Multiple short cell extensions
  - Contain fewer intermediate filaments, made from GFAP subunits

Light Microscopy
- Only the large, light (euchromatic) nucleus is visible in routine preparations.
- Astrocytes can be visualized using special stains, e.g., antibodies against GFAP.

MEMO-BOX
- "Astron" is Greek for star: Astrocytes are star-shaped cells.
- FIbrous astrocytes:
  - Most common in whIte substance
  - Fibrous as they contain numerous Intermediate filaments

Oligodendrocytes

Structure
- Small cell
- Few, thin branching cell extensions
- Small, dark (heterochromatic) nucleus

Divided into
- Interfascicular oligodendrocytes:
  - In white matter
  - Located in rows between axons
  - Functionally similar to the Schwann cells of the PNS
- Satellite (perineuronal) oligodendrocytes:
  - In gray matter
  - Located adjacent to the nerve cell bodies
  - Functionally similar to the satellite cells of the PNS

Function
- Interfascicular oligodendrocytes:
  - Form myelin sheaths in CNS:
    1. Each branch of a cell extension makes contact with an axon.
    2. Ensheaths the axon and wraps around the axon multiple times (as a rolled up paper).
    3. Multiple compactly packed layers of oligodendrocyte plasma membrane surround the axon, forming a segment of a myelin sheath.

- ◦ Myelination is similar to that of Schwann cells, with some differences (Table 14.5).
- • Satellite oligodendrocytes:
  - ◦ Regulate the microenvironment around nerve cell bodies.

Light Microscopy
Only the small, dark (heterochromatic) nucleus is visible in routine preparations.

Table 14.5 Differences in myelination between Schwann cells and interfascicular oligodendrocytes

	Schwann cell	Interfascicular oligodendrocyte
Number of axons, on which myelin segments are formed	Each cell ensheaths one axon	Each cell ensheaths ≥1 axon
Segments of myelin sheath per axon	Each cell forms one segment	Each cell forms multiple segments, one per cell extension branch
Gaps between myelin sheath segments (nodes of Ranvier)	Small	Large
Envelops unmyelinated axons	Yes	No, unmyelinated axons in CNS are bare, i.e., not enveloped by glial cells

MEMO-BOX
- • "Oligo" is Greek for few and "dendron" is Greek for tree → oligodendrocytes have few, branched cell extensions.
- • Interfascicular oligodendrocytes: Located in whIte substance and form myelIn sheaths in the CNS.

Microglia

General
- • Smallest glial cell of the CNS.
- • Part of mononuclear phagocyte system (Chap. 7).
- • Motile cells.
- • Can proliferate and become activated in response to damage or disease in the CNS.

Structure
- Small cell
- Short, thin cell extensions
- Small, elongated, dark (heterochromatic) nucleus

Function

The immune cell of the CNS:
- Tissue damage or disease → microglia are activated into reactive microglia, with the functions:
  - Phagocytosis of, e.g., bacteria and damaged cells
  - Antigen presentation

Light Microscopy

Only the small, elongated, dark (heterochromatic) is visible in routine preparations.

Ependymal Cells

General

Line the fluid filled cavities of the CNS:
- The ventricles of the brain
- The central canal of the spinal cord

Structure
- Simple cuboidal/columnar epithelium
- Luminal surface is covered with:
  - Cilia: most abundant in ependymal cells outside of choroid plexus
  - Microvilli: most abundant in ependymal cells of choroid plexus
- Lacks basement membrane → rest directly on end feet of astrocyte cell extensions

Function
- Production of cerebrospinal fluid in the choroid plexuses (Chap. 16)
- Facilitation of cerebrospinal fluid movement via cilia

GLIAL CELLS OF THE PERIPHERAL NERVOUS SYSTEM

Schwann Cells

General (Fig. 14.4, Table 14.6)
- Schwann cells ensheath all axons in the PNS.
- Functionally similar to the interfascicular oligodendrocytes of the CNS.

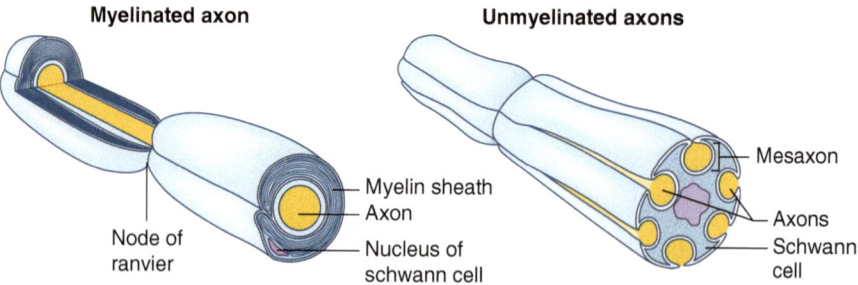

Fig. 14.4 Ensheathment of axons by Schwann cells: cross sections through peripheral nerve fibers, showing the structure of the Schwann cells and axons of myelinated and unmyelinated nerve fibers

Satellite Cells

General
- Surround the nerve cell bodies in ganglia.
- Functionally similar to the satellite (perineuronal) oligodendrocytes of the CNS.

Structure
- Small cuboidal cell
- Small, dark (heterochromatic) nucleus

Function
- Electrical insulation of the nerve cell bodies
- Controls microenvironment around nerve cell bodies in ganglia.

Light Microscopy
Only the small, dark (heterochromatic) nucleus is visible in routine preparations.

Table 14.6 Schwann cells

	Schwann cells of unmyelinated nerve fibers	Schwann cells of myelinated nerve fibers
Ensheath	Thin axons, ⊘ <1 μm: • Each Schwann cell envelops multiple thin axons forming a Remak bundle → unmyelinated axons • Chains of Schwann cells ensheath the axons along their path in the PNS • There are no gaps between the adjacent Schwann cells	Thick axons, ⊘ ≥1 μm: • Each Schwann cell forms a segment of the myelin sheath around a single thick axon → myelinated axon • Chains of Schwann cells (myelin sheath segments) ensheath the axon along the path in the PNS • ≈1 μm gaps (nodes of Ranvier) are found between adjacent Schwann cells
Structure		
• Length	200–400 μm, elongated parallel to the axons	300–1500 μm, elongated parallel to the axon
• Nucleus	Elongated and central	Peripheral and ovoid, located midways in cell
• Ensheathment of axon via	Multiple pocket-shaped invaginations (mesaxons) of the cell membrane, each containing one to a few axons	Multiple, densely packed layers of the cell membrane (myelin sheath) surrounding a single axon
• Cytoplasm	Located centrally in the cell	Located peripherally, around the nucleus and in the two ends of the cell
• External lamina (similar to a basal lamina)	+	+
Function	Ensheath thin axons (⊘ <1 μm) and package them into Remak bundles: • Separate axons from each other • Separate axons from the surrounding tissues	Form a myelin sheath around thick axons (⊘ ≥1 μm): • Increase conducting speed in axon • Separate axon from the surrounding tissues

Light microscopy	• Nucleus is visible
	• Multiple dark axons are seen within the cell
		• Routine preparation:
		  ○ Nucleus is visible
		  ○ Lipids of myelin sheath leach out → seen as "cloudy" empty space surrounding the central darker axon
		  ○ Lipids can be preserved using frozen sections or fixed and stained, e.g., with osmium tetroxide which stains the myelin sheath black/brown

Ensheathment process	Schwann cell forms multiple pocket-shaped invaginations (mesaxons) of the cell membrane, each surrounding one to a few axons	1. Schwann cell invaginates an axon into its center and spirals around it (as a rolled up paper) 2. Multiple compactly packed layers of cell membrane surround the axon, forming a myelin sheath

Guide to Practical Histology: Nerve Tissue

General

Contains nerve cells (neurons):

- Nerve cell bodies:
  - Are only found in the central nervous system and in ganglia.
  - Have a distinct morphology:
    - Large, central, light nucleus with a single central nucleolus → the nucleus resembles an eye.
    - Basophilic clumps are seen in the cytoplasm surrounding the nucleus.

Location

Makes up the major part of the nervous system, see (Chap. 16)

References

2, 5, 6, 25, 33, 34, 40.

Part IV
Histology of Organs

Chapter 15
Musculoskeletal System

General
- Perform movement of body parts, e.g.:
  - ○ Limbs during walking
  - ○ Diaphragm during respiration
- Movements are controlled via:
  - ○ The central nervous system (mostly voluntary)
  - ○ Reflex arches (involuntary)
- The movement facilitates other processes, e.g.:
  - ○ The venous blood return, via the skeletal muscle pump and the respiratory pump (Chap. 17).

Function
Movement of body parts via:
- Skeletal parts, which act as rigid lever arms
- Joints, which act as pivot points
- Ligaments, which keep skeletal parts in place
- Skeletal muscles, which exert force on skeletal parts through tendons

© Springer International Publishing Switzerland 2017
A. Rehfeld et al., *Compendium of Histology*, DOI 10.1007/978-3-319-41873-5_15

Consists of
- Skeleton:
  - Bones
  - Cartilages
  - Joints
  - Ligaments
- Skeletal muscles
- Tendons

Skeleton

General
- The skeleton is formed by bones and cartilages.
- Skeletal parts are connected through joints and ligaments.

Consist of
Three principal tissues:
- Bone tissue (Chap. 9)
  - Main component of adult skeleton
- Cartilage (Chap. 8):
  - Main component of fetal skeleton
  - Found in adult skeleton as, e.g.:
    - Individual cartilages:
      - Form fracture-resistant parts of the skeleton, e.g., in the ear and the respiratory tract.
    - Cartilage parts of bones:
      - Epiphyseal growth plates (removed at end of puberty)
      - Articular cartilage on articulating bone surfaces
- Dense connective tissue (Chap. 7):
  - Outer part of periosteum (Chap. 9)
  - Ligaments

Divided into
- Skeletal parts:
  - Bones
  - Cartilages
- Connections between skeletal parts:
  - Joints
  - Ligaments

BONES

General
Form the major part of the adult skeleton.

Function
- Supporting organs:
  - Facilitate movement: Acts as lever arms for muscles, using joints as pivots.
  - Bolster against gravity.
  - Protect inner organs.
  - Contain bone marrow (Chap. 10).
- Take part in calcium and phosphate homeostasis, through Ca^{2+} and PO_4^{3-} storage.

Consist of
- Bone tissue (Chap. 9):
  - Compact bone tissue.
  - Spongy bone tissue.
  - The proportion of compact and spongy bone tissue in bones varies. An example is given for a long bone (Fig. 15.1):
    - Diaphysis (shaft):
      - Compact bone tissue: makes up the main part
      - Spongy bone tissue: thin inner layer lining the medullary cavity
    - Epiphyses (ends):
      - Compact bone tissue: Thin outer layer.
      - Spongy bone tissue: Make up main part.
    - Metaphyses (the junctions between diaphysis and epiphyses):
      - Compact bone tissue: Thin outer layer, which thickens towards the diaphysis.
      - Spongy bone tissue: Make up main part.
- Medullary spaces:
  - Spaces within bone
  - Filled with bone marrow (Chap. 10)
- Cartilage (Chap. 8):
  - Covers articulating surfaces as articular cartilage
  - Forms epiphyseal growth plates in long bones (until end of puberty)
- Periosteum (Chap. 9):
  - Covers outer surfaces, except areas with articular cartilage.
- Endosteum (Chap. 9):
  - Lines all inner surfaces.

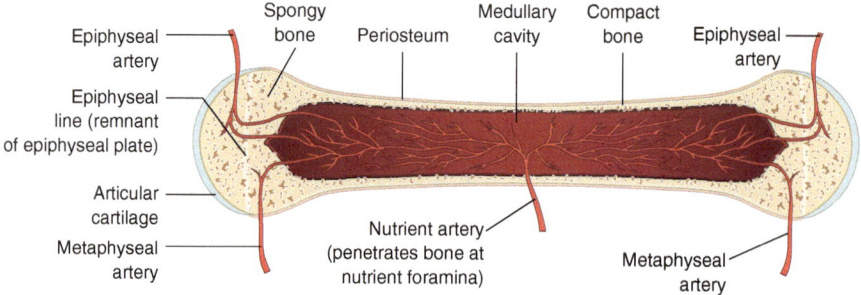

Fig. 15.1 The organization of bone tissue and large blood vessels of a mature long bone

Divided into
Bones are classified into four groups according to shape:
- Long bones:
  - Longer in one axis
  - For example, femur
- Short bones:
  - Equal length and ⊘
  - For example, carpal bones
- Flat bones:
  - For example, cranial bones
- Irregular bones:
  - For example, vertebrae

Vessels of Bones

General
- Blood vessels are found in all parts of the bone, except in the articular cartilage.
- Lymph vessels are only found in the periosteum.
- An example of the blood supply for a long bone is described here (Table 15.1, Fig. 15.1).

Function
Nourish the bone and the inner part of articular cartilage.

Nerves of Bones

General
- Larger nerves are found in the periosteum:
  - These nerves are responsive to pain.
- Small branches follow blood vessels into the Haversian canals of the bone tissue.

Table 15.1 Blood supply of a long bone

Blood vessel		Path
One to two nutrient arteries ↓		Transverse the bone at the mid-diaphysis, through the nutrient foramina, i.e., the hole through which the periosteal bud entered during bone formation
Two central longitudinal arteries ↓		• Each artery runs towards its own epiphysis • Anastomoses with branches from numerous metaphyseal and epiphyseal arteries
Many radiating artery branches ↓ ↓		Run towards the periphery of the medullary space

Capillaries	Blood vessels in Haversian and Volkmann's canals ↓	• Capillaries: run towards the sinusoids
		• Blood vessels in Haversian and Volkmann's canals:
		  ○ Run through the bone tissue to the outer surface of the bone
		  ○ Anastomoses with blood vessels of periosteum

Sinusoids ↓		• Anastomoses with each other in the periphery • Send out extensions towards the central vein
One central longitudinal vein		Follow the path of the central longitudinal arteries and nutrient arteries

CARTILAGES

General
- Cartilage makes up the major part of the fetal skeleton, forming miniature models of the adult bones:
  - Most of the cartilages are replaced by bone tissue through endochondral ossification (Chap. 9).
- Form fracture-resistant parts of the skeleton, e.g., in the ear and the respiratory tract.

Function
Semirigid, flexible, and resistant to fractures

Consist of
- Hyaline cartilage, e.g., in respiratory tracts
- Elastic cartilage, e.g., in external ear

JOINTS (ARTICULATIONS)

Structure

Junctions between two or more skeletal parts.

Function
- Connect skeletal parts.
- Allow movement of skeletal parts in relation to each other.
- Some joints act as pivots.

Divided into
- Synarthroses: Immobile/slightly movable
- Synovial joints (diarthroses): Permit movement

Synarthroses

General
- Immobile/slightly movable
- Without joint cavity

Divided into
- Syndesmoses:
  - Skeletal parts connected by connective tissue
  - For example, cranial sutures
- Synchondroses:
  - Skeletal parts connected by hyaline cartilage
  - For example, between ribs and the sternum
- Synostoses:
  - Skeletal parts connected by bone tissue formed via ossification of syndesmoses and synchondroses
  - For example, ossified epiphyseal discs
- Symphyses:
  - Fibrocartilage sandwiched between hyaline cartilages covering skeletal parts
  - For example, pubic symphysis and intervertebral discs

Synovial Joints

Function

Permit movement

Structure
- Articulating skeletal surfaces are:
  - Covered by articular cartilage.
  - Separated by a joint cavity with synovial fluid.
  - Encapsulated by a joint capsule.

- Synovial membrane covers all non-articulating inner surfaces in the joint cavity.
- Intra-articular structures of fibrocartilage, e.g., articular menisci and discs, are found in some joints.

Consist of
- Articular cartilage
- Joint capsule
- Synovial membrane
- Synovial fluid

Articular cartilage

Structure
- 2–5 mm thick
- Covers articulating surfaces of bone
- Not surrounded by a perichondrium
- Avascular
  - Cells are nourished by diffusion from synovial fluid and blood vessels in underlying bone.
  - Compression and decompression of ground substance → pumping action → aids diffusion, especially in deep regions.

Function
- Resists compression
- Bears weight
- Smooth, low-friction articular surface
- Distributes force to underlying bone

Consists of
- Hyaline cartilage
- Fibrocartilage, only in the joints of the clavicle and mandible

Divided into (Table 15.2)
- Superficial zone, towards the free articular surface
- Intermediate zone
- Deep zone
- Calcified zone, towards the underlying bone

Joint capsule

General
Surrounds the joint.

Structure
- Dense connective tissue attached to the involved bone parts.
- Continuous with periosteum of the involved bones.

- Capsule contains local thickenings, capsular ligaments.
- Penetrated by blood vessels and nerves.
- Contains mechanoreceptors, which resemble Ruffini's and Pacinian corpuscles (Chap. 20).

Table 15.2 Zones of articular cartilage

Zone	Extracellular matrix	Chondrocytes
Superficial zone	Collagen fibrils in bundles parallel to the surface	Chondrocytes elongated with the long axis parallel to the surface
Intermediate zone	Collagen fibrils obliquely orientated in relation to surface	Round chondrocytes
Deep zone	Collagen fibrils perpendicular to surface	Round chondrocytes in columns perpendicular to the surface
Calcified zone	Deposition of calcium phosphate crystals → calcified extracellular matrix	No chondrocytes

Function
Protection of joints:
- Bendable
- Tough and resistant to overstretching, especially the capsular ligaments.
- If the capsule is overstretched, the mechanoreceptors are activated → reflex muscle contraction, which protect the joint from further overstretching.

Synovial membrane

General
- Lines interior surface on:
  - All non-articulating surfaces in joint cavities
  - Bursae
  - Tendon sheaths
- One of the few exceptions of a non-epithelial tissue lining a cavity

Structure
- Specialized connective tissue membrane.
- Well-vascularized with fenestrated capillaries → facilitates exchange between blood and synovial fluid.
- Numerous folds and villi extend into the joint cavity → increase inner surface area → large area for production of synovial fluid.

Consist of
- Extracellular matrix
- Synovial cells

Synovial cells

Structure
Form a membrane of 1–2 cell layers.

Divided into
- Type A synovial cells
  - Macrophage-like, derived from monocytes
  - Remove debris from synovial fluid
- Type B synovial cells:
  - Fibroblast-like
  - Produce components of:
    - Extracellular matrix
    - Synovial fluid, e.g., hyaluronan

Synovial fluid

General
Fills the cavity of:
- Synovial joints
- Bursae
- Tendon sheaths

Structure
Clear, viscous, yellowish fluid.

Function
Lowers the friction between articulating surfaces.

Consists of
- Ultrafiltrate of blood plasma
- Additional substances:
  - For example, hyaluronan → increases viscosity of the synovial fluid

LIGAMENTS

General
Connect skeletal parts

Function
- Robust, but flexible
- Keep skeletal parts in place, relative to each other
- Contribute to the stability of joints

Consist of
- Dense regular connective tissue (Chap. 7), with thick bundles of parallel collagen fibers
- Dense elastic connective tissue (Chap. 7), with thick bundles of parallel elastic fibers: only in elastic ligaments, e.g., ligamenta flava

Skeletal Muscles

General
- Connected to the skeleton through tendons.
- Contraction of skeletal muscles is controlled via:
  - The central nervous system (mostly voluntary)
  - Reflex arches (involuntary), e.g.:
    - Stretch reflex
    - Golgi tendon reflex

Function
Movement of skeletal parts

Consist of
- Skeletal muscle tissue (Chap. 13)
- Connective tissue containing blood vessels and nerves
- Sensory receptors
  - Muscle spindles
  - Golgi tendon organs

Connective Tissue Sheaths of Skeletal Muscles

Structure
- Contains:
  - Blood vessels
  - Lymph vessels
  - Nerves
- Continuous with tendons, which attach the muscle to bone

Function
Transduce the contractile force of skeletal muscle tissue to the tendon.

Divided into (Table 15.3, Fig. 15.2)
- Epimysium
- Perimysium
- Endomysium

Table 15.3 Connective tissue sheaths of skeletal muscles

Layer	Connective tissue	Location
Epimysium	Dense irregular connective tissue	Surrounds the entire muscle
Perimysium	Dense irregular connective tissue	Surrounds groups of muscle cells forming fascicles
Endomysium	Delicate mesh of reticular fibers	• Surrounds the individual muscle cells • Located just outside the external lamina

Sensory Receptors of Skeletal Muscles

General
- Proprioceptors
- Monitor the tension of the tendon and stretch of the muscle
- Take part in reflex arches

Divided into
- Muscle spindles
- Golgi tendon organs

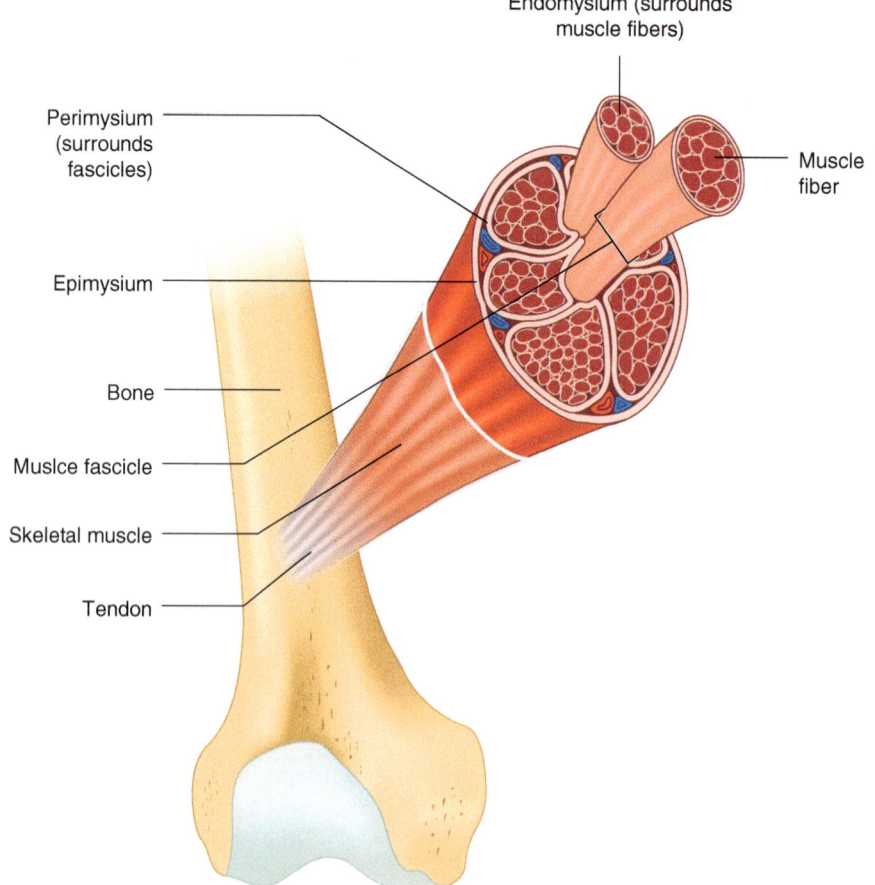

Fig. 15.2 Skeletal muscle structure with the connective tissue sheaths of skeletal muscles shown

Muscle spindle

Structure (Fig. 15.3)
- Encapsulated fusiform element:
  - ⊘ < 1 mm
  - Up to 2 mm long
- Located within skeletal muscle tissue.
- Found in all skeletal muscles.

Function
Proprioception:
- Stimulated by stretching of the muscle
- Part of the stretch reflex:
  - Initiate contraction via motor neurons if the muscle is stretched.
  - Keep muscle length steady.
  - For example, used to maintain posture.

Consists of
- Connective tissue capsule:
  - Modified perimysium.
  - Surrounds spindle cells.
- Spindle cells:
  - Two different types of small modified skeletal muscle cells.
  - Are stretched concurrent with surrounding muscle tissue.
- Afferent (sensory) nerve fibers:
  - Penetrate the capsule and spiral around both types of spindle cells.
  - Stimulated by stretching of the spindle cells.
- Efferent (motor) nerve fibers:
  - Penetrate the capsule and innervate one of the spindle cell types:
    - Enable contraction in this type of spindle cell.
    - Contractive state of these spindle cells regulates the sensitivity of the muscle spindle by setting the threshold force needed to stretch it.

Fig. 15.3 Muscle spindle in longitudinal section

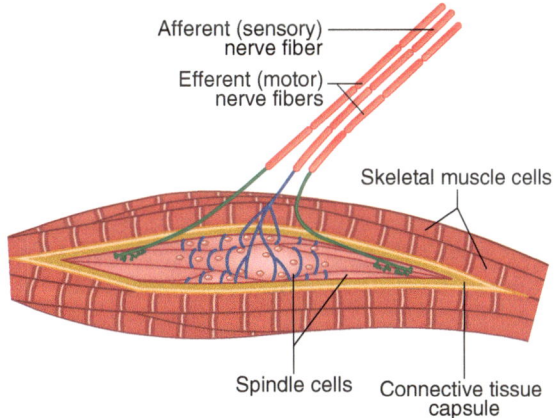

Golgi tendon organ

Structure
- Encapsulated element.
- Located at the junction between skeletal muscle tissue and tendon.

Function
Proprioception:
- Monitors the force of muscle contraction, by sensing the tension within the tendon.
- Part of the Golgi tendon reflex:
  - Inhibit contraction via motor neurons if the tension of the tendon is excessive.
  - Protects the tendon against overstretching and rupture.

Consists of
- Connective tissue capsule
- Small bundle of collagen fibers within the capsule
  - Connects to skeletal muscle fibers at one end and merges with the collagen fibers of the tendon at the other end.
  - Are stretched concurrent with the collagen fibers of the tendon.
- A single afferent (sensory) nerve fiber:
  - Penetrates the capsule, branches, and spirals around the collagen fibers.
  - Stimulated by stretching of the collagen fibers.

Tendons

General
Connect the skeletal muscles to the skeleton.

Function
- Transduce the contractile force of the skeletal muscles to the skeleton.
- Have a strong resistance to force in the direction of the parallel collagen fibers.

Consist of
Dense regular connective tissue (Chap. 7), with thick bundles of parallel collagen fibers

Aponeuroses
General
Broad, flat tendons:
- Contains bundles of parallel collagen fibers arranged in multiple layers.
- Fibers are arranged orthogonally in adjacent layers.

Connective Tissue Sheaths of Tendons
Structure
Contain:
- Blood vessels
- Lymph vessels
- Nerves

Divided into (Table 15.4)
- Epitendineum
- Peritendineum
- Endotendineum

Table 15.4 Connective tissue sheaths of tendons

Layer	Connective tissue	Location
Epitendineum	Dense irregular connective tissue	Surrounds the entire tendon
Peritendineum	Dense irregular connective tissue	Surrounds groups of fascicles
Endotendineum	Dense irregular connective tissue	Surrounds groups of collagen fiber bundles forming fascicles

Guide to Practical Histology: Musculoskeletal System

General
- Skeleton consists of:
  - Bones:
    - Bone tissue (Chap. 9)
    - Cartilage parts (Chap. 8)
    - Bone marrow (Chap. 10)
    - Periosteum of connective tissue (Chap. 7)
  - Cartilages:
    - Cartilage (Chap. 8)
  - Joints (see below)
  - Ligaments:
    - Dense regular connective tissue (Chap. 7)
- Skeletal muscles:
  - Skeletal muscle tissue (Chap. 13)
  - Sensory organs of skeletal muscle (see below)
- Tendons:
  - Dense regular connective tissue (Chap. 7)

JOINTS

Synovial Joint

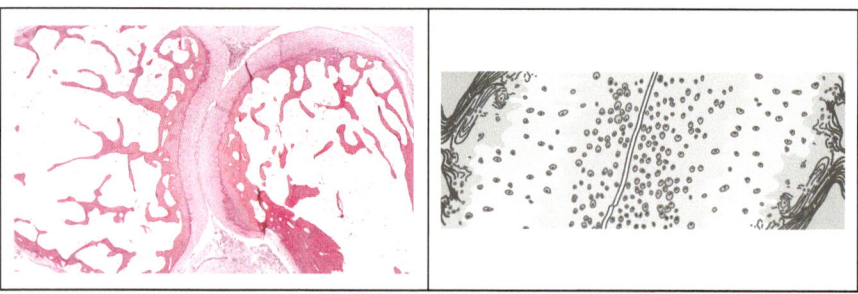

Left: photomicrograph of articular cartilage covered bone of synovial joint. Magnification: Low. Stain: HE (Courtesy of professor Jørgen Tranum-Jensen, University of Copenhagen). *Right*: Simplified illustration of articular cartilage covered bone of synovial joint

Characteristics
- Bone tissue part or parts covered with articular cartilage (most commonly hyaline cartilage).
- Adjacent to articular cartilage is a large white (empty) space (joint cavity).

Symphysis

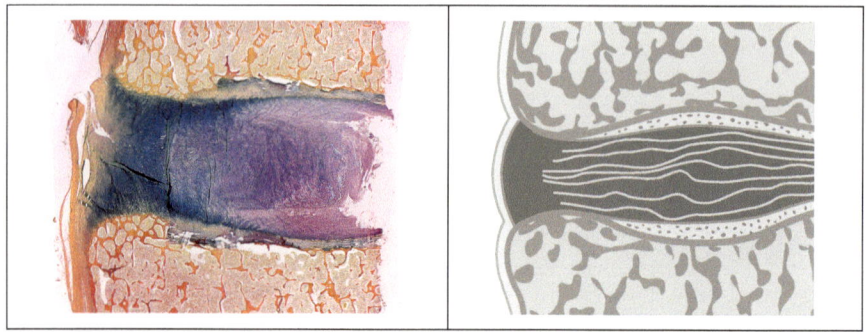

Left: photomicrograph of symphysis between vertebrae. Magnification: macroscopic. Stain: Van Gieson and Alcian Blue (Courtesy of professor Jørgen Tranum-Jensen, University of Copenhagen). *Right*: Simplified illustration of symphysis between vertebrae

Characteristics
Fibrocartilage sandwiched between hyaline cartilage covered bone parts.

Location
For example, seen between vertebrae

SENSORY ORGANS OF SKELETAL MUSCLES

Muscle Spindle

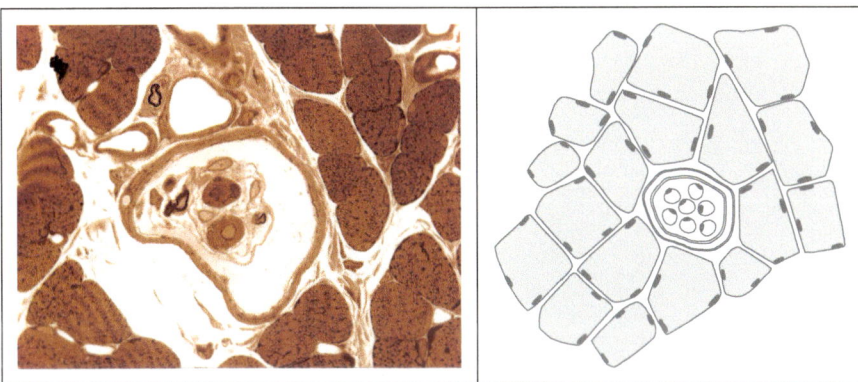

Left: photomicrograph of muscle spindle. Magnification: high. Stain: paraphenylenediamine (Courtesy of professor Jørgen Tranum-Jensen, University of Copenhagen). *Right*: Simplified illustration of muscle spindle

Characteristics
- A thin capsule of connective tissue containing:
  - A few thin muscle fibers surrounded by a white (empty) space
- Located within skeletal muscle tissue
- Often seen in near relation to cross sections of nerves.

References

5, 7, 25, 32, 33, 34, 44, 45.

Chapter 16
The Nervous System

Contents

General

Organ system mainly composed of nerve tissue

Function

- Enables the body to rapidly respond to changes in the external and internal environment
- Controls activity of organs in corporation with the endocrine system, which communicates more slowly

© Springer International Publishing Switzerland 2017
A. Rehfeld et al., *Compendium of Histology*, DOI 10.1007/978-3-319-41873-5_16

Consists of
- Nerve tissue (Chap. 14)
- Connective tissue (Chap. 7)

Divided into
The nervous system can be divided into parts, both anatomically and functionally.

Anatomically divided into

- Central nervous system (CNS):
  - Brain:
    - Cerebrum
    - Cerebellum
    - Brain stem
  - Spinal cord
- Peripheral nervous system (PNS):
  - Peripheral nerves
    - Cranial nerves
    - Spinal nerves
  - Ganglia
    - Sensory ganglia
    - Autonomic ganglia
      - Sympathetic ganglia
      - Parasympathetic ganglia

Functionally divided into

- Somatic nervous system
  - Conscious, voluntary control
    - Except reflex arcs, which are involuntary
  - Sensory and motor innervation to all body parts except internal organs
- Autonomic nervous system
  - Unconscious, involuntary control
  - Sensory and motor innervation to internal organs
  - Divided into:
    - Sympathetic nervous system
    - Parasympathetic nervous system
    - Enteric nervous system (Chap. 21)

Central Nervous System

General
- The part of the nervous system inside the brain and spinal cord
- Surrounded by connective tissue sheaths, called meninges
- Contains fluid filled cavities:
  - Ventricular system of the brain
  - Central canal of the spinal cord

Divided into
- Brain:
  - Cerebrum
  - Cerebellum
  - Brain stem
- Spinal cord

Consists of
- Gray matter:
  - Cell bodies of:
    - Nerve cells
    - Glial cells
  - Neuropil (meshwork of cell extensions):
    - Nerve cell extensions:
      - Axons +/− myelination
      - Dendrites
    - Glial cell extensions
- White matter:
  - Glial cells
  - Axons, primarily myelinated:
    - Solitary
    - In bundles (tracts)

Light microscopy
- Gray matter:
  - Unstained: Gray (due to numerous nuclei)
  - HE: Basophilic
- White matter:
  - Unstained: White (due to high content of myelin)
  - HE: Pale acidophilic

CEREBRUM

Structure
- Two cerebral hemispheres
  - Connected by:
    - The corpus callosum
    - Diencephalon, the central core of the cerebrum
- Located within the cranium

Function
Higher brain functions, e.g.:
- Initiation of motor output to, e.g., skeletal muscles
- Processing of sensory input from, e.g., the visual system

Consists of
- Gray matter:
  - Cerebral cortex (cortex cerebri)
    - Outermost layer, covering the white matter
  - Nuclei:
    - Areas of gray matter located within the white matter
    - For example, the basal ganglia and the thalamic nuclei
- White matter:
  - Located centrally in the cerebral hemispheres
  - Forms tracts in the corpus callosum and the diencephalon

Cerebral cortex

General
Highly folded via:
- Folds (gyri)   ⎫
- Grooves (sulci)   ⎬ Increase surface area
                     ⎭

Structure
- Granular layers:
  - Most afferent nerve fibers form synapses with neurons in these layers
  - Well-developed in the sensory parts of the cerebral cortex
- Pyramidal layers:
  - Most efferent nerve fibers originate from neurons in these layers
  - Well-developed in motoric parts of the cerebral cortex

Consists of

Six layers (from surface → center):

1. Molecular layer:
   - Few neurons
   - Many axons and dendrites, connecting cortical areas
2. External granular layer:
   - Small pyramidal neurons
   - Numerous stellate neurons
3. External pyramidal layer:
   - Small and medium pyramidal neurons
4. Internal granular layer:
   - Densely packed stellate neurons
   - Small pyramidal neurons
   - Most afferent nerve fibers form synapses with neurons in this layer
5. Internal pyramidal layer:
   - Large pyramidal neurons
   - Giant pyramidal neurons (Betz cells), only seen in primary motor cortex
   - Most efferent nerve fibers originate from neurons in this layer
6. Multiform layer:
   - Small pyramidal and multiform neurons
   - Many nerve fibers

Divided into

- Neocortex:
  ○ Major part of cerebral cortex
  ○ Covers almost the entire surface of cerebrum
  ○ Contains six cell layers
- Allocortex:
  ○ Areas of the cerebral cortex with only 3 or 4 cell layers
  ○ For example, hippocampus

CEREBELLUM

Structure

- Two cerebellar hemispheres
- Connected by vermis
- Located in the posterior fossa of the cranium

Function
- Maintenance of balance and posture
- Coordination of voluntary movements

Consists of
- Gray matter
  - Cerebellar cortex (cortex cerebelli)
    - Outermost layer, covering the white matter
  - Nuclei
    - Areas of gray matter located within the white matter
    - For example, the dentate nucleus
- White matter
  - Located centrally

Cerebellar cortex

General
Very highly folded via folds (folia) → increase surface area

Structure
- Main types of neurons:
  - Purkinje cells
  - Granule cells
- Additional interneurons:
  - Golgi cells
  - Stellate cells
  - Basket cells

Consists of
Three layers (from surface → center) (Table 16.1):
- Molecular layer
- Purkinje cell layer
- Granule cell layer

BRAIN STEM

General
- Elongated structure
- Connects:
  - Cerebrum
  - Cerebellum
  - Spinal cord
- Contains the nuclei of cranial nerves III–XII

Table 16.1 Layers of the cerebellar cortex

Layer (from surface → center)	Purkinje cell part	Granule cell part	Thickness	Staining
1. Molecular layer	Dendritic trees, which branch within a plane, perpendicular to the folia	Parallel fibers (axons), running parallel to the folia	Thick	Pale acidophilic
2. Purkinje cell layer	Large nerve cell bodies	Axons	A single layer of cell bodies of Purkinje cells	Basophilic
3. Granule cell layer	Axons	Small nerve cell bodies	Thick	Basophilic

Function
- Autonomic reflexes
- Regulates awareness
- Sensory and motoric action of the cranial nerves III–XII

Divided into
- Midbrain: Connects to cerebrum
- Pons: Connects to cerebellum
- Medulla oblongata: Continuous with spinal cord

Consists of
- Gray matter:
  - Nuclei of cranial nerves are seen surrounded by white matter
  - Remaining areas of gray matter are not clearly separated from white matter
- White matter

SPINAL CORD

Structure
- Long cylindrical structure
  - ≈45 cm long
  - Ovoid, ⊘ 6–13 mm
- Located within the spinal canal
- Continuous with the brain stem

Function
- Carries sensory and motoric information between the PNS and the CNS
- Contains motor neurons of reflex arcs

Divided into
31 segments, each giving rise to a pair of spinal nerves:
- 8 cervical segments
- 12 thoracic segments
- 5 lumbar segments
- 5 sacral segments
- 1 coccygeal segment

Consists of
- Gray matter
  - Located centrally around the central canal
  - Butterfly shaped on cross section
- White matter
  - Surrounds the gray matter

MENINGES

Structure
Connective tissue covering the CNS

Consists of (Fig. 16.1)
- Dura mater, outermost layer
- Arachnoid, middle layer
- Pia mater, inner layer

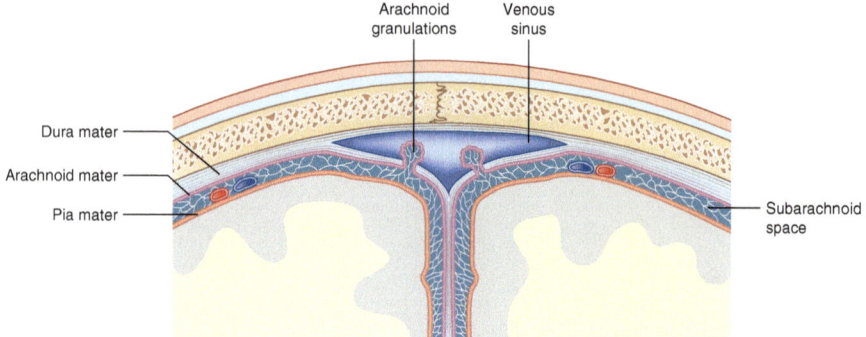

Fig. 16.1 The meninges of the brain, showing arachnoid granulations into a venous sinus

Dura Mater

General
Outermost meningeal layer

Structure
- Thick layer of dense connective tissue containing:
  - Blood vessels
  - Lymph vessels
  - Sensory nerves
- Outer surfaces are covered with simple squamous epithelium
- Form sheetlike folds:
  - Contain venous sinuses (spaces lined with endothelium), which receive blood from the veins of the brain
  - For example, falx cerebri, which separates the two cerebral hemispheres

Divided into
- Intracranial dura
  - Surrounds the brain
  - Consist of two layers:
    - Outer periosteal layer
      - Continuous with the periost of the cranium
    - Inner meningeal layer
      - Continuous with the spinal dura
- Spinal dura
  - A sack surrounding the spinal cord
  - Continuous with the inner meningeal layer of the intracranial dura

Arachnoid

General
- Middle meningeal layer
- Separated from pia mater by the subarachnoid space

Structure
- Loose connective tissue covered with epithelium
- Connected with pia mater via numerous trabeculae running through subarachnoid space forming a network

Consist of
- Simple squamous epithelium (outer layer)
- Thin core of loose connective tissue
- Simple squamous epithelium (inner layer)

Subarachnoid space

General
- Contains cerebrospinal fluid that:
  - Fills into subarachnoid space through holes in the fourth ventricle
  - Is resorbed into the bloodstream through small protrusions of arachnoid (arachnoid granulations), into the venous sinuses of dura mater (Fig. 16.1).
- Contains blood vessels, which give off branches that penetrate pia mater to enter the CNS.

Pia mater

General
- Innermost meningeal layer
  - Connected with arachnoidea via numerous trabeculae running through subarachnoid space (weblike appearance)
- Separated from the underlying glia limitans, formed by end feet of astrocyte cell extensions, by the subpial space:
  - Contains a dense capillary network

Structure
- Thin layer, with the same composition as the arachnoid
- Lines the surface of the CNS, following the grooves and ridges
- Continuous with the connective tissue sheath (tunica adventitia) of blood vessels entering the CNS

VENTRICULAR SYSTEM

General
- Interconnected spaces within the central nervous system
- Continuous with the central canal of the spinal cord
- Contains cerebrospinal fluid:
  - Empties into subarachnoid space through holes in the fourth ventricle

Structure
- Lined with ependymal cells
- Communicate with:
  - The subarachnoid space through holes in the fourth ventricle
  - The central canal of the spinal cord, which is continuous with the fourth ventricle

Function
Production of cerebrospinal fluid in choroid plexuses (see below)

Consists of
- Two lateral ventricles (a right and a left ventricle)
- Third ventricle
- Fourth ventricle

Choroid plexuses

General
- Areas in the ventricles where the cerebrospinal fluid is produced
- Each of the four ventricles contains a choroid plexus

Function
Production of cerebrospinal fluid, 0.5 l per day:
- Formed by transport of blood plasma constituents through the ependymal cells

Consist of
- Ependymal cell layer:
  - Bulges into the lumen of the ventricle, forming villi
  - Covered with luminal microvilli → increase surface area
  - Cells are connected with tight junctions, forming the blood–cerebrospinal fluid barrier:
    - Blocks the intercellular pathway between the ependymal cells → constituents of the cerebrospinal fluid must be transported through the ependymal cells to reach the ventricular system
- Pia mater
  - In direct contact with the ependymal cells in the choroid plexus
  - Subpial space contains fenestrated capillaries, which form loops within the villi

Cerebrospinal Fluid

General
Formed in the choroid plexuses

Structure
- Clear, colorless fluid
- Located in:
  - The ventricular system of the brain
  - The central canal of the spinal cord
  - The subarachnoid space

Function
- Communicates with the interstitial fluid of the CNS, as ependymal cells outside the choroid plexuses do not contain tight junctions
- Removes waste products from the CNS

- Provides buoyancy:
  - Makes the brain and spinal cord "float" in the cerebrospinal fluid of the subarachnoid space
  - Protects the brain and spinal cord against mechanical trauma

Consists of
- Water, 99 %
- Electrolytes
- Small amounts of protein
- Few cells

CENTRAL CANAL

General
Contains cerebrospinal fluid

Structure
- Central space within the spinal cord
- Continuous with the fourth ventricle of the ventricular system
- Lined with ependymal cells

BLOOD–BRAIN BARRIER

General
Barrier separating the nerve tissue of the CNS from selected substances in the blood

Structure
- Found throughout the CNS
- Except in the circumventricular organs, where the capillaries are fenestrated, e.g., in the choroid plexuses

Function
- Selective transport of:
  - Large (>500 Da) or water-soluble (hydrophilic) substances
    - These must be selectively transported through endothelium to reach the CNS
    - In contrast, small, lipid-soluble (hydrophobic) substances can freely pass endothelium by passive diffusion
- Protects CNS from, e.g.:
  - Fluctuations in electrolytes ⎤
  - Hormones   ⎬ Homeostasis of the microenvironment in the CNS
  - Metabolites   ⎦

Consists of
- Inner part:
  - ○ Tight junctions between endothelial cells of the capillaries:
    - ▪ Blocks the intercellular pathway
    - ▪ Forms a barrier between:
      - • The arterial blood
      - • The nerve tissue of the CNS
    - ▪ Regulated by the end feet of astrocyte cell extensions, which cover basement membrane of endothelium
- Outer part:
  - ○ Tight junctions between cells in the arachnoid:
    - ▪ Forms a barrier between:
      - • The venous blood of the venous sinuses of dura mater
      - • The cerebrospinal fluid in the subarachnoid space

BLOOD SUPPLY OF THE BRAIN

Arterial Blood Supply of the Brain

General
- The blood supply comes from contralateral anterior and posterior parts
- Forms an anastomosis called the cerebral arterial circle

Divided into
See Table 16.2.

Cerebral arterial circle (Circle of Willis)
General
- A circular anastomosis of cerebral arteries (Fig. 16.2)
- Connects the blood supply from the paired vertebral and internal carotid arteries

Table 16.2 Blood supply of the brain

	Anterior part		Posterior part
Extracranial blood vessels	Internal carotid artery (paired)		Vertebral artery (paired)
• Enters the cranium through	Carotid canal		Foramen magnum
Intracranial blood vessels	Internal carotid artery (paired)		Vertebral artery (paired)
			Basilar artery (single)
• Terminal branches	Anterior cerebral artery (paired)	Medial cerebral artery (paired)	Posterior cerebral artery (paired)

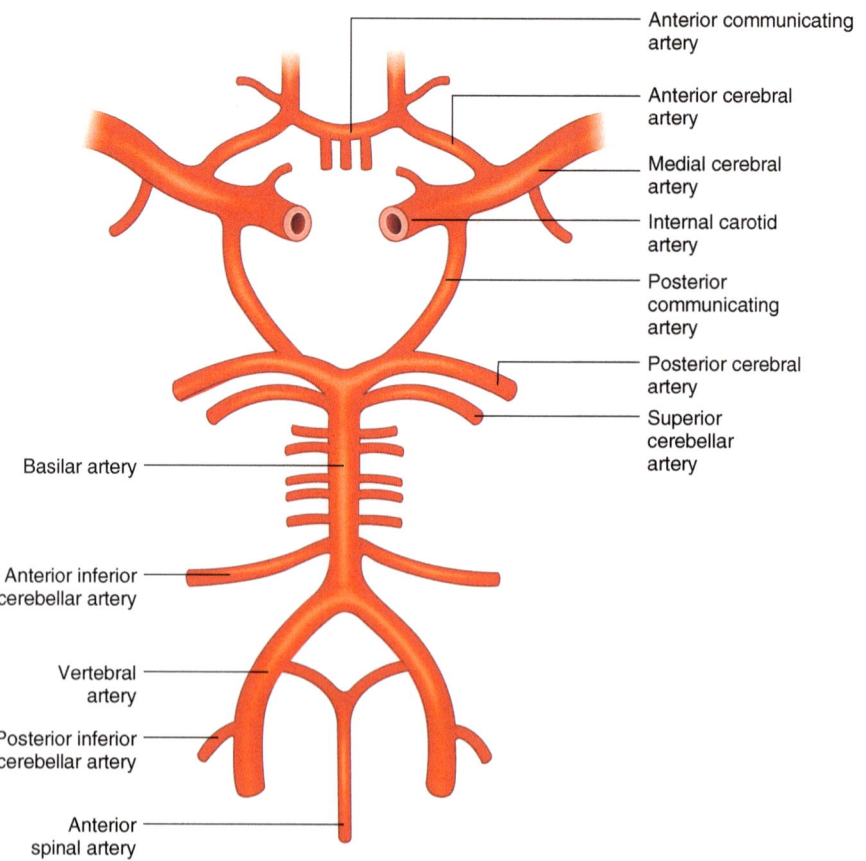

Fig. 16.2 The cerebral arterial circle

Consists of
- Anterior cerebral artery (paired)
  - A terminal branch from the internal carotid artery
- Anterior communicating artery
  - Connects the paired anterior cerebral arteries
- Internal carotid artery (paired)
- Posterior cerebral artery (paired)
  - A terminal branch from the basilar artery
- Posterior communicating artery (paired)
  - Connects the posterior cerebral artery with the internal carotid
- Basilar artery

Venous Drainage of the Brain

General
Does not follow the cerebral arterial system

Consists of
- Veins:
  - Drains to the venous sinuses of dura mater
  - Contains:
    - No valves
    - No muscle tissue in wall
- Venous sinuses of dura mater:
  - Cavities within the two layers of dura mater
  - Form a connected network
  - Lined with endothelium
  - Contain no valves
  - Receives:
    - Blood from the veins of the brain
    - Cerebrospinal fluid from the subarachnoid space, through small protrusions of arachnoid (arachnoid granulations)
  - Empties to the internal jugular vein (paired)

Divided into
- Veins
  - Superficial veins
  - Profound veins
- Venous sinuses, e.g.:
  - Superior sagittal sinus
  - Inferior sagittal sinus
  - Sigmoid sinus (paired)

BLOOD SUPPLY OF THE SPINAL CORD

Arterial Blood Supply of the Spinal Cord

General
- Supplied by three longitudinal arteries running parallel with the spinal cord
- The three longitudinal arteries are reinforced via anastomoses with multiple segmental arteries

Divided into
- Anterior spinal artery
  - A fusion of two branches from the vertebral arteries (paired)
  - Descend anterior to the spinal cord

- Right posterior spinal artery
  - Branch from the right vertebral artery
  - Descend on the right side of the spinal cord
- Left posterior spinal artery
  - Branch from the left vertebral artery
  - Descend on the left side of the spinal cord

Venous Drainage of the Spinal Cord

General
- Spinal veins:
  - Drains to a venous plexus in the vertebral canal, which empty into intervertebral veins
  - Contain no valves.

Peripheral Nervous System

General
The part of the nervous system outside the brain and spinal cord

Divided into
- Peripheral nerves
  - Cranial nerves
    - Cranial nerves I and II are often considered a part of the central nervous system.
  - Spinal nerves
- Ganglia
  - Sensory ganglia
  - Autonomic ganglia:
    - Sympathetic ganglia
    - Parasympathetic ganglia

PERIPHERAL NERVES

Structure
- Bundles of nerve fibers
- Nerves branch distally → smaller nerves → single nerve fibers
- Nerve fibers have a wavy path within the nerve, which allows stretching of nerves during movement, without rupturing of the nerve fibers

Function

Transmission of:
- Efferent (motor) impulses from the CNS to effector cells
- Afferent (sensory) impulses from sensory receptors to the CNS

Divided into

- Cranial nerves:
  - Twelve pairs:
    - Cranial nerves I and II:
      - Originate from the brain
      - Often considered a part of the central nervous system
    - Cranial nerves III to XII:
      - Originate from the brain stem
- Spinal nerves:
  - Thirty-one pairs:
    - Originate from the spinal cord, one pair from each segment

Consist of

- Nerve fibers:
  - Axon(s):
    - A single myelinated axon
    - Multiple unmyelinated axons
  - Schwann cells enveloping axon(s)
- Connective tissue (Table 16.3):
  - Surrounds the nerve fibers
  - Contains vessels and sensory nerves

Table 16.3 Connective tissue of peripheral nerves

Layer	Connective tissue type	Location	Blood vessels and sensory nerves	Lymph vessels
Epineurium	Dense irregular connective tissue	Surrounds the entire nerve	+	+
Perineurium	Specialized connective tissue with 1–6 layers of perineural cells: • Squamous cells • With an external lamina on both surfaces	• Surrounds bundles (fascicles) of nerve fibers • Forms the blood–nerve barrier, through tight junctions between the perineural cells	+	−
Endoneurium	Loose connective tissue	Surrounds single nerve fibers	−	−

FUNCTIONAL DIVISION OF NERVE FIBERS

General

Nerves consist of a combination of nerve fibers:

- Efferent (motor) nerve fibers:
  - Carry impulses away from the CNS
  - Divided into:
    - Visceral efferent nerve fibers
    - Somatic efferent nerve fibers
- Afferent (sensory) nerves fibers:
  - Carry impulses towards the CNS
  - Divided into:
    - Visceral afferent nerve fibers
    - Somatic afferent nerve fibers

Efferent (Motor) Nerve Fibers

Visceral efferent nerve fibers

Structure

- Unmyelinated axons (postganglionic nerve fibers) of the neurons in the autonomic ganglia:
  - Preganglionic nerve fibers are generally lightly myelinated
- End in close relation to:
  - Cardiac muscle
  - Smooth muscle
  - Glandular epithelium
- Do not form synapses

Function

Transmits impulses as a part of the autonomic nervous system → involuntary control

Somatic efferent nerve fibers

Structure

- Myelinated axons
- Form neuromuscular junctions (synapses) with skeletal muscle cells

Function

Transmits impulses as a part of the somatic nervous system → voluntary control

Afferent (Sensory) Nerve Fibers

General

Myelination of afferent nerve fibers depend on sensory modality, e.g.:

- Nerve fibers of muscle spindles are myelinated
- Nerve fibers transmitting slow pain are unmyelinated

Visceral afferent nerve fibers

Function
- Part of the autonomic nervous system
- Receive sensory impulses from sensory receptors, called interoceptors:
  - Located in internal organs
  - For example, sinus caroticus (Chap. 17)

Somatic afferent nerve fibers

Function
- Part of somatic nervous system
- Receive sensory impulses from sensory receptors:
  - Proprioceptors:
    - Located in:
      - Skeletal muscles (Chap. 15)
      - Tendons (Chap. 15)
      - Joints (Chap. 15)
  - Exteroceptors:
    - Located in:
      - Skin (Chap. 20)
      - Eye (Chap. 28)
      - Ear (Chap. 29)
      - Nose (Chap. 18)
      - Tongue (Chap. 21)

Sensory Receptors

General
Specialized to respond to various stimuli

Function
Convert stimuli into afferent nerve impulses

Divided into
- Free (nonencapsulated) nerve endings (Chap. 20)
- Encapsulated nerve endings:
  - Nerve endings surrounded by a connective tissue capsule.
  - Divided into:
    - Mechanoreceptors (Chap. 20)
    - Thermoreceptors (Chap. 20)
    - Proprioceptors (Chap. 15)

Functional classification of sensory receptors

Divided into
- Exteroceptors
  - React to stimuli of external environment

- Interoceptors
  - React to stimuli within the internal organs
- Proprioceptors
  - Sense body position, muscle tone, and movement

GANGLIA

General
- Aggregations of nerve cell bodies in the PNS
- The only location of nerve cell bodies outside the CNS

Divided into (Table 16.4)
- Sensory ganglia:
  - Contain pseudounipolar, sensory neurons:
    - Do not receive synapses within the ganglion
  - Found in association with all spinal nerves and some cranial nerves
- Autonomic ganglia:
  - Contain multipolar, motor neurons:
    - Receive synapses within the ganglion
  - Divided into:
    - Sympathetic ganglia
    - Parasympathetic ganglia

Table 16.4 Ganglia

	Sensory ganglia	Autonomic ganglia
Neurons		
• Anatomical type	Pseudounipolar neurons	Multipolar neurons
• Functional type	Sensory neuron	Motor neuron
• Cell body ⊘	15–100 μm	15–60 μm
• Nucleus	Central	Eccentric
• Surrounded by satellite cells	Yes	Yes
• Receive synapses in ganglion	No	Yes

Nerve fibers	Fill up spaces between neurons:
	• Myelination depends on the sensory modality, e.g.:
	  ◦ Nerve fibers of muscle spindles are myelinated
	  ◦ Nerve fibers transmitting slow pain are unmyelinated
		Fill up spaces between neurons:
		• Preganglionic nerve fibers are generally lightly myelinated
		• Postganglionic nerve fibers are unmyelinated

Capsule of dense connective tissue, continuous with the epi- and perineurium of nerves	Present	• Present • Except for ganglia located in the wall of internal organs (intramural ganglia)

Guide to Practical Histology: Nervous System

CENTRAL NERVOUS SYSTEM

Cerebrum

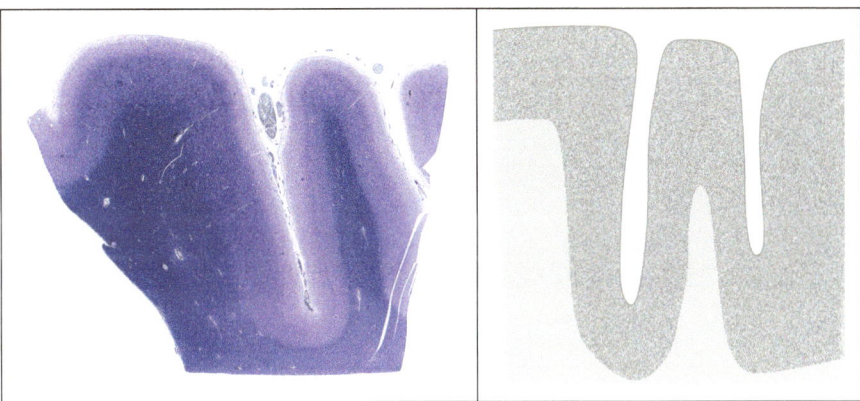

Left: photomicrograph of cerebral cortex. Magnification: macroscopic. Stain: Klüver–Barrera (Courtesy of professor Jørgen Tranum-Jensen, University of Copenhagen). *Right*: simplified illustration of the cerebral cortex

Cerebral cortex

Characteristics

Macroscopically:

- Consists of two layers:
  - Gray matter (cortex):
    - A basophilic outermost layer
    - Contains characteristic large triangular nerve cell bodies:
      - Very large nerve cell bodies (Betz cells) are seen in primary motor cortex.
      - In the visual cortex, a macroscopic visible line of Gennari (large bundle of axons) runs parallel to the surface.
  - White matter:
    - A pale eosinophilic core underneath the cortex
- The border between gray and white matter is distinct.

Can be mistaken for

Cerebellar cortex:

- Surface is more folded.
- Contains three distinct layers macroscopically:
  - ○ A pale eosinophilic superficial layer
  - ○ A basophilic middle layer
  - ○ A pale eosinophilic core of white matter

Cerebellum

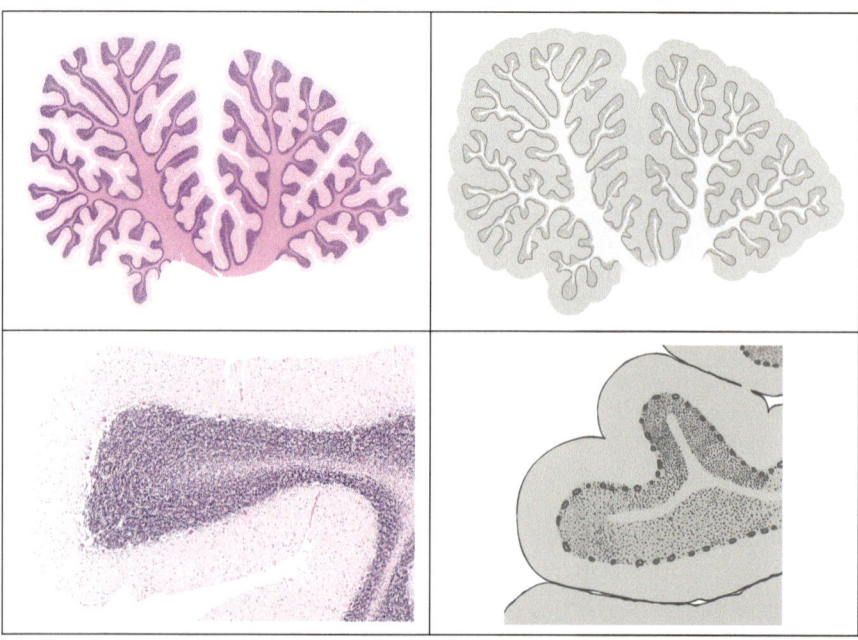

Top left: photomicrograph of cerebellar cortex. Magnification: macroscopic. Stain: HE (Courtesy of professor Jørgen Tranum-Jensen, University of Copenhagen). *Top right*: simplified illustration of the cerebellar cortex. *Bottom left*: photomicrograph of branch of cerebellar cortex. Magnification: Low. Stain: HE (Courtesy of professor Jørgen Tranum-Jensen, University of Copenhagen). *Bottom right*: simplified illustration of branch of cerebellar cortex

Cerebellar cortex

Characteristics

- Macroscopic:
  - ○ Surface is highly folded (resembles a piece of cauliflower)
  - ○ Distinct borders are seen between the superficial eosinophilic layer, the middle basophilic layer, and the central eosinophilic core.
- Microscopic: Each branch of the "cauliflower" consists of:
  - ○ Gray matter (cortex):

- Molecular layer:
  - Thick pale eosinophilic superficial layer
- Purkinje cell layer:
  - A row of large round nerve cell bodies (Purkinje cells)
- Granule cell layer:
  - Thick basophilic layer towards the white matter
  - White matter:
    - Central pale eosinophilic core

Can be mistaken for

Cerebral cortex:
- Surface is less folded.
- Contains two distinct layers macroscopically:
  - A basophilic superficial layer
  - A pale eosinophilic core of white matter

Spinal Cord

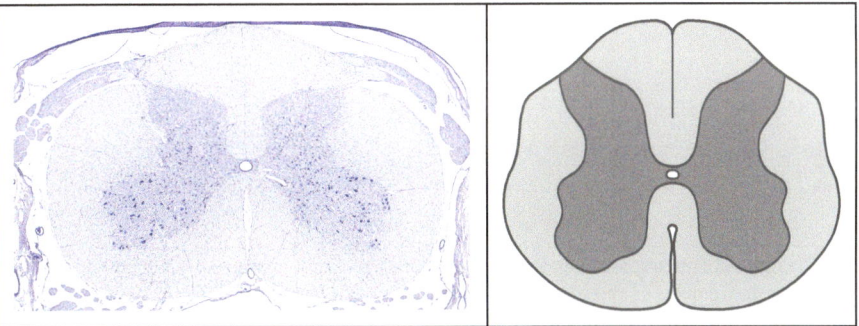

Left: photomicrograph of spinal cord. Magnification: macroscopic. Stain: toluidine blue (Courtesy of professor Jørgen Tranum-Jensen, University of Copenhagen). *Right*: simplified illustration of the spinal cord

Characteristics

Cross section:
- Macroscopic: An oval structure, with a dark butterfly (gray matter) in the center.
- Microscopic:
  - Gray matter contains large nerve cell bodies.
  - A central small white space (central canal), lined with simple cuboidal epithelium (ependymal cells), is seen.

PERIPHERAL NERVOUS SYSTEM

Peripheral Nerve

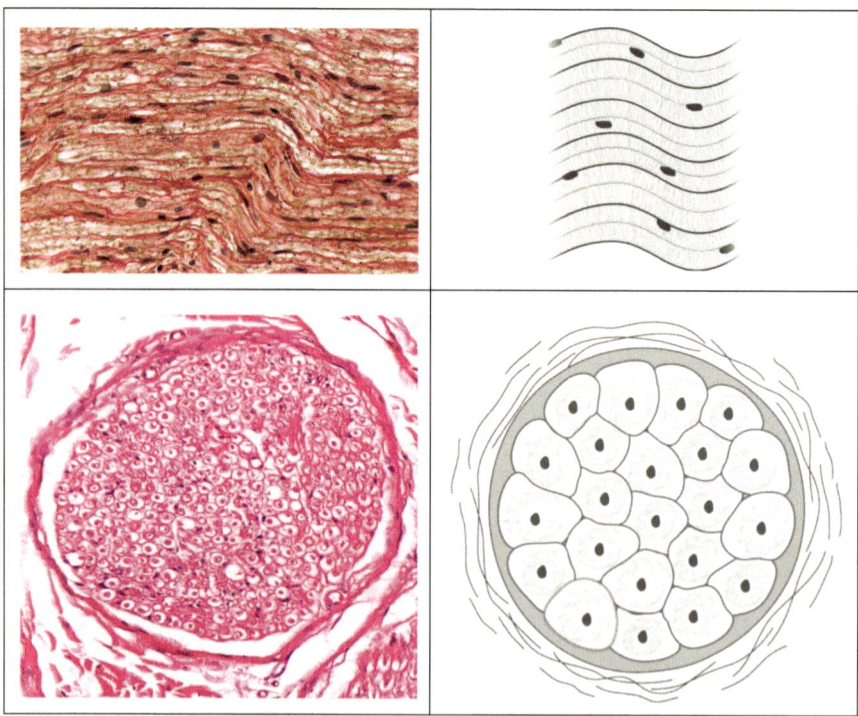

Top left: photomicrograph of longitudinal sectioned peripheral nerve. Magnification: high. Stain: Van Gieson (Courtesy of professor Jørgen Tranum-Jensen, University of Copenhagen). *Top right*: simplified illustration of longitudinal sectioned peripheral nerve. *Bottom left*: photomicrograph of cross sectioned peripheral nerve. Magnification: high. Stain: HE (Courtesy of professor Jørgen Tranum-Jensen, University of Copenhagen). *Bottom right*: simplified illustration of cross sectioned peripheral nerve

Characteristics
- Larger nerves are often seen together with large blood vessels.
- Often both cross, oblique, and longitudinal sections are seen in the same specimen, as the nerve has a wavy path:
  - Longitudinal section:
    - Nerve fibers are highly wavy:
      - Dark lines (axons)
      - Pale, weakly eosinophilic, "cloudy" areas (remnants of myelin sheath) surround the myelinated axons.

- Scattered nuclei of Schwann cells and fibroblasts.
- Dense connective tissue surrounds bundles of nerve fibers as well as the entire nerve.
  - Cross section:
    - With cross sectioned myelinated nerve fibers (resemble eyes):
      - Central dark dot (axon)
      - Pale, weakly eosinophilic, "cloudy" rings (remnants of myelin sheath)
    - Dense connective tissue surrounds the entire nerve and divides the nerve fibers into bundles.
    - Scattered dark nuclei of Schwann cells and fibroblasts.

Special staining
- Van Gieson:
  - Stains collagen fibers of dense connective tissue red
  - Stains remnants of myelin sheath yellow
- Osmium tetroxide:
  - Fixates and stains myelin black/brown.
  - Cross sections of nerve fibers are seen as dark rings (myelin sheaths) surrounding a lighter center (axon).

Can be mistaken for
Longitudinal section:
- Smooth muscle:
  - The smooth muscle fibers:
    - Shorter and less wavy
    - More eosinophilic
    - More densely packed and have indistinct cell borders
  - Nuclei are of similar sizes, in contrast to in nerves, where the nuclei are of the different sizes.

Sensory Ganglia

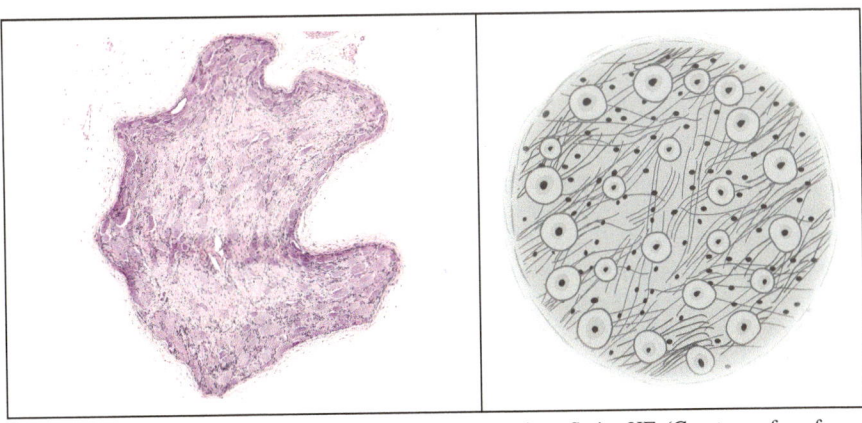

Left: photomicrograph of spinal ganglion. Magnification: low. Stain: HE (Courtesy of professor Jørgen Tranum-Jensen, University of Copenhagen). *Right*: simplified illustration of spinal ganglion

Characteristics
- Surrounded by an eosinophilic capsule of dense connective tissue.
- Nerve cell bodies are larger and more numerous in the periphery of the ganglion:
  - Macroscopic: Seen as a dark area, underneath the eosinophilic capsule.
- Most nerve fibers are seen centrally in ganglion:
  - Macroscopic: Seen as a central light area.
- Nerve cell bodies:
  - Are of different sizes
  - Contain a central nucleus
  - Are surrounded by small cuboidal satellite cells

Can be mistaken for
Autonomic ganglia:
- Nerve cell bodies:
  - Are of more similar size
  - Contain a peripheral nucleus
  - Arranged equally in the whole ganglion

Autonomic Ganglia

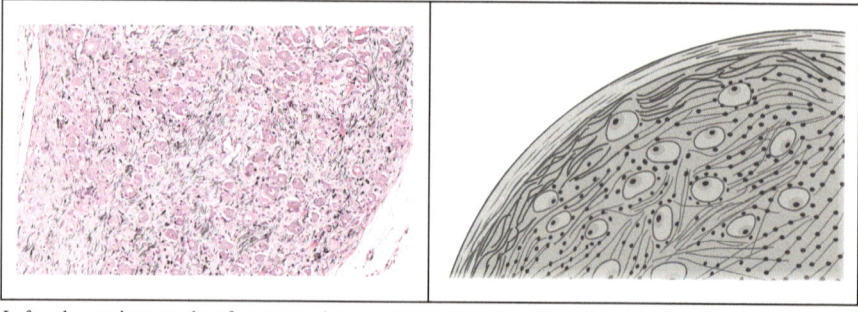

Left: photomicrograph of autonomic ganglion. Magnification: low. Stain: HE (Courtesy of professor Jørgen Tranum-Jensen, University of Copenhagen). *Right*: simplified illustration of autonomic ganglion

Characteristics
- Surrounded by an eosinophilic capsule of dense connective tissue.
  - Some autonomic ganglia are located in the wall of internal organs and lack a capsule.
- Nerve cell bodies:
  - Arranged equally in the whole ganglion
  - Are of relative similar size
  - Contain a peripheral nucleus
  - Surrounded by small cuboidal satellite cells
- Nerve fibers run between nerve cell bodies.

Can be mistaken for

Sensory ganglia:
- Nerve cell bodies:
  - ○ Are larger and more numerous peripherally in ganglion
  - ○ Are of different size
  - ○ Contain a central nucleus

References

5, 10, 11, 18, 22, 25, 33, 34, 40, 45.

Chapter 17
The Cardiovascular System

Contents

General
- Forms two transport systems:
  - The blood vascular system, which transports blood
  - The lymphatic vascular system, which transports lymph
- The pumping action of the heart drives the flow of blood through the blood vascular system.

© Springer International Publishing Switzerland 2017
A. Rehfeld et al., *Compendium of Histology*, DOI 10.1007/978-3-319-41873-5_17

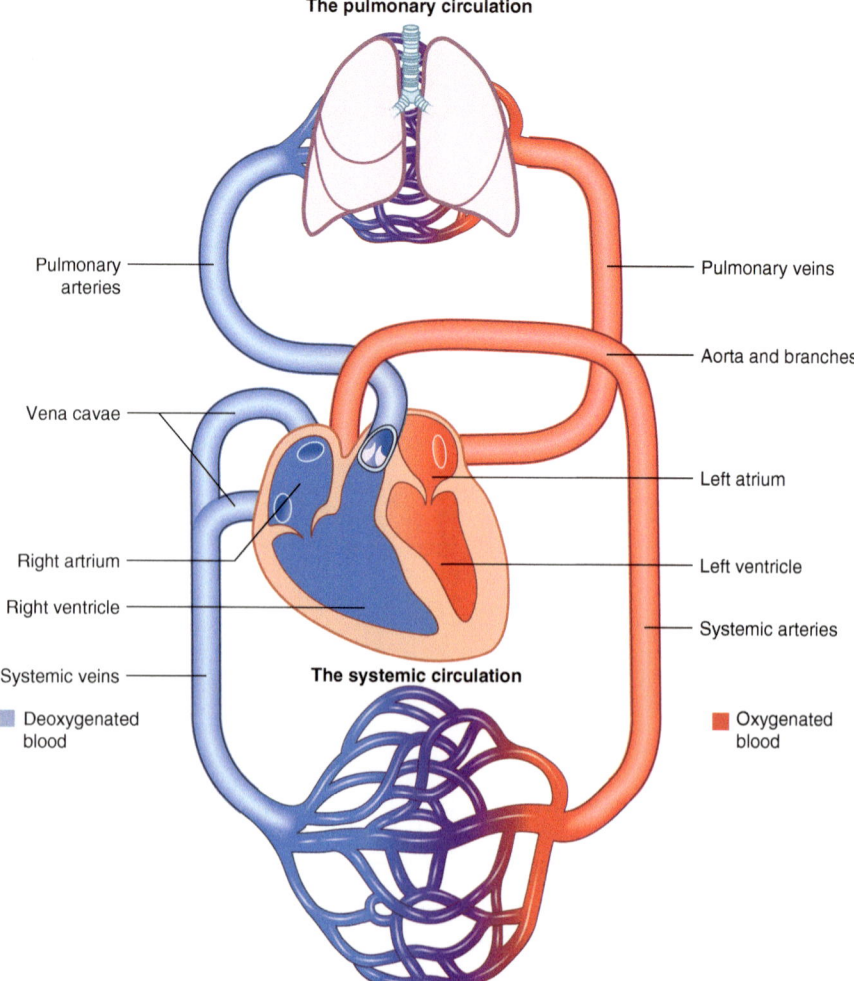

Fig. 17.1 The heart and blood vascular system, showing the systemic and pulmonary circulations, connected by the heart

Function
Transport system:
- Heart and blood vascular system (Fig. 17.1):
    - Transportation of blood between the heart and tissues, within two separate circulations connected by the heart:
        - The systemic circulation
            - The nutritive blood supply of all tissues
            - Transports oxygenated blood from the left ventricle of the heart to tissues

- The pulmonary circulation
  - The functional, non-nutritive, blood supply of the lungs
  - Transports deoxygenated blood from the right ventricle of the heart to the alveolar capillaries of the lungs, where the blood is oxygenated
- Lymphatic vascular system:
  - Transportation of excess fluid from tissues back to the blood
  - Important part of the immune system (Chap. 19)

Consists of
- Heart (cor, cardia)
- Vascular systems:
  - Blood vascular system:
    - Arteries
    - Arterioles
    - Capillaries
    - Venules
    - Veins
  - Lymphatic vascular system:
    - Lymph capillaries
    - Lymphatic vessels
    - Lymphatic ducts

The Heart

Structure
- $6 \times 9 \times 12$ cm, 250–350 g
- Muscular, hollow organ
- Surrounded by the pericardium
- Located to the left in the middle mediastinum

Function
- Pumping blood:
  - The left ventricle pumps oxygenated blood into the systemic circulation.
  - The right ventricle pumps deoxygenated blood into the pulmonary circulation.
- Endocrine secretion:
  - Natriuretic peptides, with blood pressure lowering effect
    - Atrial natriuretic peptide (ANP)
    - Brain natriuretic peptide (BNP)

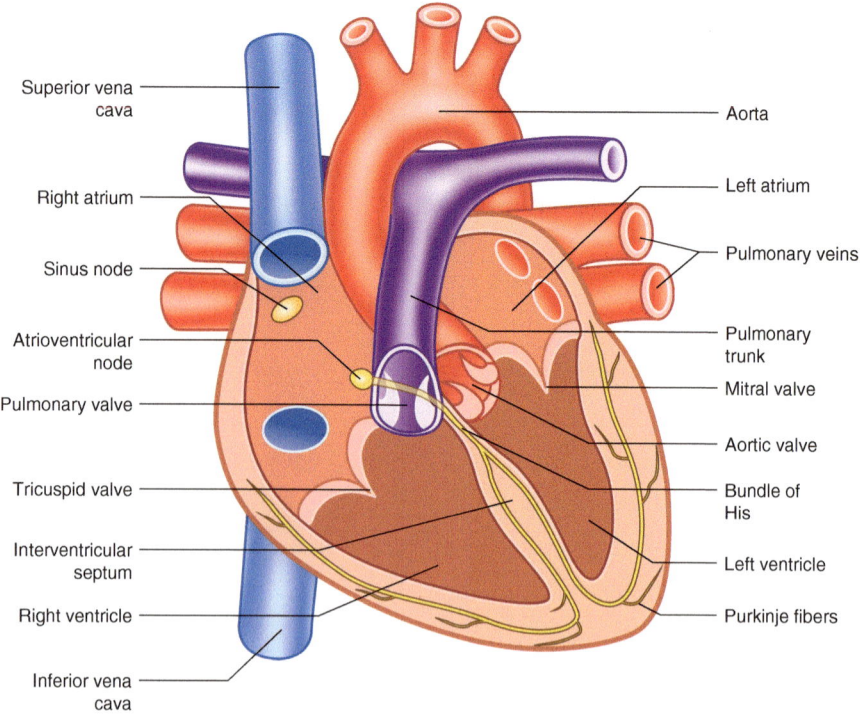

Superior vena cava

Right atrium

Sinus node

Atrioventricular node

Pulmonary valve

Tricuspid valve

Interventricular septum

Right ventricle

Inferior vena cava

Aorta

Left atrium

Pulmonary veins

Pulmonary trunk

Mitral valve

Aortic valve

Bundle of His

Left ventricle

Purkinje fibers

Fig. 17.2 The heart: Divided into four chambers, and containing four valves. The impulse propagating system consists of the SA node, AV node, the bundle of His, and the Purkinje fibers

Divided into (Fig. 17.2)

- Atria
  - Two receiving chambers:
    - Left atrium
    - Right atrium
  - A small conical pouch (auricle) projects from each atrium.
  - The left and right atria are separated by a thin interatrial septum (septum interatriale):
    - The septum consists of a membranous and muscular part.
    - The septum is covered with endothelium on both sides.
- Ventricles
  - Two discharging chambers:
    - Left ventricle
    - Right ventricle
  - The left and right ventricles are separated by a thick interventricular septum (septum interventriculare):
    - The septum consists of a membranous and muscular part
    - The septum is covered with endothelium on both sides

Consists of
- Cardiac muscle
- Connective tissue of the heart
- Conducting system of the heart

THE CARDIAC MUSCLE

General

The wall of the heart and the major parts of the interatrial and interventricular septae are primarily composed of cardiac muscle tissue (Chap. 13).

The Cardiac Wall

Structure
- The layers of the wall are continuous with the layers of the walls of the afferent and efferent blood vessels.
- In the ventricles, papillary muscles project from the wall and into the lumen.

Consists of
- Endocardium
  - The luminal layer of the wall
  - Thicker in the atria than in the ventricles
- Myocardium
  - Thicker in the ventricles than in the atria
  - Thicker in the left ventricle than in the right ventricle
- Epicardium
  - The visceral layer of the serous pericardium

Light Microscopy
- Endocardium
  - Endothelium
    - Simple squamous epithelium: flattened, polygonal cells on a basal lamina
  - Subendothelial layer
    - Thin layer of connective tissue
  - Myoelastic layer
    - Dense connective tissue with elastic fibers and smooth muscle cells
  - Subendocardial layer
    - Loose connective tissue, vessels and nerves
    - Not present in papillary muscles and chordae tendinae
    - Contains the Purkinje fibers
    - Continuous with the connective tissue of the myocardium
- Myocardium
  - Cardiac muscle cells
    - Cylindrical, sometimes branched, cells arranged end-to-end
    - 1-2 light, ovoid nuclei, located centrally
    - Cross-striations
    - Granules in atrial cardiac muscle cells
      - Contain precursors to natriuretic peptides
    - Intercalated discs at cell junctions:
      - Gap junctions that transmit action potentials (depolarizations)
      - Adhering junctions (fascia adherens) and desmosomes that transmit contractile forces.
  - Dense connective tissue
    - With abundant elastic fibers in the atria, and few elastic fibers in the ventricles
    - Abundant blood vessels
- Epicardium
  - Mesothelium
    - Simple squamous epithelium: flattened, polygonal cells on a basal lamina
  - Submesothelial layer
    - Loose connective tissue with vessels, nerves and abundant adipose tissue

CONNECTIVE TISSUE OF THE HEART

Divided into
- Valves
- Chordae tendineae
- Fibrous skeleton (cardiac skeleton)

Valves

Function
Prevent backflow of the blood

Divided into (Fig. 17.2)
- Atrioventricular (AV) valves
  - Located between the atria and ventricles
    - Left side of the heart: Mitral (bicuspid) valve, with two cusps
    - Right side of the heart: Tricuspid valve, with three cusps
- Semilunar valves
  - Located between the ventricles and efferent vessels
    - Left ventricle and ascending aorta: Aortic valve
    - Right ventricle and pulmonary trunk: Pulmonary valve

Light Microscopy
- Core of dense connective tissue
  - Continuous with the connective tissue of the surrounding fibrous rings
- Endothelium covering the core
- Avascular

Chordae Tendineae

Structure
- Fibrous, threadlike strings.
- Extending from the ventricular surface of the AV valves and from the free edge of the AV valves to the papillary muscles.
- Covered with endothelium.

Function
Prevent the AV valves from protruding into the atria as the ventricles contract, i.e., prevents blood from flowing back into the atria.

Fibrous Skeleton

Function
- Provide attachment for:
  - Atrial and ventricular myocardium
  - Valves
- Isolation:
  - Prevents electrical impulses from running freely between atria and ventricles

Consists of
- Four fibrous rings (annuli fibrosi), surrounding the valve openings (orifices)
- Two fibrous trigones, connecting the four fibrous rings
  - Right and left fibrous trigone (trigonum fibrosum dextrum et sinistrum)
- The membranous parts of interventricular and interatrial septae

Light Microscopy
Dense irregular connective tissue

CONDUCTING SYSTEM OF THE HEART

General
Due to gap junctions between cardiac muscle cells, the heart contracts as a unit (syncytium):
1. The atria first empty into the ventricles.
2. The ventricles then empty into the aorta and pulmonary arteries.

Function (Table 17.1)
Initiation and conduction of rhythmic impulses (depolarizations) in the myocardium → rhythmic contractions of the heart.

Consists of (Fig. 17.2)
- Sinoatrial (SA) node
- Atrioventricular (AV) node
- AV bundle (bundle of His), which branches into:
  - Right bundle branch
  - Left bundle branch, which branches into:
    - Anterior fascicle
    - Posterior fascicle
- Purkinje fibers, which branch from the bundles and fascicles.

Light Microscopy
See Table 17.1.

Table 17.1 Conducting system of the heart

	Location	Consists of	Function	Light microscopy
Sinoatrial (SA) node	• Subepicardial • Near the junction of the right atrium and the superior vena cava	Modified cardiac muscle cells, called nodal muscle cells	Pacemaker function: modified cardiac muscle cells of the SA node control the heart rate, since they generate the impulses with the highest frequency	Both the SA node and the AV node consist of nodal muscle cells: • Smaller than the standard cardiac muscle cells • Fewer myofibrils • Fewer and less developed intercalated discs
Atrioventricular (AV) node	• Subendocardial • In the septal wall of the right atrium	Modified cardiac muscle cells, called nodal muscle cells	Deceleration of the impulse from atria to ventricles → allows the atria to empty into the ventricles before the ventricles contract	
AV bundle (bundle of His)	• Bundle of His runs through the right fibrous trigone • The right and left bundle branches run in the interventricular septum	Modified cardiac muscle cells	• Conduction of the impulse from the AV node to the myocardium of the ventricles • The bundle of His is the only muscular connection between the atria and the ventricles	Both the bundle of His and the Purkinje fibers consist of modified cardiac muscle cells: • Thicker and paler than standard cardiac muscle cells • Fewer myofibrils, located peripherally in the cells • Large, spherical nuclei • Abundant glycogen
Purkinje fibers	In the subendocardial layer of the ventricles	• Modified cardiac muscle cells • Are distally connected to standard cardiac muscle cells, to which they transmit the impulses	Conduct the impulse faster than the standard cardiac muscle cells → the impulse quickly reaches the entire ventricular myocardium and the ventricles contracts as a unit	

Regulation of the heart rate

- The cardiac muscle cells have different intrinsic frequencies:
  - ○ Highest in the atria (60–100/min), which controls the heart rate
  - ○ Lowest in the ventricles (30–45/min)
- The intrinsic heart rate, and the force of contraction, is modulated by:
  - ○ The autonomic nervous system
    - ▪ Sympathetic nervous system → increases heart rate (tachycardia) and force of contraction
    - ▪ Parasympathetic nervous system → decreases heart rate (bradycardia) and force of contraction
  - ○ Catecholamines from the adrenal medulla
    - ▪ Epinephrine (adrenaline) and norepinephrine (noradrenaline) → increases the heart rate (tachycardia)
  - ○ The heart rate is also modulated by several other substances, e.g., thyroid hormones.

Impulse propagation pathway

1. SA node
2. Atrial cardiac muscle cells
3. AV node (slows down the impulse)
4. Bundle of His
   - ▪ Right bundle branches
   - ▪ Left bundle branches
     - • Left anterior fascicle
     - • Left posterior fascicle
5. Purkinje fibers
6. Ventricular heart muscle cells.

PERICARDIUM

General

A double-layered sac containing the heart and the roots of the large vessels entering and exiting the heart.

Consists of
- Fibrous pericardium
- Serous pericardium:
  - Parietal layer
    - - Separated by the pericardial cavity - -
  - Visceral layer, i.e., the epicardium

Pericardial cavity

Structure
- A (potential) space between the two layers of the serous pericardium
- Contains a small amount of serous fluid

Function
Enables the heart to contract with minimum friction.

BLOOD SUPPLY OF THE HEART

Structure
- Coronary arteries run in the epicardium and give off smaller branches, which run perpendicular into the myocardium where they form a well-developed capillary network.
- The coronary arteries are functional end arteries, i.e., they do not form functional anastomoses.

Function
Blood supply of the cardiac wall
- During the diastole the myocardium relaxes, allowing blood to fill into the myocardial vessels.

Consists of
- Arteries, originating from ascending aorta:
  - Right coronary artery (RCA)
    → Posterior interventricular artery (PIV, PDA)
  - Left coronary artery (LMS, LCA)
    → Left anterior descending artery (LAD)
    → Left circumflex artery (LCX)
- Veins:
  - Cardiac veins (vv. cordis) → coronary sinus (sinus coronarius) → right atrium.
  - Veins run parallel to the coronary arteries.

RECEPTORS FOR CARDIOVASCULAR REFLEXES

General
- Specialized sensory receptors that supply centers in the brain stem with information on blood pressure, pO_2, pCO_2, and pH.
- Cardiovascular reflexes are important for regulation of cardiac output and respiratory rate.

Consist of
- The carotid sinus (sinus caroticus)
- Carotid and aortic bodies

The Carotid Sinus (Sinus Caroticus)

Structure
- Bilateral baroreceptors in the wall of the initial part of the common carotid arteries (aa. carotides communes).
- Functionally similar receptors are located in the aortic arch.

Function
- Monitors of the arterial blood pressure
- Sends information to vasomotor centers in the brain stem
  - Sensory nerve endings respond to stretching of the vessel wall and send impulses via cranial nerve IX (the glossopharyngeal nerve) to centers in the medulla oblongata.

Consists of
Modified blood vessel wall:
- Tunica media contains less smooth muscle and more elastic fibers.
- Tunica adventitia is thick, rich in elastic fibers, and abundant in sensory nerve endings.

The Carotid Body (Glomus Caroticum)

Structure
- Bilateral chemoreceptors in the bifurcation of the common carotid arteries (aa. carotides communes), on the outer surface of the arteries.
- Functionally similar receptors, called glomus aorticum, are located in the aortic arch.

Function
- Senses the pO_2, pCO_2, and pH of the blood
- Sends information to respiratory and vasomotor centers in the brain stem:
  1. Glomus cells respond to changes in pO_2, pCO_2 and pH of the blood.
  2. Glomus cells release neurotransmitters to the associated nerve fibers.
  3. Impulses travel via cranial nerve IX (the glossopharyngeal nerve) to centers in the medulla oblongata.

Consists of
- Cells
  - Type I: Glomus cells
    - Cords of epitheloid cells with vesicles containing neurotransmitters
    - Derived from the neural crest
  - Type II: Supporting cells
- Nerve fibers
- Capillary network

Blood Vascular System

General
Forms a network of blood vessels between the heart and tissues:
- Arteries originate from the ventricles of the heart and end in capillary beds.
- Veins originate from capillary beds and end in the atria of the heart.

Structure
The wall of blood vessels consist of three tunics (layers) (luminal → peripheral):
- Tunica intima:
  - Endothelium on a basal lamina
  - Subendothelial loose connective tissue
- Tunica media:
  - Circularly arranged smooth muscle cells:
    - The only cell type in the layer
    - Produce the extracellular components of tunica media
  - Ground substance with collagen and elastic fibers
- Tunica adventitia:
  - Loose connective tissue with collagen and elastic fibers
    - Merges with the surrounding connective tissue
  - In large vessels, the tunica adventitia contains:
    - Blood and lymph vessels (vasa vasorum)
    - Nerves (nervi vasorum)

Divided into
Can be devided anatomically and functionally into parts.

Anatomically divided into

- Macrovascular system:
  - Arteries
  - Veins
- Microvascular system:
  - Arterioles
  - Capillaries
  - Venules

Functionally divided into

Two separate circulations connected by the heart:
- The systemic circulation
- The pulmonary circulation
  - Have a thinner wall, due to lower blood pressure here

MEMO-BOX
The layers of the blood vessel wall are remembered by **A**cute **M**yocardial **I**nfarct (**AMI**):
- Tunica **A**dventitia
- Tunica **M**edia: The **M**iddle layer → the smooth **M**uscle cell is the only cell type here.
- Tunica **I**ntima: The "**I**ntimate" layer, closest to lumen.

ARTERIAL PART OF THE BLOOD VASCULAR SYSTEM

Arteries and Arterioles

General
- The blood vessels between the ventricles of the heart and the capillary beds
- Have thick walls, since they conduct blood at a high pressure

Structure
- Arterial wall:
  - Thick, compared to the wall of veins.
  - An internal and external elastic membrane distinctly separates the three tunics of the wall.
  - Gets gradually thinner and changes in composition, as the larger arteries branch into smaller arteries:
    - Relatively less elastic components
    - Relatively more smooth muscle tissue
- Arteriolar wall:
  - Only 1–2 layers of smooth muscle cells in tunica media.

Function
- Distribution of blood
- Regulation of blood pressure:
  - Affected by the degree of the constriction of the blood vessels, which is regulated by:
    - Sympathetic nerve fibers → vasoconstriction
    - Hormones and local mediators → vasoconstriction or vasodilation.

Divided into (Table 17.2)
- Arteries
  - Large arteries (elastic arteries)
    - The largest arteries, e.g., aorta
  - Medium arteries (muscular arteries)
    - Most of the named arteries are of this type, e.g., the radial artery.
    - Have a thick wall compared to the luminal ⊘.
  - Small arteries
    - The branches of the medium arteries, e.g., the common digital arteries.
- Arterioles:
  - The smallest branches of the arterial system
  - Capillaries originate from both:
    - Arterioles
    - Metarterioles, which are the terminal branches of arterioles.

Table 17.2 Overview of arteries and arterioles

	Large arteries	Medium arteries	Small arteries	Arterioles
Luminal ⌀	>10 mm	10–2 mm	2–0,1 mm	100–10 μm
Tunica intima	Endothelium with tight junctions			
	Basal lamina			
	Subendothelial loose connective tissue with smooth muscle cells	Subendothelial loose connective tissue (thin layer)	–	
• Thickness of tunica intima	Thick	Thin		
Internal elastic membrane	+ The innermost elastic lamina of tunica media	+ Distinct and wavy	+	±
Tunica media	Multiple layers of smooth muscle cells	>10 layers of smooth muscle cells	3–10 layers of smooth muscle cells	1–2 layers of smooth muscle cells
	Ground substance with: • Multiple concentric, fenestrated elastic lamellae • Collagen fibers • Elastic fibers	Ground substance with: • Collagen fibers • Elastic fibers		
• Thickness of tunica media	Thick			Thin
External elastic membrane	+ The outermost elastic lamina of tunica media	+	±	–
Tunica adventitia	Loose connective tissue with: • Collagen fibers • Elastic fibers • Blood and lymph vessels (vasa vasorum) 　○ Only in arteries with a luminal ⌀ ≥ 0.5 mm • Nerves (nervi vasorum)			Loose connective tissue
• Thickness of tunica adventitia	Thin, <½ the thickness of tunica media	Thick, approximately as thick as tunica media		Very thin

(continued)

Table 17.2 (continued)

	Large arteries	Medium arteries	Small arteries	Arterioles

Blood supply	• Tunica intima and the inner half of media are nourished from the lumen
	  ○ Diffusion is facilitated by the fenestrations of the elastic lamellae
	• Outer half of media and adventitia are nourished from the blood vessels of adventitia
		• Arteries with a luminal ◌≥0.5 mm:
		  ○ Tunica intima and inner half of media are nourished from the lumen
		  ○ Outer half of media and adventitia are nourished from the blood vessels of adventitia
		• Arteries with a luminal ◌<0.5 mm:
		  ○ All layers are nourished from lumen
				All layers are nourished from lumen

Function	Are called "windkessel" vessels as they: • Diminish fluctuations in blood pressure → uniform blood flow ○ Takes place as elastic components distend during high pressure (systole) and recoil during lower pressure (diastole)	Are called distribution vessels as they: • Regulate the blood flow to tissues		Are called resistance vessels as they: • Maintain/regulate systemic blood pressure • Reduce local blood pressure, before blood enters capillary beds • Regulate blood flow to capillary beds

Metarterioles

General
• Small, terminal branches of the arterioles
• End directly in the postcapillary venules.

Structure (Fig. 17.3)
• Without an internal elastic membrane.
• The distal part of metarteriole lacks smooth muscle and is called a "thoroughfare channel."
• Multiple capillaries originate from metarteriole, surrounded by precapillary sphincters.

Function (Fig. 17.3)
Act as thoroughfare channels:
• Constriction of the associated precapillary sphincters:
  ○ Blood bypasses the capillary bed and flows directly to the postcapillary venule.

CAPILLARIES

General
- The smallest branches of the vascular system
- Form anastomosing networks (capillary beds) in tissues
  - The blood flow to a capillary bed is regulated by the degree of constriction in:
    - Precapillary sphincters
    - Arterioles and metarterioles
    - Capillaries of the capillary bed (via pericyte contraction, see below)
- Originate from arterioles and metarterioles, surrounded by precapillary sphincters
- Are called exchange vessels, together with the postcapillary venules.

Structure
- Luminal ⊘ 4–10 μm
- Thin wall, only consisting of a tunica intima:
  - Endothelium
  - Basal lamina
  - Pericytes, enclosed within the basal lamina

Divided into (Table 17.3)
- Continuous capillaries
- Fenestrated capillaries
- Discontinuous capillaries (sinusoids)

Function
- Exchange of:
  - Solutes between blood and tissues, e.g., O_2, nutrients, and hormones
  - Fluid (blood filtrate) between blood and tissues
    - The amount of fluid exchanged depends on capillary type and amount of tight junctions between endothelial cells.
    - The fluid exchange primarily takes place in the direction from blood to tissues.
- Some capillaries have specialized functions, e.g., filtration of erythrocytes in the sinusoids of the spleen (Chap. 19).

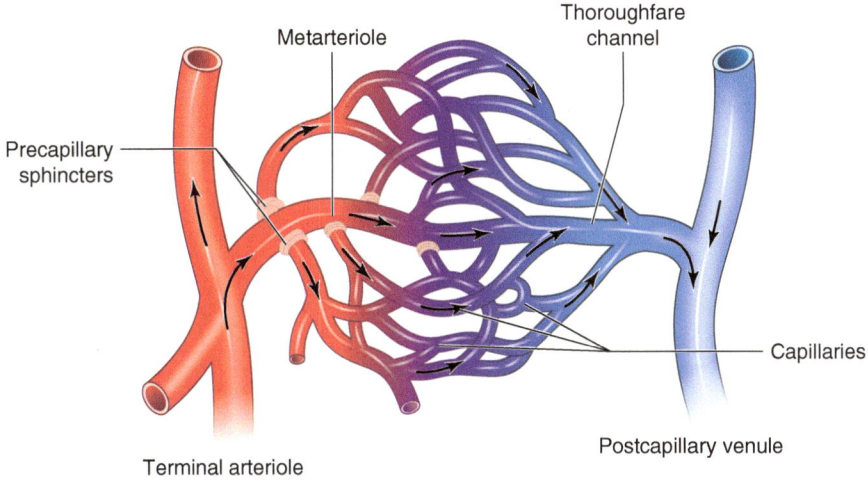

Precapillary sphincters open

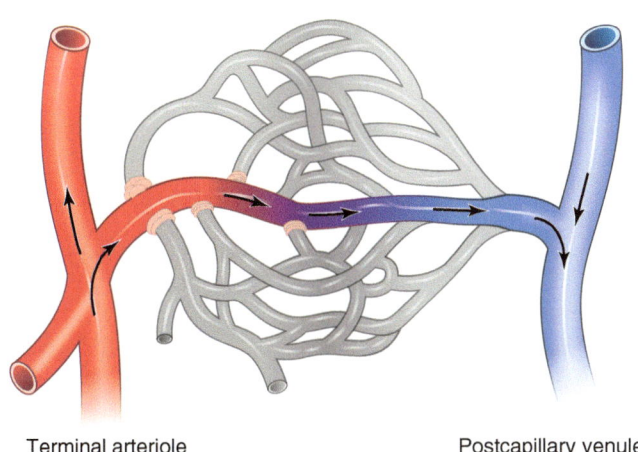

Precapillary sphincters closed

Fig. 17.3 A capillary bed. Top part shows the blood flow, when precapillary sphincters are open. Bottom part shows the blood flow, when precapillary sphincters are closed, and blood is shunted through the metarteriole

Facilitation of exchange in capillaries

Exchange in capillaries is facilitated by:
- The thin capillary wall → short diffusion distance between blood and tissues.
- Narrow luminal ⊘ → short diffusion distance for O_2 and CO_2 between erythrocytes and capillary wall.
- The increased permeability of fenestrated and discontinuous capillaries.

Pericytes

General
- Cells surrounding the endothelium of capillaries and postcapillary venules
- Scattered along the vessel wall
- Enclosed within the basal lamina of the endothelium.

Structure
- Flattened cell
- Large dark nucleus
- Cell extensions branch and wrap around the endothelium

Function
- Mesenchymal multipotent stem cell, giving rise to, e.g., endothelial cells and smooth muscle cells during wound healing.
- Contractile cell → regulate capillary blood flow
- Provide structural support for capillaries and postcapillary venules

Table 17.3 Capillary types

	Continuous capillaries	Fenestrated capillaries	Discontinuous capillaries (sinusoids)
Luminal ⊘	4–10 µm	4–10 µm	Irregular: • Up to 40 µm • Fills out spaces between cellular cords
Endothelium	• 0.2 µm thick • Multiple invaginations and vesicles, ⊘ 70 nm (a sign of active transcytosis)	• 0.2 µm thick • Flattened areas, 0.1 µm thick, with 70 nm fenestrations (formed when vesicles simultaneously fuse with both surfaces) • A diaphragm of glycocalyx covers each fenestration	• 0.2 µm thick • Large fenestrations without diaphragms • Gaps between the endothelial cells
Basal lamina	Continuous	Continuous	Discontinuous/absent
Tight junctions	+	+	−
Location	Most common type, e.g., in muscle tissue	For example, found in endocrine tissue	Only in: • Liver • Spleen • Bone marrow

MEMO-BOX
- **CONTINUOUS** capillaries: only capillary type with a **CONTINUOUS** wall, i.e., lacking fenestrations and gaps.
- **DISCONTINOUS** capillaries: have a **DISCONTINOUS**/absent basal lamina

VENOUS PART OF THE BLOOD VASCULAR SYSTEM

Postcapillary Venules

General
- The smallest branches of the venous system.
- Drain blood from the capillary beds.
- Similar in structure and function to capillaries.
- Are called exchange vessels, together with capillaries.

Structure
- Luminal ⌀ 10–50 μm
- Thin wall, only consisting of a tunica intima:
  - Endothelium with loosely arranged tight junctions → easy passage for fluid
  - Basal lamina
  - Pericytes, enclosed within the basal lamina
- Special high endothelial venules (HEV) with cuboidal endothelium are found in lymph nodes (Chap. 19).

Function
- Exchange (similar to capillaries):
  - The fluid exchange primarily takes place in the direction from tissues to blood.
  - Facilitated by:
    - The loosely arranged tight junctions between the endothelial cells
    - The lower intravascular pressure as compared to in the capillaries
- Site of leukocyte migration out of the blood and into tissues (Chap. 7).

Veins and Muscular Venules

General
- The blood vessels between postcapillary venules and the atria of the heart.
- Have thin walls, since they conduct blood at a low pressure.
- Valves are found in muscular venules, small veins, and medium veins, which transport blood against gravity, e.g., those of the limbs.
- The venous blood flow is enhanced by:
  - Skeletal muscle pump:
    - Contraction of skeletal muscles in limbs force venous blood in adjacent veins towards the heart, as valves block retrograde flow.
  - Respiratory pump:
    - Contraction of diaphragm during respiration generates pressure changes in the thorax and abdomen, which facilitate venous blood flow towards the heart.

Structure
- Wall of muscular venules:
  - Only 1–2 layers of smooth muscle cells in tunica media.
- Wall of veins:
  - Thin, compared to the walls of arteries.
  - The tunics of the venous wall are not distinctly separated since the internal and external elastic membranes are absent/less defined.
  - Contains more connective tissue and less smooth muscle than in arteries.
  - Gradually thickens and changes composition, as the smaller veins converge into larger veins.

Function
- Transport of blood towards the heart
- Contain about 60 % of the total blood volume, which is why they are called capacitance vessels:
  - Innervated by sympathetic nerve fibers: Increased sympathetic activity → vasoconstriction → reduces capacity, e.g. during blood loss.

Divided into (Table 17.4)
- Muscular venules
- Veins
  - Small veins
  - Medium veins:
    - Most named veins are of this type, e.g., the median cubital vein
  - Large veins:
    - The largest veins, e.g., the superior vena cava

Light Microscopy
- The lumen is large and due to the thin wall often collapsed in specimens.
- Medium veins are often found adjacent to a medium artery.

Valves

General
- Found in muscular venules, small veins, and medium veins, which transport blood against gravity, e.g., those of the limbs.
- Lack in the veins of the thorax, abdomen, spinal canal, and brain.

Table 17.4 Overview of veins and muscular venules

	Muscular venules	Small veins	Medium veins	Large veins
Luminal ⊘	50–100 µm	0.1–1 mm	1–10 mm	>10 mm
Tunica intima	Endothelium with tight junctions			
	Basal lamina			
	–		Subendothelial loose connective tissue (thin layer) with few smooth muscle cells	Subendothelial loose connective tissue (thick layer) with few smooth muscle cells
• Thickness of tunica intima	Thin			Thick
Tunica media	1–2 layers of smooth muscle cells	2–3 layers of smooth muscle cells	3–5 layers of smooth muscle cells	3–15 layers of smooth muscle cells
	Ground substance with: • Collagen fibers • Elastic fibers			
• Thickness of tunica media	Thin			
Tunica adventitia	Loose connective tissue with: • Collagen fibers • Elastic fibers			Loose connective tissue with: • Collagen fibers • Elastic fibers • Longitudinally arranged bundles of smooth muscle cells • Blood and lymph vessels (vasa vasorum) • Nerves (nervi vasorum)
• Thickness of tunica adventitia	Thick			Very thick (several times the thickness of tunica media)
Valves	• In blood vessels, which transport blood against gravity, e.g., those of the limbs • Prevent retrograde flow of blood in these blood vessels			-
Function	Collect blood from postcapillary venules and transport it to small veins	Transport blood to medium veins	Transport blood to larger veins	Return blood to the atria of the heart
	Capacitance vessels: Contain about 60 % of the total blood volume			

Structure
Folds of tunica intima, with a connective tissue core:
- Free border of fold:
  - Projects into the lumen
  - Points in the direction of the blood flow (towards the heart)
- Located pairwise across to each other in the vessel wall (bicuspid valves)

Function
- Restrict retrograde flow of blood.
- Act in cooperation with the skeletal muscle pump, to enhance venous blood flow.

Consist of
- Pocket-shaped folds of tunica intima
- Thin core of connective tissue

ENDOTHELIUM

General
Innermost lining of blood and lymph vessels.

Function
- Forms a selective permeability barrier (see below)
- Regulates blood flow and vascular resistance (see below)
- Regulates hemostasis (see below)
- Endocrine function:
  - Secrete various growth factors.
- Regulate immune response:
  - Express adhesion molecules, used when leucocytes migrate out of blood vessels and into tissues (Chap. 7).
  - Secrete various interleukins.

Light Microscopy
- Simple squamous epithelium
- Endothelial cells:
  - Flat and polygonal
  - Elongated in the direction of the blood flow.

The selective permeability barrier of endothelium

Divided into

Permeability of endothelium depends on the type of molecule:
- Permeable to:
  - Fat-soluble molecules
  - Small, uncharged water-soluble molecules

  ⎱ Transverse the plasma membrane by simple diffusion

- Selectively permeable to:
  - Large water-soluble molecules
  - Charged water-soluble molecules

  ⎱ Can only cross the endothelium via paracellular and transcellular pathway

Function

Large or charged water-soluble molecules can only cross endothelium via:
- Paracellular pathway:
  - Regulated by tight junctions
  - Transport of, e.g., H_2O
- Transcellular pathway, using:
  - Channel proteins
    - Transport of, e.g., ions
  - Carrier proteins
    - Transport of, e.g., glucose
  - Pinocytotic vesicles
    - Transport of fluid (plasma) with solutes
  - Receptor-mediated endocytosis
    - Transport of, e.g., insulin.

The regulatory role of endothelium on blood flow and blood pressure

Endothelium regulates blood flow and vascular resistance → regulate systemic and local blood pressure:
- Secretes substances, acting on the smooth muscle of the blood vessel wall:
  - Vasodilators, e.g., NO
  - Vasoconstrictors, e.g., endothelins
- Secretion is regulated by, e.g.:
  - Mechanoreceptors, affected by blood flow and pressure
  - Chemoreceptors, affected by the blood content of O_2 and CO_2.

The regulatory role of endothelium on hemostasis

Endothelium takes part in the regulation of hemostasis (Chap. 12):
- Maintain a barrier between platelets of the blood and the subendothelial connective tissue → prevent platelet plug formation

- Secretion of:
  - Anticoagulants: inhibit coagulation
  - Antithrombogenic agents: inhibit platelet aggregation
  - Prothrombogenic agents:
    - Stimulate platelet aggregation.
    - Secretion is induced by, e.g., damage to endothelium.

VASCULAR SPECIALIZATIONS

Consist of
- Portal systems
- Arteriovenous anastomoses

Portal Systems

Structure
Blood vessels (veins or arterioles) interposed between two capillary beds.

Consists of
- Venous portal systems
  - The hepatic portal system (v. portae hepatis) (Chap. 22)
  - The hypophyseal portal system (Chap. 24)
- Arterial portal system
  - The efferent arterioles of the kidneys (Chap. 23)

Arteriovenous Anastomoses (Arteriovenous Shunts)

General
- A direct connection between an arteriole and a venule, bypassing the capillary bed.
- Found numerously in the skin (called glomus bodies), e.g., of the fingers, toes, ears, and nose, as well as in the erectile tissue of the penis and clitoris.
- The smooth muscle tissue in the wall of the arteriole regulates the blood flow through the anastomose:
  - Relaxation of the smooth muscle tissue → blood bypasses the capillary bed and flows directly to a venule.
  - Contraction of the smooth muscle tissue → blood flows through the capillary bed.
    - In contrast, contraction of ordinary arterioles decreases blood flow to the capillary bed.

Function

Regulation of blood flow, taking part in, e.g.:
- Thermoregulation:
  - Blood bypassing the capillary beds of the skin conserves heat.
  - Blood flowing through the capillary beds of the skin dissipates heat.
- Erection:
  - Closing the arteriovenous shunt leads blood into the cavernous tissue → erection.

Consist of
- Arteriole
  - Often coiled
  - Tunica media contains a thick layer of smooth muscle tissue
  - Surrounded by a connective tissue capsule
  - Richly innervated
- Venule

Lymphatic Vascular System

General
- Component of the immune system (Chap. 19)
- Pathway of lymph from intercellular space:
  1. Lymph capillaries
  2. Afferent lymphatic vessels
  3. Lymph nodes
  4. Efferent lymphatic vessels
  5. Thoracic duct/right lymphatic duct
  6. Large veins at the base of the neck

Function
- Drainage of excess fluid (2–3 l/day) from the intercellular space:
  - Transports the fluid (lymph) back to the blood.
  - The flow of lymph is driven by compression from adjacent skeletal muscles.
- Transportation of solutes and cells to the blood, e.g.:
  - From the secondary lymphoid organs:
    - Lymphocytes and immunoglobulins
  - From the small intestine:
    - Absorbed cholesterol and fatty acids (chyle)
  - From the intercellular space in general:
    - Plasma proteins lost with the blood filtrate in capillaries and postcapillary venules

Lymph Capillaries

General
- Originate as blind-ended vessels in the intercellular space.
- Found in:
  ○ Most tissues with blood vessels
  ○ Numerous in the dermis of the skin, lamina propria of mucous membranes, and underneath serous membranes, e.g., pleura
- Lack in:
  ○ Tissues without blood vessels, e.g.:
    ▪ Cartilage
  ○ Some tissues with blood vessels, e.g.:
    ▪ Bone tissue, bone marrow, and the inner ear

Structure
- Larger than blood capillaries, with a luminal ⌀ up to 100 μm.
- Thin, highly permeable wall, consisting of:
  ○ Endothelium without tight junctions → easy passage for fluid
  ○ Discontinuous basal lamina → easy passage for fluid
- Anchoring filaments between the basal lamina of the endothelium to the surrounding collagen fibers → keep the lymph capillaries open, even during high pressure in the surrounding tissue.

Function
Drainage of fluid with cells and solutes, from intercellular space.

Lymphatic Vessels

Structure
- Similar to small veins:
  ○ Thinner walls, than the small veins.
  ○ Contain valves:
    ▪ Resemble those of veins.
    ▪ More numerous than in veins.
- Pass through lymph nodes:
  ○ Several afferent lymphatic vessels
    ↓
  ○ Lymph node
    ↓
  ○ One efferent lymphatic vessel

Function
- Transport lymph to the lymphatic ducts
- Contractions of the smooth muscle tissue in the wall → peristaltic movements, which aid the transport

Lymphatic Ducts

General
Formed as the efferent lymphatic vessels converge

Structure
Similar to medium veins:
- Smooth muscle in both circular and longitudinal layers in tunica media.
- The thoracic duct contains valves.

Function
Return lymph to the blood vascular system:
- Empty into the large veins at the root of the neck, at the junctions between the internal jugular veins and the subclavian veins.

Divided into
- Thoracic duct
- Right lymphatic duct

Guide to Practical Histology: The Cardiovascular System

THE HEART

General
The only organ that contains cardiac muscle tissue

Atrial and Ventricular Wall

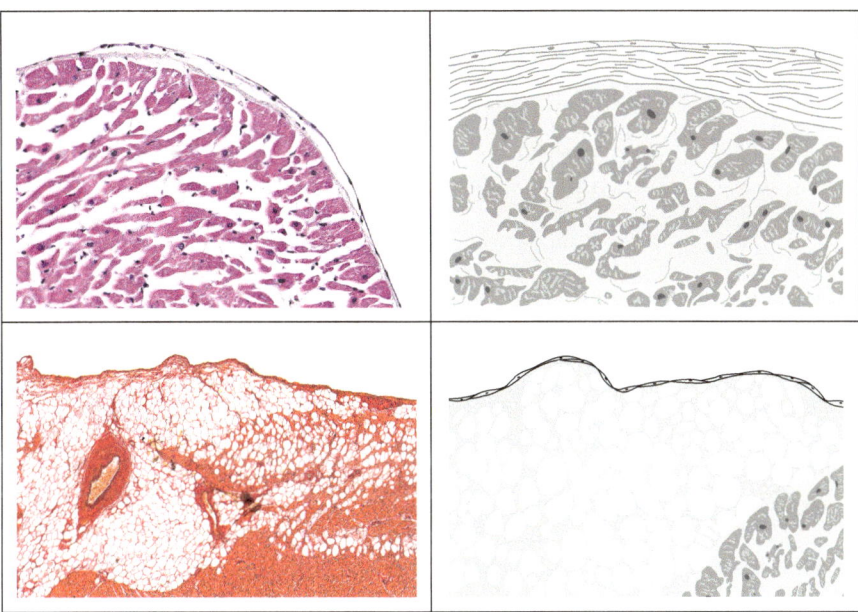

Top panel, left: photomicrograph of the luminal part of the cardiac wall. Magnification: low. Stain: HE. (Courtesy of associate professor Steen Seier Poulsen, University of Copenhagen). *Top panel, right*: simplified illustration of the luminal part of the cardiac wall. *Bottom panel, left*: photomicrograph of the visceral pericardium. Magnification: low. Stain: Sirius Red. (Courtesy of associate professor Steen Seier Poulsen, University of Copenhagen). *Bottom panel, right*: Simplified illustration of the visceral pericardium

Characteristics

Luminal → superficial:

- Endocardium: endothelium on a layer of dense connective tissue
- Myocardium:
  - Cardiac muscle tissue
  - Dense connective tissue and numerous capillaries
- Epicardium:
  - Loose connective tissue containing adipose tissue, blood vessels, and nerves
  - Simple squamous epithelium (mesothelium)

Can be mistaken for

Interatrial and interventricular septae:

- Endocardium on both sides
- Lack the epicardium

Interatrial and Interventricular Septae

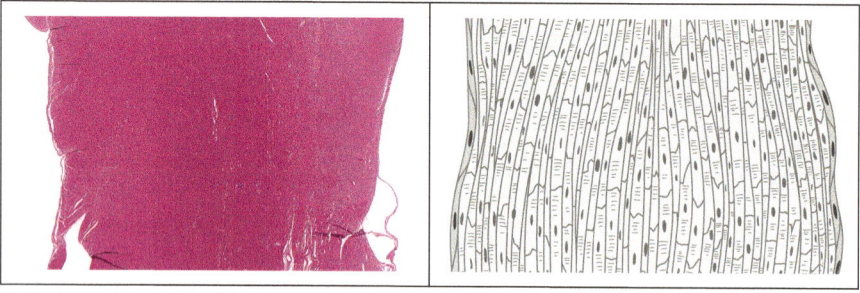

Left: photomicrograph of the interventricular septum. Magnification: low. Stain: HE (Courtesy of associate professor Steen Seier Poulsen, University of Copenhagen). *Right*: simplified illustration of the interventricular septum

Characteristics
- A core of myocardium:
  - ◦ Cardiac muscle tissue, dense connective tissue, and numerous capillaries.
- Both sides are covered with endothelium resting on a layer of dense connective tissue (endocardium).

Can be mistaken for
Atrial and ventricular wall:
- Endocardium only seen on one side of the myocardium
- Visceral epicardium, with adipose tissue seen on the other side

Cardiac Valves

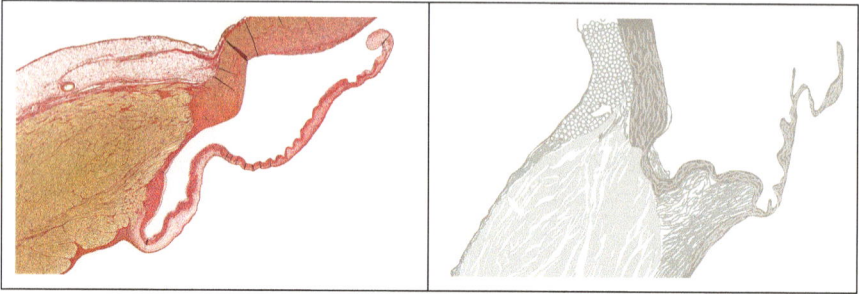

Left: photomicrograph of the aortic orifice, the aortic wall above, right, the aortic valve to the right, and the ventricular wall on the bottom, left. Magnification: low. Stain: Sirius Red (Courtesy of associate professor Steen Seier Poulsen, University of Copenhagen). *Right*: simplified illustration of the semilunar valve

Characteristics
- A core of dense connective tissue, covered with endothelium
- With relation to the myocardium:
  - Cardiac muscle tissue, dense connective tissue, and numerous capillaries

Divided into
- Atrioventricular valves:
  - Seen in relation to the fibrocartilage of the fibrous trigonum
- Aortic and pulmonary valves:
  - Seen in relation to an elastic artery wall (aorta or pulmonal trunk)

ARTERIES

General
- Have a thick wall compared to the ⊘ of their lumen
- Keep a circular shape in cross section after preparation, in contrast to veins, which have thinner walls and are often collapsed.

Large (Elastic) Artery

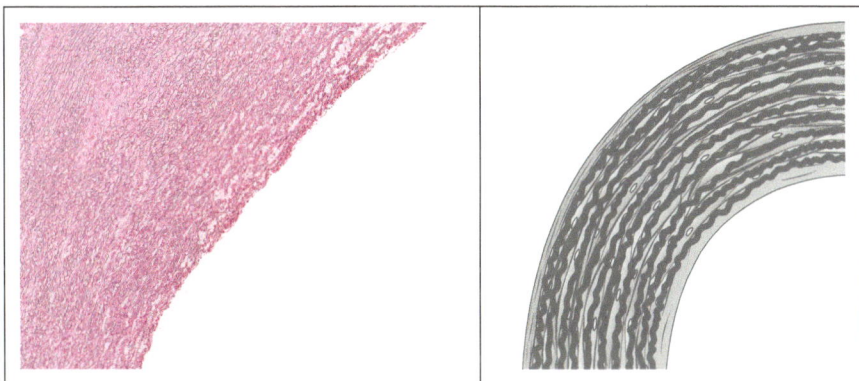

Left: photomicrograph of large artery. Magnification: low. Stain: HE (Courtesy of professor Jørgen Tranum-Jensen, University of Copenhagen). *Right*: simplified illustration of large artery

Characteristics
- Macroscopic:
  - A part of, or a whole ring-shaped structure
- Microscopic:
  - Innermost layer is smooth.
  - The wall contains multiple thick, wavy concentric elastic lamellae.
    - The elastic fibers are strongly refractive and "flash" when focusing in and out of the focal plane.

Special Staining
- Orcein: Elastic fibers are stained red/brown and lose their refractive properties.
- Weigert's (resorcin–fuchsin): Elastic fibers are stained blue/black and lose their refractive properties.

Medium (Muscular) Artery

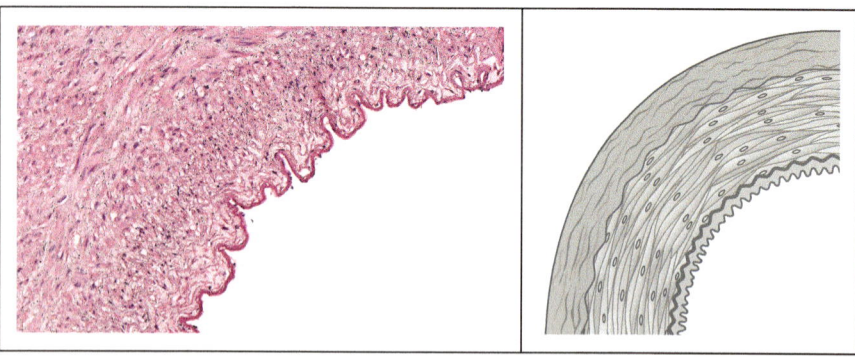

Left: photomicrograph of medium artery. Magnification: low. Stain: HE (Courtesy of professor Jørgen Tranum-Jensen, University of Copenhagen). *Right*: simplified illustration of medium artery

Characteristics
- Macroscopic:
  - A ring-shaped structure
  - Often seen together with one to two collapsed ring-shaped structures (veins)
- Microscopic:
  - Innermost layer is highly wavy.
  - Just below endothelium, a single, highly wavy, strongly refractive elastic membrane is seen.
  - More profoundly, smooth muscle tissue is seen.

Arterioles

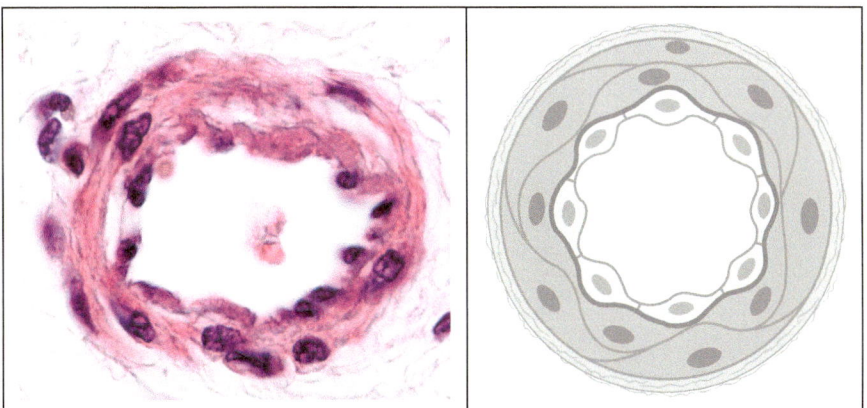

Left: photomicrograph of arteriole. Magnification: high. Stain: HE (Courtesy of professor Jørgen Tranum-Jensen, University of Copenhagen). *Right*: simplified illustration of arteriole

Characteristics
- A single, highly wavy, strongly refractive elastic membrane is normally seen below the endothelium.
- More profound, 1–2 layers of smooth muscle cells are seen.

Can be mistaken for
Muscular venules:
- Do not have an elastic membrane below endothelium
- Contain a thicker layer of surrounding connective tissue (tunica adventitia)

CAPILLARIES

Continuous and Fenestrated Capillaries

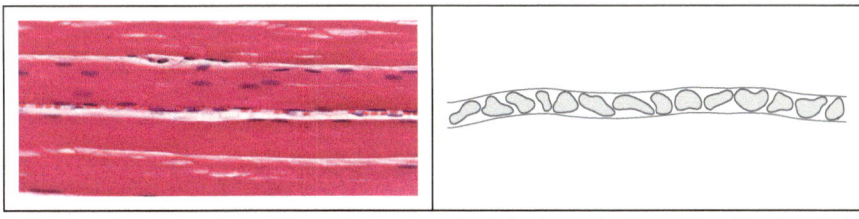

Left: photomicrograph of a capillary of constant ⊘ in skeletal muscle tissue. Magnification: high. Stain: HE (Courtesy of professor Jørgen Tranum-Jensen, University of Copenhagen). *Right*: simplified illustration of constant ⊘

Characteristics
- Narrow white spaces of constant ⊘
- Contain multiple eosinophilic erythrocytes

Discontinuous Capillaries (Sinusoids)

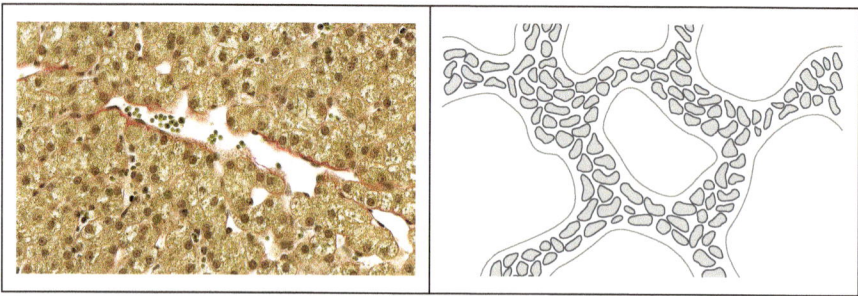

Left: photomicrograph of a sinusoid of the liver. Magnification: high. Stain: Sirius Red (Courtesy of associate professor Steen Seier Poulsen, University of Copenhagen). *Right*: simplified illustration of a sinusoid

Characteristics
- White spaces of varying ⊘
- Contain multiple eosinophilic erythrocytes
- Only found in the liver, spleen, and bone marrow

References

4, 5, 9, 14, 25, 27, 30, 33, 34, 38, 42, 45.

Chapter 18
The Respiratory System

Contents

General
- Anatomically divided into:
  - Upper respiratory tract
  - Lower respiratory tract
- Functionally divided into:
  - Conductive part (airways)
  - Respiratory part
  - Ventilation mechanism

© Springer International Publishing Switzerland 2017
A. Rehfeld et al., *Compendium of Histology*, DOI 10.1007/978-3-319-41873-5_18

Function
- Conduction of air, from the external environment to the sites of gas exchange
- Ventilation of air
- Filtration, warming, and humidification of the inhaled air
- Gas exchange, respiration:
  - Oxygen (O_2) from air to blood
  - Carbon dioxide (CO_2) from blood to air
    - CO_2 plays a role in the regulation of the pH homeostasis (bicarbonate buffer system), together with the kidneys.
- Sense of smell (olfaction) in the nasal cavities
- Production of sounds (speech) in the larynx and upper respiratory tract

Functionally divided into

- Conductive part:
  - Upper respiratory tract
    - Nasal cavities (cavum nasi)
    - Paranasal sinuses (sinus paranasales)
    - Nasopharynx
    - Oral cavity (cavum oris)
    - Oropharynx
    - Laryngopharynx
  - Lower respiratory tract
    - Larynx
    - Trachea
    - Bronchi
    - Bronchioles ($\rightarrow$ terminal bronchioles) ⎤
- Respiratory part: ⎬— Lungs (Pulmones)
    - Respiratory bronchioles
    - Alveolar ducts (ducti alveolares)
    - Alveoli   ⎦
- Ventilating mechanism
  - Elastic tissue of the lungs
  - Bones and cartilage of the thoracic cage
  - Skeletal muscles
    - Diaphragm (m. diaphragma)
    - Intercostal muscles (mm. intercostales)
    - Accessory respiratory muscles

Respiratory Epithelium

General
- Lines the conductive part of the respiratory system
- Exceptions are:
  - The nasal vestibule
  - The olfactory region
  - The oral cavity and the oropharynx
  - Few areas in the larynx, e.g., the vocal cords

Consists of
- Ciliated, pseudostratified columnar epithelium
- Six cell types:
  - Ciliated cells
  - Goblet cells
  - Brush cells
  - Small granule cells (Kulchitsky cells)
  - Basal cells
  - Intraepithelial lymphocytes, most commonly T lymphocytes

Light Microscopy
See Table 18.1.

Upper Respiratory Tract

Consists of
- Nasal cavities
- Paranasal sinuses
- Nasopharynx
- Oral cavity (Chap. 21)
- Oropharynx (Chap. 21)

Table 18.1 Cells of the respiratory epithelium

Cell	Function	Light microscopy	Abundance

Ciliated cells	Transport of mucus and entrapped particles towards the pharynx: ciliary movements are responsible for this "mucociliary clearance"	• Tall, columnar cells
		• Extend through the full height of the epithelium
		• Cilia:
		  • Seen as hairlike projections on luminal cell surface
		  • 250–300 per cell
		• Dark line in the apical cytoplasm, underneath the cilia, due to accumulated basal bodies
			Most abundant

Goblet cells	Mucus secretion	• Goblet shaped cells
		• Extend through the full height of the epithelium
		• Basal nuclei
		• Mucus granules in apical part of the cell
		  • Pale vacuolar region in HE
		  • Stains pink with PAS
			Numerous

Brush cells	Chemoreceptor	• Columnar cells • Apical brush border due to multiple microvilli • Each cell forms a synapse with an afferent nerve fiber, at the basal surface	Few
Small granule cells (Kulchitsky cells)	Part of the diffuse neuroendocrine system	• Secretory granules in the basal part of the cell • In HE preparation: hard to distinguish from basal cells	Few
Basal cells	Stem cells for the other epithelial cell types	Do not reach apical surface	Few
Intraepithelial lymphocytes	Part of bronchus-associated lymphatic tissue (BALT) (Chap. 19)	• Small round cells • Dark nucleus fills up most of the cytoplasm	Few

NASAL CAVITY (CAVUM NASI)

General
- Paired compartments
  - Separated by a nasal septum (septum nasi) of bone and cartilage
- Three bony protrusions (conchae, turbinates) on the lateral wall of each nasal cavity increase the surface area.

Function
- Moistens and temperates inhaled air
- Sensory organ: Sense of smell (olfaction) in the olfactory region

Divided into
- Nasal vestibule (vestibulum nasi)
  - The anterior 1½cm part of the nasal cavity
  - Lined with thin skin containing terminal hairs, vibrissae
  - Communicates anteriorly with the external environment, through the nostrils (nares)
- Main nasal cavity (cavum nasi proprium)
  - Communicates with:
    - Lateral: the nasolacrimal ducts and paranasal sinuses
    - Posterior: the nasopharynx, through the choanae
  - The mucosa is divided into two regions:
    - Respiratory region (regio respiratoria)
      - Located in:
        - The nasal septum
        - The floor of the main nasal cavity
        - The middle and inferior conchae
    - Olfactory region (regio olfactoria)
      - Located in:
        - The ceiling of the main nasal cavities
        - The superior conchae

Light Microscopy
- Nasal vestibule
  - Stratified squamous epithelium with sebaceous glands and hairs (vibrissae).
  - Posteriorly the epithelium gradually transforms into respiratory epithelium.
  - The epithelium rests on connective tissue and elastic cartilage.
- Main nasal cavity
  - Mucosa of the respiratory region
    - Respiratory epithelium on a thick basement membrane

- Lamina propria:
  - Dense irregular connective tissue with:
    - Mucoserous glands
      - Secretions moisten the inhaled air
    - Well-developed vascular network, with capillary loops close to the surface
      - Contributes to the heating of the inhaled air
  - Tightly attached to the periosteum and perichondrium of the skeleton of the nose
- Mucosa of olfactory region (see below)

Olfactory Region

Structure
- Macroscopically yellowish/brownish mucous membrane
- Located in:
  - The ceiling of the main nasal cavity
  - The superior conchae
- Approximately 10 cm^2

Function
Sense of smell (olfaction)

Consists of
- Olfactory epithelium:
  - Tall, pseudostratified epithelium
  - Three cells types (Fig. 18.1):
    - Olfactory cells
    - Sustentaculum cells
    - Basal cells
- Lamina propria
  - Rests on bone tissue

Light Microscopy
- Olfactory epithelium
  - Olfactory cells
    - Bipolar neurons, with:
      - One luminal dendrite with a knob-like ending, the olfactory vesicle
        - Long cilia with chemoreceptors radiate from the olfactory vesicle.
      - One basal, the unmyelinated axon
  - Sustentaculum cells (support cells)
    - Broad apex, narrow base
    - Apical, ovoid nuclei
    - Microvilli on the apical surface
    - Lipofuscin granules
    - Separates the olfactory cells and surrounds their dendrites and axons

- ○ Basal cells
  - ▪ Small round or cone-shaped stem cells on the basal lamina
- Lamina propria
  - ○ Loose connective tissue, continuous with periosteum
  - ○ Bundles of unmyelinated axons from the olfactory cells (fila olfactoria)
    - ▪ Run through the area cribrosa of the ethmoid bone
    - ▪ Form cranial nerve I (n. olfactorius)
  - ○ Large serous Bowman's glands
    - ▪ Secretes fluid to the olfactory surface
    - ▪ Fluid traps and dissolves odorants
  - ○ Vessels and nerves

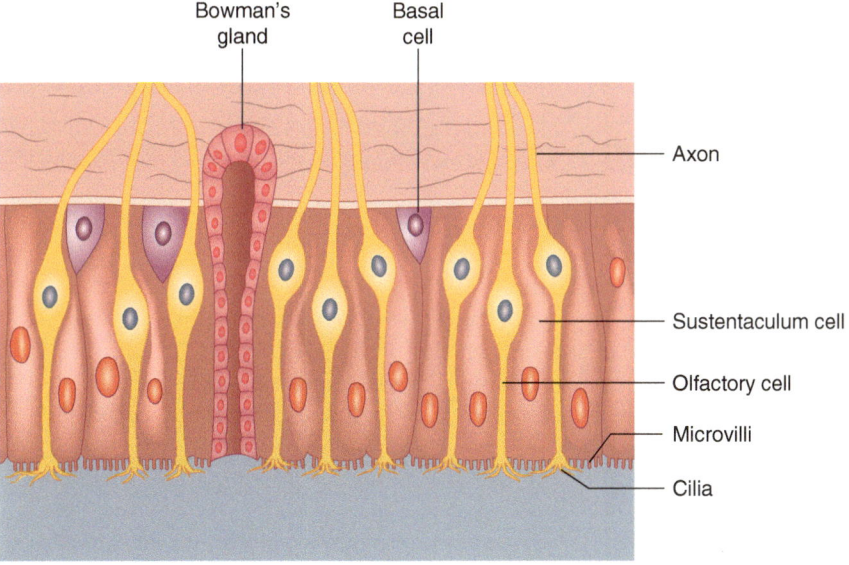

Fig. 18.1 Olfactory mucosa of the nasal cavity

THE PARANASAL SINUSES (SINUS PARANASALES)

Structure
- Paired air-filled cavities in the cranial bones.
- Connected to the nasal cavity through narrow openings.
- Mucus from epithelial goblet cells is swept towards the nasal cavities by the ciliary movements.

Function
Take part in resonation of speech

Consists of
- Frontal sinuses
- Maxillary sinuses
- Ethmoid sinuses
- Sphenoid sinuses

Light Microscopy
- The mucosa resembles the mucosa of the respiratory region of the main nasal cavities, but is less developed
- Rests on connective tissue and bone tissue

NASOPHARYNX

Structure
- The superior part of the pharynx
- Communicates with:
  - Anterior: the nasal cavities
  - Lateral: the auditory tubes (Eustachian tubes, tubae auditivae) (Chap. 29)
  - Inferior: the oropharynx (Chap. 21)
- Contains the pharyngeal tonsil (tonsilla pharyngea) (Chap. 21).
- Mucus from epithelial goblet cells is swept towards the oropharynx by the ciliary movements.

Light Microscopy
The mucosa resembles the mucosa of the respiratory region of the main nasal cavity

Lower Respiratory Tract

Consists of
- Larynx
- Trachea
- Bronchi
- Bronchioles
- Alveolar ducts
- Alveoli

LARYNX

Structure
- 4–5 cm long.
- Hollow, complex, tubular cartilage skeleton.
- Cartilage skeletal parts are joined by ligaments and laryngeal muscles.

Function
- Airway:
  - Connection between the oropharynx and trachea
- Phonation:
  - The vocal cords vibrate when air from the lungs are expelled.
  - By altering the tension of the vocal cords and the width of the space between them (rima glottidis), the pitch of the sound is changed.
  - The airways superior to the larynx modify the sounds further.
- Closing mechanisms:
  - The epiglottis folds down and closes the laryngeal opening (aditus laryngis) to prevent food and fluid from entering the lower respiratory tract. e.g., when swallowing
  - Attempted exhalation against a closed airway (maximal adduction of the vocal cords) enables intrathoracic and intra-abdominal pressure to rise.
    - This is called Valsalva's maneuver and is used during, e.g., coughing, sneezing, and weight lifting.

Consists of
- Mucosa:
  - Two pairs of lateral tissue folds project into the lumen below the laryngeal vestibule, with the free border running anteroposteriorly:
    - Vestibular folds (false vocal cords):
      - Immobile
    - - - - Ventricle: Narrow space between the vestibular folds and vocal cords - - - -
    - Vocal cords (plicae vocales):
      - Mobile
      - Each cord consists of a vocal ligament (ligament vocalia), a vocalis muscle (m. vocalis), and mucosa
- Skeleton:
  - Hyaline cartilage
    - In the main parts of the skeleton
    - For example, the thyroid and the cricoid cartilages
  - Elastic cartilage
    - For example, the epiglottis and some of the smaller laryngeal cartilages

- Intrinsic laryngeal muscles:
  - Several small skeletal muscles
  - Move the vocal cords and the cartilage skeleton
  - For example, the vocalis muscle within the vocal cords
- Ligaments

Light Microscopy
- Mucosa:
  - Epithelium
    - Stratified squamous epithelium covers areas with mechanical tear:
      - The luminal surface of the vocal ligaments
      - The main part of the epiglottis
    - Respiratory epithelium lines the rest of the larynx
  - Lamina propria
    - Loose connective tissue with abundant elastic fibers
    - Mucoserous glands
    - The vocal ligaments: parallel dense bundles of elastic fibers, within the vocal cords
- Skeleton:
  - Hyaline cartilage
  - Elastic cartilage
- Muscle:
  - Skeletal muscle fibers

TRACHEA

Structure
- 10–12 cm, $\varnothing$ 1.5–2.5 cm
- Flexible tube, with a stiff wall
- Runs from the larynx to the tracheal bifurcation, where it is divided into two main bronchi

Function
- Airway
- Traps inhaled particles in mucus on the luminal surface

Tracheal wall

Consists of
- Mucosa
- Submucosa
- Skeleton of cartilage and muscle:

  ○ 16–20 C-shaped cartilage rings
    ▪ Keeps the tracheal lumen open.
    ▪ Posterior opening is spanned by m. trachealis.
    ▪ Spaces between adjacent rings are bridged by fibro-elastic tissue.
  ○ M. trachealis
    ▪ Transverse smooth muscle fibers in the posterior opening of the cartilage rings
• Adventitia
  ○ Binds trachea to neighboring structures

Light Microscopy
• Mucosa:
  ○ Respiratory epithelium on a basement membrane
  ○ Lamina propria
    ▪ Loose connective tissue, with abundant elastic fibers and fibroblasts
    ▪ Numerous lymphocytes, plasma cells, and mast cells, all a part of Bronchus-associated lymphoid tissue (BALT) (Chap. 19)
• Submucosa:
  ○ Loose connective tissue, with elastic fibers
  ○ Mucoserous glands, secreting to the respiratory epithelium surface
  ○ Blood and lymphatic vessels
• Skeleton:
  ○ Hyaline cartilage: C-shaped rings
  ○ Smooth muscle fibers (m. trachealis)
  ○ Fibroelastic connective tissue continuous with the perichondrium surrounds the cartilage rings
• Adventitia:
  ○ Loose connective tissue and adipose tissue
  ○ Blood vessels, lymphatic vessels, and nerves

THE BRONCHIAL TREE

General
• The trachea is divided into two main bronchi at the carina, and the airways continue to divide into smaller and smaller branches.
• The branching is dichotomous, i.e., dividing into two
• Approximately 21 generations of branches in total

Structure
• Bronchi: 7–10 generations
  ○ The two main bronchi form the first generation
• Bronchioles: 14 generations
  ○ Seven generations of conductive bronchioles, including terminal bronchioles
  ○ Seven generations of respiratory bronchioles including alveolar ducts

Consists of (Fig. 18.2)

Main bronchi (primary bronchi)

↓   - - - - - - Interlobar septa - - - - - -

Lobar bronchi (secondary bronchi): each supplying a pulmonary lobe

↓   - - - - - - Intersegmental septa - - - - - -

Segmental bronchi (tertiary bronchi): each supplying a bronchopulmonary segment

↓   - - - - - - Interlobular septa - - - - - -

Bronchi

↓

Bronchioles: each supplying a pulmonary lobule

↓

Terminal bronchioles

↓

Respiratory bronchioles

↓

Alveolar ducts (ducti alveolares)

↓

Alveolar sacs (sacci alveolares)

↓

Alveoli

Fig. 18.2 The bronchial tree. From the main bronchi to the alveoli several generations of dichotomous branching take place

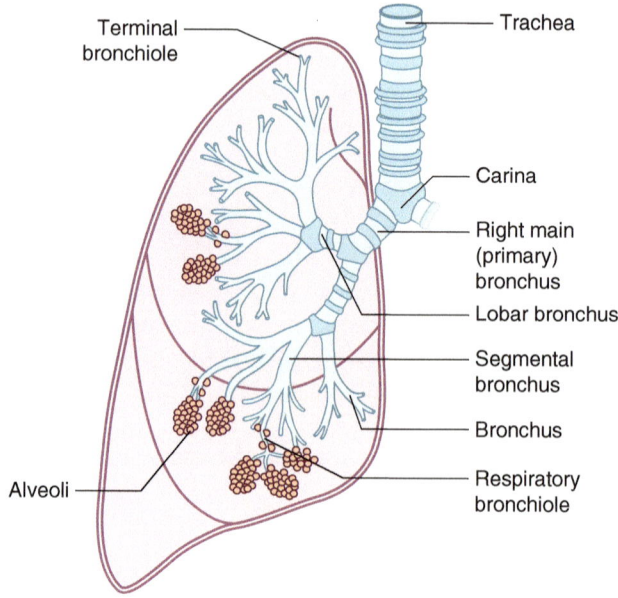

Bronchi

Structure

- Two main bronchi (primary bronchi, bronchi principales) run laterally from the tracheal bifurcation.
- Enter each lung at hilum:
  - Left main bronchus branches into two lobar bronchi, which branch into segmental bronchi.
  - Right main bronchus is shorter and wider than the left and branches into three lobar bronchi, which branch into segmental bronchi.
- The bronchial wall contains cartilage and mucoserous glands, like the trachea.
  - Cartilages are not C-shaped, but irregular.

Function

- Conduction of air
- Trap inhaled particles in mucus on the luminal surface

Light Microscopy

See Table 18.2.

Bronchioles

Structure

The bronchiolar wall contains neither cartilage, nor mucoserous glands.

Function

- Conduction of air
  - Regulated by bronchoconstriction and bronchodilation, primarily controlled by the autonomous nerve system
- Trap inhaled particles in mucus on the luminal surface
- Secretion of surfactant
  - Surfactant forms a surface fluid film that lowers the surface tension in the interface between air and epithelium
    - Prevents alveolar collapse
    - Eases the work of ventilation
  - Surfactant consists of
    - Phospholipids
    - Proteins
    - Lipids
- Gas exchange
  - In the alveoli of the respiratory bronchioles

Table 18.2 Light microscopy: bronchi → alveolar ducts

	Bronchi	Bronchioles	Terminal bronchioles	Respiratory bronchioles	Alveolar ducts
Wall thickness	——————————————— Decreasing ——————————————→				
Luminal ⊘	——————————————— Decreasing ——————————————→				
	≥1 mm	<1 mm	<1 mm	<1 mm	
Mucosa					

• Epithelium	• Respiratory epithelium
	• Height decreases as bronchi narrows
		Respiratory epithelium → Ciliated simple columnar epithelium:
		
		• Ciliated cells
		• Clara cells
		  ○ No cilia
		  ○ Rounded luminal projection
		  ○ Secretory vesicles
		
		Less ciliated cells and more Clara cells as bronchioles narrow
			Simple cuboidal epithelium:	As in terminal bronchioles, but with alveoli in the wall	• Completely lined with alveoli openings
					• Extremely flattened squamous cells, between the alveolar openings

• Lamina propria	• Loose connective tissue ○ Gradually thinner as bronchi narrows • Abundant elastic fibers • BALT	• Thin layer of loose connective tissue • Elastic fibers • BALT	• Thin layer of loose connective tissue • Elastic fibers	• Thin layer of loose connective tissue • Elastic fibers	• Thin layer of elastic and collagen fibers • Smooth muscle cells surround the alveolar opening
Submucosa	• Loose connective tissue • Abundant elastic fibers • Numerous small mucoserous glands	Gradually thinner	–	–	–
Muscularis/ cartilage	Hyaline cartilage: • Rings in main bronchi • Isolated irregular plates in the intrapulmonary bronchi • Smaller and less numerous plates as the bronchi narrows Cartilage is surrounded by: • Dense connective tissue, continuous with perichondrium • Circular layer of smooth muscle cells	• Relatively thick, circular layer of smooth muscle cells • No cartilage	• Relatively thick, circular layer of smooth muscle cells • No cartilage	• Circular layer of smooth muscle cells • No cartilage	–
Adventitia	• Dense connective tissue • Continuous with the connective tissue of adjacent structures	–	–	–	–

Divided into
- Conductive bronchioles
  - Without alveoli in the wall
- Terminal bronchioles
  - Constitutes the last generation of conductive bronchioles
  - Branches into respiratory bronchioles
- Respiratory bronchioles
  - With alveoli in their wall

Light Microscopy
See Table 18.2.

Alveolar Ducts (Ducti Alveolares)

General
- The last generation of branches in the bronchial tree
- Almost completely lined with alveolar openings
- Alveolar sacs are clusters of alveoli that are located:
  - In the distal end of the alveolar ducts
  - Scattered in the wall of the alveolar ducts

Light Microscopy
See Table 18.2.

MEMO-BOX
Cartilage and glands "follow each other" in the bronchial tree, i.e., if there is no cartilage, there are no glands:
- Bronchi contain both.
- Bronchioles contain neither.

Innervation of the Bronchial Tree

General

The bronchial tree is innervated by the autonomous nerve system:
- The parasympathetic nerve system acts through release of acetylcholine, which binds to muscarinic receptors, and stimulates:
  - Constriction of the bronchi
  - Increased mucus secretion
- The sympathetic nerve system acts through release of catecholamines, which bind to β2-receptors and stimulate:
  - Dilatation of the bronchi
  - Decreased mucus secretion

MEMO-BOX

Sympathetic nerve system (fight or flight):
It requires oxygen to fight or to flight, which is why catecholamines → bronchodilation.

Alveoli

Structure
- Balloon-shaped air-filled spaces
- ⌀ 200 μm
- 150–250 million alveoli per lung
- Total surface area of 75 m^2
- Each alveolus is surrounded by a rich capillary network

Function
- Site of gas exchange
- Secretion of surfactant

Alveolar wall (interalveolar septum)

Structure (Table 18.3)
- The thin wall between two neighboring alveolar spaces
- Penetrated by alveolar pores (10–15 μm), allowing air to spread between alveoli:
  - Collateral air distribution
  - Balancing the air pressure

Light Microscopy

See (Table 18.3).

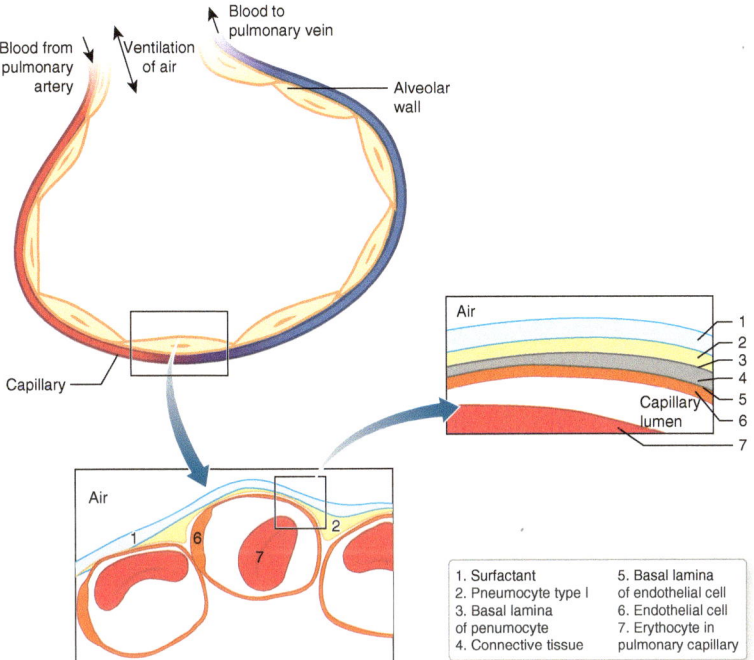

Fig. 18.3 The air–blood barrier

Air–blood barrier

General
The distance between blood and air, over which O_2 and CO_2 must diffuse (Fig. 18.3)

Structure
- 0.6 µm (0.1–1.5 µm) thick
- The connective tissue of the alveolar wall is often absent → the basal laminae of the alveolar epithelium and the capillary endothelium are often fused.

Consists of
- Surfactant
- Thin brim of cytoplasm of a type I pneumocyte
- Basal lamina of the pneumocyte
- Connective tissue (often absent)
- Basal lamina of the endothelial cell
- Thin brim of cytoplasm of an endothelial cell

Table 18.3 Alveolar wall

	Location	Function	Light microscopy
Epithelium			
• Type I pneumocytes	Cover 95 % of the internal surface area of the alveoli		• Exceptionally thin squamous cell (0.1 μm) • Flattened nucleus • Few organelles grouped near the nucleus • Tight junctions between both pneumocyte types
• Type II pneumocytes	Cover 5 % of the internal surface area of the alveoli	• Secrete surfactant • Progenitor cells for type I pneumocytes	• Irregular, pale, cuboidal cell • Large, round nucleus • rER, Golgi apparatus, and abundant apical vesicles, 1–2 μm (lamellar bodies) • Tight junctions between both pneumocyte types

• Alveolar macrophages (dust cells)	• Located on the epithelial surface and in the interseptal connective tissue
	• Leave the alveoli in two ways:
	  • Migration to the ciliated cells in the bronchioles → mucociliary transport to pharynx
	  • Migration through the alveolar wall to the bronchiolar connective tissue and into the lymphatic vessels (less common)
		Phagocytosis of:
		• Inhaled particles in alveolar space
		• Dead erythrocytes from damaged capillaries
			Dark due to:
			• Carbon from inhaled air
			• Hemosiderin from degraded hemoglobin of dead erythrocytes

Connective tissue	Below epithelium	• Elastic fibers in the wall enable alveoli to expand and recover their shape during ventilation • Contains the richest capillary network in the entire body	A thin layer of elastic and collagen fibers with: • Rich network of continuous capillaries • Scattered fibroblasts, alveolar macrophages, and lymphocytes

LUNGS (PULMONES)

General
- Paired organ, the right lung is 15–20% bigger than the left.
- Located in the thorax.
  - The two lungs are separated by the mediastinum.
- Volume: 3–6 l (of air).

Function
- Ventilation
- Air conduction
- Respiration, gas exchange

Consists of
- Parenchyma:
  - Lobes
    - Each supplied by a lobar bronchus:
      - Left lung: Two lobar bronchi → two lobes
      - Right lung: Three lobar bronchi → three lobes
    - Divided into bronchopulmonary segments
  - Bronchopulmonary segments
    - Each supplied by a segmental bronchus:
      - Left lung: nine segmental bronchi
      - Right lung: ten segmental bronchi
    - Each has their own blood supply
    - Divided into lobules
  - Lobules
    - Pyramid shaped, with apex directed towards the pulmonary hilum
    - Each supplied by a bronchiole
    - Divided into acini
  - Acini
    - 3–5 acini per lobulus
    - Consist of:
      - One terminal bronchiole
      - Lung tissue ventilated by the terminal bronchiole
  - Respiratory bronchiolar unit
    - Smallest functional unit of the lung
    - Consists of:
      - One respiratory bronchiole
      - Associated alveolar ducts and alveoli

- Stroma:
  - Connective tissue separates the portions of the lung.
    - Interlobar septa: between the lobes
    - Intersegmental septa: between the bronchopulmonary segments
    - Interlobular septa: between the lobules
  - Contains the majority of the blood and lymphatic vessels of the lungs.
  - In the periphery the connective tissue is continuous with subpleural connective tissue.

Blood Supply of the Lungs

General
The lungs have a functional circulation and a nutritive circulation.
- Pulmonary circulation:
  - Functional vessels
  - Transports deoxygenated venous blood from the right ventricle of the heart (low pO_2, high pCO_2) to the capillary network in the alveolar walls
- Bronchial circulation:
  - Nutritive vessels
  - Transports oxygenated arterial blood from aorta (high pO_2, low pCO_2) to the pulmonary tissue.
  - Anastomoses with branches of the pulmonary circulation at the level of the respiratory bronchioles → capillary networks of the bronchial circulation drains to the veins of the pulmonary circulation

Structure
- Branches of
  - The pulmonary artery
  - The bronchial arteries   Accompany the bronchi and bronchioles,
  - Lymphatic vessels   sharing their adventitia
  - Nerves
- Branches of the pulmonary veins run individually in connective tissue between portions of the lung (interlobular → intersegmental)
  - Near the hilum the veins follow the bronchial tree
- Due to low pressure in the pulmonary circulation, the walls of the pulmonary blood vessels are relatively thin, compared with the blood vessels of the systemic circulation

Consists of
- Pulmonary circulation:
  1. Pulmonary trunk (truncus pulmonalis)
  2. Left and right pulmonary artery (a. pulmonalis sinister et dexter)
  3. Lobar branches
  4. Segmental branches
  5. Smaller branches
  6. Rich capillary networks in the alveolar walls
  7. Venules
  8. Veins
  9. Four pulmonary veins (vv. pulmonales)
  10. The left atrium of the heart
- Bronchial circulation:
  1. Bronchial arteries from aorta (rr. bronchiales)
  2. Branches
  3. Capillary networks
  4. Drained by pulmonary venules, as well as the azygos vein (v. azygos) and the hemiazygos vein (v. hemiazygos)

Pleura

Structure
- Serous membrane covering the external surface of the lungs and their surroundings
- The two layers of pleura are separated by the pleural cavity (cavum pleurae)
  - A potential space
  - Contains a small amount of serous fluid

Function
The fluid in the pleural cavity minimizes friction → eases ventilation movements.

Consists of
- Parietal layer (pleura parietalis): on mediastinum and the inside of the thoracic wall
  - - Separated by the pleural cavity - -
- Visceral layer (pleura pulmonalis, pleura visceralis): on the external surface of the lung

Light Microscopy
- Mesothelium:
  - Simple squamous epithelium on a basal lamina
- Submesothelial connective tissue:
  - Dense connective tissue with elastic fibers.
  - The connective tissue of pleura visceralis is continuous with the interlobular connective tissue of the lungs.

Guide to Practical Histology: The Respiratory System

General
- Many parts of the respiratory system are lined with respiratory epithelium:
  - Pseudostratified columnar epithelium with ciliated cells and goblet cells.
- Bronchi, bronchioles and alveoli are often seen in the same specimen.
- Some of the diffuse and follicular lymphatic tissue of the lower respiratory tract is black due to inhaled carbon particles (anthracotic lymphatic tissue).

Olfactory Region

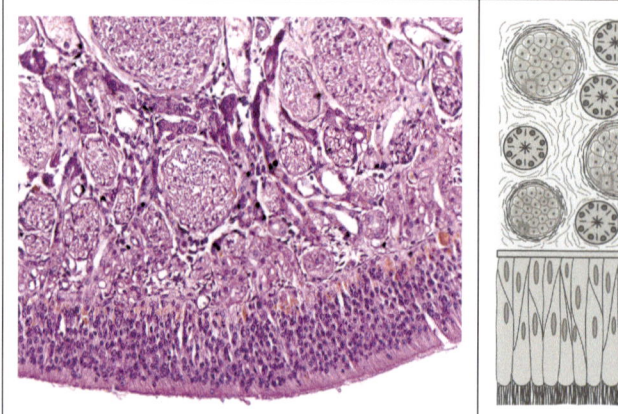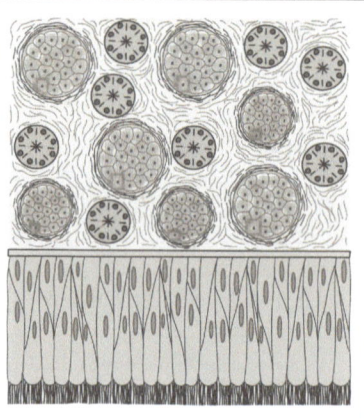

Left: photomicrograph of the olfactory mucosa. Magnification: high. Stain: HE (Courtesy of associate professor Steen Seier Poulsen, University of Copenhagen). *Right*: simplified illustration of the olfactory mucosa

Characteristics
Distinct layers in the mucosa:
- Epithelium:
  - A high, well-arranged pseudostratified columnar epithelium
- Lamina propria:
  - Connective tissue with serous exocrine glands
  - Nerve fibers from the olfactory cells

Epiglottis

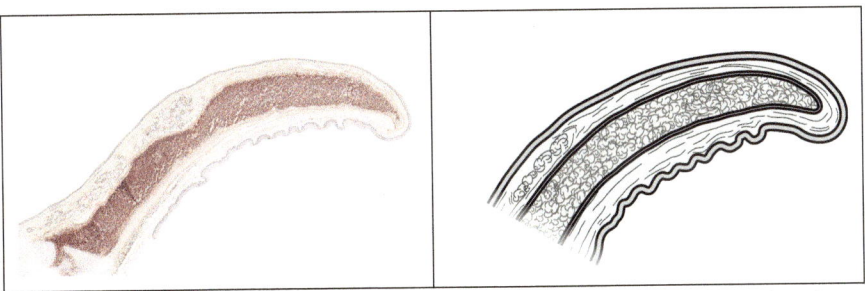

Left: photomicrograph of the epiglottis. Magnification: low. Stain: HE (Courtesy of professor Jørgen Tranum Jensen, University of Copenhagen). *Right*: simplified illustration of the epiglottis

Characteristics
- Macroscopic: resembles a claw/hook
- Microscopic:
  - A core of elastic cartilage
  - Mucosa:
    - Respiratory epithelium lines one side of the cartilage.
    - Nonkeratinized squamous epithelium lines the other side of the cartilage.
    - Seromucous exocrine glands are scattered in the connective tissue under the epithelium.

Can be mistaken for
Soft palate:
- Core of skeletal muscle tissue
- Without elastic cartilage

Trachea

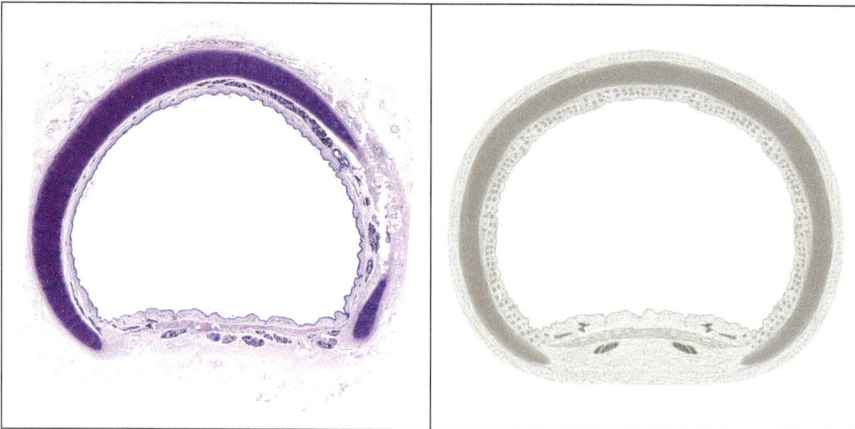

Left: photomicrograph of the trachea. Magnification: low. Stain: Alcian Blue-PAS (Courtesy of associate professor Steen Seier Poulsen, University of Copenhagen). *Right*: simplified illustration of the trachea

Characteristics
- Cross section:
  - Hyaline cartilage in "horseshoe C-shape."
  - The two ends of the horseshoe are joined by smooth muscle tissue.
  - Lumen lined with respiratory epithelium.
- Longitudinal section:
  - A row of regular "islets" of hyaline cartilage.
  - Islets are connected by connective tissue.
  - Lumen lined with respiratory epithelium.

Can be mistaken for
Longitudinal section of a bronchus:
- Has smooth muscle tissue between the "islets" of cartilage

THE BRONCHIAL TREE

Bronchi

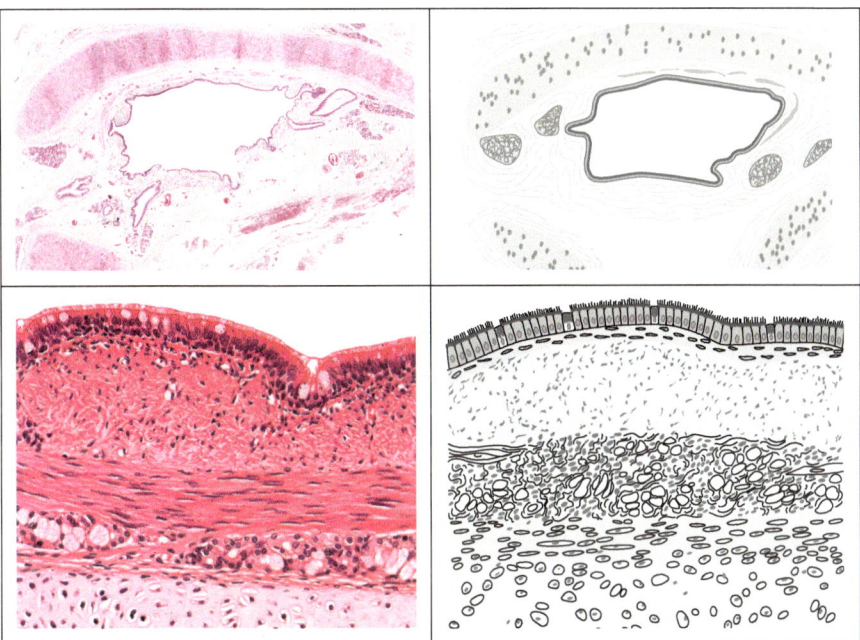

Top panel, left: photomicrograph cross section of a bronchus. Magnification: low. Stain: HE (Courtesy of professor Jørgen Tranum Jensen, University of Copenhagen). *Top panel, right*: simplified illustration of a bronchus. *Bottom panel, left*: photomicrograph of the luminal part of a bronchial wall. Magnification: high. Stain: HE (Courtesy of professor Jørgen Tranum Jensen, University of Copenhagen). *Bottom panel, right*: simplified illustration of the luminal part of a bronchial wall

Characteristics

Cross section:
- Irregular ring-shaped structure:
  - Luminally lined with respiratory epithelium
  - Wall contains loose connective tissue with mucous glands
  - Surrounded by
    - Smooth muscle tissue
    - "Islets" of hyaline cartilage

Can be mistaken for
- Longitudinal section of the trachea:
  - No smooth muscle tissue is seen between the "islets" of hyaline cartilage.
- Bronchioles:
  - Smaller ⌀ than bronchi
  - No mucous glands or cartilage in their wall

Bronchioles

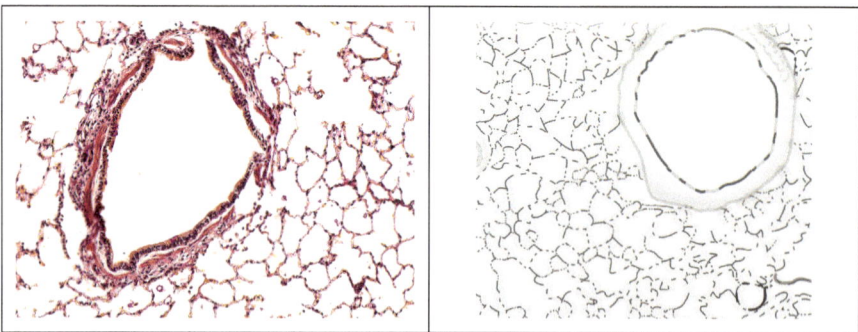

Left: photomicrograph of lung tissue with a bronchiole and alveoli. Magnification: high. Stain: PAS (Courtesy of associate professor Steen Seier Poulsen, University of Copenhagen). *Right*: simplified illustration of lung tissue with a bronchiole

Characteristics
Cross section:
- Ring-shaped structure within lung tissue:
  - Lumen is lined with ciliated pseudostratified or simple columnar epithelium
  - Surrounded by several layers of smooth muscle cells.

Can be mistaken for
Bronchi:
- Larger ⌀ than bronchioles
- Have mucous glands and hyaline cartilage in their wall

Alveoli

Characteristics
- White spaces separated by thin walls with numerous capillaries:
  - The wall is lined with simple squamous epithelium on both sides.
- Often seen together with:
  - Bronchioles
  - Bronchi (sometimes)

Can be mistaken for
Mammary gland (lactating):
- Contains thicker connective tissue strands between the alveolar end pieces (which resembles lung alveoli).
- The epithelium is cuboidal.
- The lumina may contain eosinophilic secretions (milk)

References

5, 25, 31, 33, 34, 45.

Chapter 19
The Immune System and the Lymphatic Organs

The Immune System

General
- The immune system is represented throughout the entire body.
- The system consists of lymphatic cells/tissues/organs, lymphatic vessels, and circulating lymph.

Function
The immune system constitutes a defense against:
- External pathogens, e.g., infectious agents such as bacteria and viruses
- Altered cells within the body, e.g.:
  - Tumor cells
  - Cells infected by virus

© Springer International Publishing Switzerland 2017
A. Rehfeld et al., *Compendium of Histology*, DOI 10.1007/978-3-319-41873-5_19

Divided into

Represented by two lines of defense (working together/in parallel):

- The innate immune system
- The adaptive (specific) immune system:
  - Cell-mediated immune response
  - Humoral (antibody-mediated) immune response

Consists of

Anatomically the immune system consists of:

- A diverse population of immune cells, seen:
  - Solitary in nonlymphatic tissues
  - Aggregated in lymphatic tissues:
    - Within areas of loose connective tissue
    - Without a surrounding capsule
  - Aggregated in specialized lymphatic organs:
    - Primary lymphatic organs
    - Secondary lymphatic organs
- The lymph, where the immune cells are in constant recirculation between:
  - Blood
  - Connective tissue and extracellular fluid
  - Secondary lymphatic organs
- The lymphatic vessels:
  - Transport lymph, with cells and pathogens from the interstitial spaces, through secondary lymphatic organs, to the blood circulation (Chap. 17).

The Innate Immune System

General

- A nonspecific, first line of defense
- Rapid response

Consists of

- First line of defense
  - Physical barriers, e.g., the skin
  - Chemical defense, e.g., low pH in the stomach
  - Biological defense, e.g., the resident microbiota of the intestines
- Secretions to epithelial surfaces and blood, e.g., lysozymes, complement, and interleukins
- Immune cells:
  - Granulocytes
  - Monocytes
  - Macrophages
  - Natural killer lymphocytes (NK cells)
  - Mast cells

The Adaptive Immune System

General
- More specific, second line of defense
- Ability to "learn," and therefore divided into:
  - Primary immune response
    - Slow response
    - Upon first exposure to an antigen
    - Memory cells develop, for later "secondary immune responses"
  - Secondary immune response
    - Faster, larger, and more specific response
    - When subsequently encountering the same antigen

Consists of
- Cell-mediated immune response
  - T lymphocytes
  - Antigen-presenting cells
- Humoral (antibody-mediated) immune response
  - Primary immune response
    - T and B lymphocytes
    - Antigen-presenting cells
  - Secondary immune response
    - Memory cells (T and B lymphocytes)
    - Antigen-presenting cells

CELLS OF THE IMMUNE SYSTEM

Consist of
- Leukocytes:
  - Lymphocytes:
    - T lymphocytes
    - B lymphocytes
    - Natural killer lymphocytes (NK cells)
  - Non-lymphocytes (Chap. 7):
    - Granulocytes
      - Neutrophils
      - Basophils
      - Eosinophils
    - Monocytes
    - Macrophages
    - Mast cells

- Supporting cells:
  - Dendritic cells ⎫
  - Follicular dendritic cells ⎬ Antigen-presenting cells
  - Langerhans cells ⎮
  - Epithelioreticular cells ⎭
  - Reticular cells

Lymphocytes

General
- Naive lymphocytes are mature immunocompetent lymphocytes that not yet have been exposed to an antigen.
- Lymphocytes are found in two pools:
  - Recirculating pool
    - Major pool
    - Circulate between: blood vascular system → lymphatic tissue → lymphatic vascular system → blood vascular system
    - Makes surveillance of different body compartments possible
  - Non-recirculating pool
    - A minor part of the lymphocytes do not recirculate, but are destined for a specific tissue.

Consist of
- T lymphocytes
  - 60–80 % of recirculating lymphocytes
- B lymphocytes
  - 20–30 % of recirculating lymphocytes
- Natural killer lymphocytes (NK cells)
  - 5–10 % of recirculating lymphocytes

Function
See Table 19.1.

Light Microscopy
- T and B lymphocytes are morphologically identical in light microscope:
  - ⊘ approximately 7 µm.
  - Spherical, intensely basophilic nucleus fills up the cell.
  - Thin brim of surrounding basophilic cytoplasm.

- NK cells
  - ⊘ 15 μm
  - Granules in cytoplasm
  - Kidney-shaped nucleus
- Subgroups of lymphocytes can be identified in immune-cytochemical sections, by staining for different surface proteins, called "cluster of differentiation" (CD) markers.

Table 19.1 Function of lymphocytes

Cell	Common name	Function
T lymphocytes		
• Helper CD4 T lymphocytes	Th cells: • Th1 • Th2	• Stimulation of inflammation (Chap. 7), via cytokines • Activation of cells, via cytokines: ○ Macrophages ○ Cytotoxic T lymphocytes ○ B lymphocytes → promote the differentiation into plasma cells • Secondary immune response: a subset differentiates into memory helper T lymphocytes
• Cytotoxic CD8 T lymphocytes	Killer T cells (CTL's)	• Removal of virus infected cells (cell-mediated immunity) • Secondary immune response: A subset differentiates into memory cytotoxic T lymphocytes • Require help (activation) from Th1 cells
• Regulatory T lymphocytes	Suppressor T cells	• Suppression of disproportionate immune responses • Regulation of tolerance to self-antigens (prevents autoimmunity)
• Gamma/delta T lymphocytes		• Similar to cells of the innate immune system • Located in epidermis and mucosal epithelium
B lymphocytes		
• B lymphocytes		• Differentiate into plasma cells • Secondary immune response: a subset differentiates into memory B lymphocytes • Require help (activation) from Th2 cells
• Plasma cells		Secretion of antibodies
Natural killer lymphocytes	NK cells	Kill altered/infected cells

Cytokines

General
- Paracrine mediators, secreted by immune cells
- Cytokines are small peptides or glycopeptides

Function
- Coordination of the actions of the innate and the adaptive immune system
- Regulation of, e.g.:
  - Lymphocyte proliferation and activation
  - Cell movement (chemotaxis)
  - Inflammation (Chap. 7)

Antigen-Presenting Cells

General
- An antigen is any molecule that stimulates the adaptive immune system.
  - Soluble, or as a part of an intact cell or a larger element
  - Usually a protein, glycoprotein, or polysaccharide
- Antigen-presenting cells (APCs) have major histocompatibility complex (MHC II) molecules on their surface (see later).
  - Except follicular dendritic cells, which, on their surface, trap antigen bound to antibodies or complement

Function
Presentation of antigens to T and B lymphocytes, which is essential in the activation of the adaptive immune system:
1. Uptake:
   Antigen-presenting cell ingests material with antigens, by one of:
   - Receptor-mediated endocytosis
   - Phagocytosis
   - Pinocytosis
2. Processing:
   Intracellular antigen processing
3. Presentation:
   The MHC II molecule on the surface of the antigen-presenting cell presents the antigen, i.e., fragments of the ingested material
4. Activation:
   Cells of the adaptive immune system (T and B lymphocytes) react when non-self-antigens are presented.

Consist of
- Cells of the mononuclear phagocyte system, e.g.:
  - Macrophages
  - Dendritic cells
  - Langerhans cells (dendritic cells of the skin)
- B lymphocytes
- Epithelioreticular cells of the thymus
- Follicular dendritic cells
  - No MHC II molecules
  - Bind antibody–antigen complexes to their surface without previous processing
  - Only located in lymphatic follicles, where they present antigens to B lymphocytes

Major Histocompatibility Complex Molecules

General

Major histocompatibility complex (MHC) molecules present antigens on cell surfaces.

Divided into
- MHC I molecules:
  - On the surface of all nucleated cells and blood platelets.
- MHC II molecules:
  - Only on the surface of antigen-presenting cells

Function
- MHC I molecules:
  - Presentation of antigens (fragments of proteins) of proteins synthesized in the cytoplasm of the specific cell
  - Make T lymphocytes able to recognize the specific cell as:
    - "Self" and not altered, or
    - "Not self" and/or altered (by cancer or virus)
- MHC II molecules:
  - Presentation of antigens of extracellular derived proteins to T and B lymphocytes and thereby activation of these cells

Lymphatic Organs and Tissues

LYMPHATIC ORGANS

General
- Organs involved in the immune response
- Consist of lymphatic tissue

Divided into
- Primary lymphatic organs
  - Thymus
  - Bone marrow (Chap. 10)
- Secondary lymphatic organs
  - Lymph nodes
  - Spleen
  - Mucosa-associated lymphatic tissue (MALT)
  - Skin-associated lymphatic tissue (SALT):
    - Lymphocytes and antigen-presenting cells of the skin are sometimes referred to as SALT.

Function
- Primary lymphatic organs:
  - Antigen-independent maturation of lymphocytes into immunocompetent lymphocytes:
    - T and B lymphocytes are produced in the red bone marrow and further matured in:
      - Thymus (T lymphocytes)
      - Bone marrow (B lymphocytes)
- Secondary lymphatic organs:
  - Antigen-dependent activation of immunocompetent lymphocytes into:
    - Effector lymphocytes
    - Memory cells

MEMO-BOX
T lymphocytes mature in **Thymus**
B lymphocytes mature in **Bone marrow**

LYMPHATIC TISSUE

General
- Specialized connective tissue
- Seen as aggregations of lymphocytes, which are defined, but not encapsulated
- All secondary lymphatic organs consist of the two different types of lymphatic tissue

Divided into
- Diffuse lymphatic tissue
- Follicular lymphatic tissue (nodular lymphatic tissue)

Consists of
Both diffuse and follicular lymphatic tissue consists of:
- Parenchyma:
  - Immunocompetent lymphocytes
  - Antigen-presenting cells
- Stroma:
  - Reticular connective tissue:
    - Reticular fibers
    - Reticular cells

Diffuse Lymphatic Tissue

Consists of
- Parenchyma
  - T lymphocytes
  - Plasma cells
  - Dendritic cells (antigen presenting)
  - Macrophages (antigen presenting)
- Stroma
  - Reticular connective tissue

Follicular Lymphatic Tissue (Nodular Lymphatic Tissue)

Structure

Contains lymphatic follicles:
- Sharply defined groups of (mainly) lymphocytes
- Not surrounded by a capsule

Consists of
- Parenchyma
    - B lymphocytes
    - Follicular dendritic cells ⎫
    - Macrophages   ⎬ Arranged in lymphatic follicles
    - Few T lymphocytes (CD4) ⎭
- Stroma
    - Reticular connective tissue

Lymphatic follicles (lymphatic nodules)

Divided into
- Primary lymphoid follicle (nodule)
    - Small aggregation of cells
- - - - - Antigen stimulation - - - - -
- Secondary lymphoid follicle (nodule) (Fig. 19.1)
    - Larger aggregation of activated cells
    - Gradually dissolves after 2–3 weeks

Function

Houses the antigen-dependent activation of naive immunocompetent B lymphocytes

Consist of
- Primary lymphatic follicles:
    - B lymphocytes
    - Follicular dendritic cells
- Secondary lymphatic follicles:
    - Germinal center:
        - Activated, proliferating B lymphocytes:
            1. Centroblasts: large mitotically active cells →
            2. Centrocytes: of variable size, with irregular nuclei →
            3. Plasmablasts (plasma cell precursor) or memory cells
        - Follicular dendritic cells
            - Major antigen-presenting cell of the follicles
            - Mesenchymal origin
        - Th2 lymphocytes (CD4)
        - Macrophages
    - Mantle (corona):
        - Naive B lymphocytes pushed aside

Light Microscopy

Secondary lymphatic follicle:

- Germinal center:
  - Light part in the center of the follicle
  - Larger, less basophilic B lymphocytes (undergoing proliferation)
  - Follicular dendritic cells
    - Difficult to distinguish in routine preparations
    - With dendritic cell extensions
  - Macrophages with apoptotic B lymphocyte debris in the cytoplasm
- Mantle:
  - Dark, peripheral border of small basophilic lymphocytes

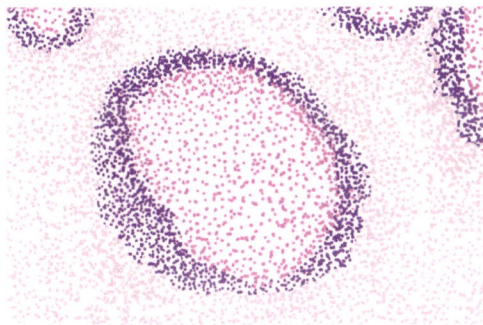

Fig. 19.1 Secondary lymphatic follicle. With a light, central germinal center and a surrounding dark mantle

Activation of B lymphocytes

1. A primary lymphatic follicle develops as B lymphocytes and follicular dendritic cells aggregate.
2. Antigens are presented to B lymphocytes by the follicular dendritic cells. Th2 lymphocytes assist in activation of the B lymphocytes that recognize an antigen.
3. A secondary lymphatic follicle is formed from the primary lymphoid follicle as:
   - An activated B lymphocyte proliferates and forms a clone of cells that are able to produce antibodies against the same antigen.
   - Specific events take place in the clone:
     - Somatic hypermutation: Mutation of immunoglobulin (antibody) genes → further variations of the immunoglobulin structure.
     - Affinity maturation: The cell with the immunoglobulin that binds most firmly to the antigen differentiates into effector B lymphocytes, and the remaining cells of the clone undergo apoptosis.
     - Class shift recombination: During differentiation of the plasma cells, the cells shift from mainly producing IgM to IgG and IgA (see later).

4. Differentiation to:
   - Effector B lymphocytes (plasma cells)
   - Memory B cells
5. The main part of the B lymphocytes undergo apoptosis

Antibody

General (Table 19.2)
- Antibodies are also called immunoglobulins
- Constitutes a part of the B-cell receptor (BCR)
- Secreted by plasma cells.
- Antibodies neutralize or mark invading pathogens, for destruction by different methods.

Table 19.2 Classes of antibodies/immunoglobulins

	IgG	IgM	IgE	IgA	IgD
Function	• Activation of phagocytosis • Neutralization of antigens	• Produced during initial response against antigen • Forms major part of the B-cell receptor	• Defense against parasites • Allergic reactions	Protection of mucosal membranes	Forms major part of the B-cell receptor
Location	• Plasma • Intercellular fluid • Fetal circulation	• Plasma • Intercellular fluid • Surface of B lympho-cytes (as a monomer)	Bound to surface of mast cells and basophils	• Exocrine secretions • Plasma • Intercellular fluid	• Plasma • Intercellular fluid • Surface of B lymphocytes
Abundance in plasma	80%	5–10%	<0.5%	10–15%	<0.5%
Form	Monomer	Regularly in a pentameric form, joined by a J chain	Monomer	A dimeric form, joined by a J chain	Monomer

Structure (Fig. 19.2)
Y-shaped glycoprotein, with a:
- Fc region
  - At the tip of the base of the Y
  - Can bind to Fc receptors on, e.g.,
    - Surface of macrophages and neutrophils
    - Surface of basophils and mast cells

- Variable region
  - At each tip of the upper ends of the Y
  - Contains the antigen binding site

Consists of
- Two identical heavy chains
- Two identical light chains

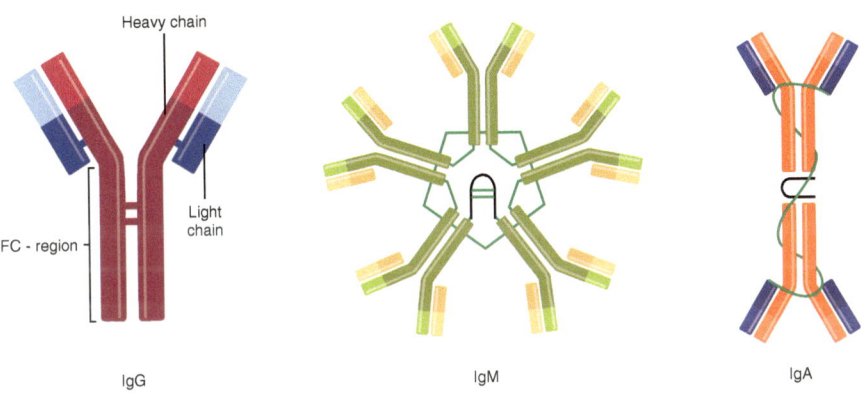

Fig. 19.2 Antibodies. A Y-shaped structure with two heavy chains and two light chains. Antibodies (immunoglobulins) exist in different classes; IgG, IgM, and IgA are the most common

THYMUS

General
- Primary lymphatic organ.
- Located in the superior, anterior part of mediastinum.
- The thymus goes through involution:
  - Lymphatic tissue is gradually replaced by adipose tissue.
  - Involution starts in puberty.

Structure
- 10 g (in adults)
- Two lobes
- Thin capsule of connective tissue surrounds the two lobes
  - Sends septa into the parenchyma, to the corticomedullary border, dividing the two lobes into partly separated lobules.
  - Septa contain blood vessels, efferent lymphatic vessels, and nerves.
- The thymic stroma is formed entirely from epithelioreticular cells (Table 19.3)
  - Differs from the reticular connective tissue stroma of other lymphatic tissues and organs

Function

Maturation of T lymphocytes → tolerance towards "self" (central tolerance)

Consists of
- Cortex
  - T lymphocytes
  - Epithelioreticular cells (thymic epithelial cells, epithelial reticular cells)
  - Numerous macrophages
- Medulla
  - T lymphocytes
  - Epithelioreticular cells
  - Macrophages
  - Dendritic cells (thymic interdigitating cells)

Light Microscopy
- Cortex: heavily basophilic due to numerous lymphocytes
  - Epithelioreticular cells (Table 19.3)
    - Large, spherical/ovoid light nucleus
    - Light, eosinophilic cytoplasm
  - T lymphocytes
    - Densely packed
  - Macrophages
    - Numerous, hard to distinguish in routine preparations
- Medulla: lighter than cortex, due to less and larger lymphocytes
  - Epithelioreticular cells (Table 19.3)
    - Large, spherical/ovoid, light nucleus
  - Dendritic cells (thymic interdigitating cells)
    - Hard to distinguish in routine preparations
  - T lymphocytes
    - Larger than in cortex, with pale nuclei
  - Macrophages
  - Hassall's corpuscles (Table 19.3)
    - 20–100 μm
    - Onion-like structure of flattened cells

Table 19.3 Epithelioreticular cells

	Cell shape	Cell adhesions	Location	Function
Type I	Squamous	• Desmosomes • Tight junctions	• Line the connective tissue of the capsule and septa • Surround the microvasculature	• Isolate developing T lymphocytes from the stroma
Type II	• Stellate • Cell extensions with keratin filaments	Desmosomes link cell extensions of adjacent cells	• Throughout the cortex • Form a cellular reticulum	• Present "self-" and "foreign" antigens (on MHC I and MHC II molecules) to maturing T lymphocytes
Type III	• Squamous • Sheet-like cell extensions	Tight junctions	Located at the interface between cortex and medulla	• Present "self-" and "foreign" antigens (on MHC I and MHC II molecules) to maturing T lymphocytes • Contributes to a functional corticomedullary barrier, together with the type IV cells
Type IV	• Squamous • Sheet-like cell extensions	Tight junctions	Located between cortex and medulla, close to the type III cells	Contributes to a functional corticomedullary barrier, together with the type III cells
Type V	• Stellate • Cell extensions with keratin filaments	Desmosomes link cell extensions of neighboring cells	• Throughout the medulla • Form a cellular reticulum	• Support T lymphocytes, dendritic cells, and macrophages • Express "self-antigens" (on both MHC I and MHC II molecules) together with dendritic cells, as a part of the negative selection
Type VI	• Flattened cells, compactly packed in concentric layers, like layers of an onion • Keratohyalin granules	Desmosomes	Form Hassall's corpuscles in medulla	• Not fully understood • Produce interleukins involved in T lymphocyte development

Development/Maturation of T Lymphocytes

General
- T lymphocytes mature during their passage from cortex to medulla.
- The process takes approximately two weeks.
- 2 % of the T lymphocytes pass both positive and negative selection.
- 98 % of the T lymphocytes undergo apoptosis and are phagocytized by macrophages.

Formation (Fig. 19.3)
1. Invasion
   - During fetal life precursor cells (pre-T lymphocytes) from the bone marrow invade and settle in the thymic tissue.
   - The pre-T lymphocytes are "double negative," i.e., express neither CD4 nor CD8 on their surface.
2. Proliferation
   - Pre-T lymphocytes proliferate and express T-cell receptor (TCR) as well as CD4 and CD8 on their surface.
     - Different pre-T lymphocytes express different TCRs.
     - The pre-T lymphocytes are "double positive," i.e., express both CD4 and CD8.
3. Positive selection:
   - Pre-T lymphocytes, which TCR does not recognize and bind to an "antigen + MHC I-complex" or "antigen + MHC II-complex" of the cortical epithelioreticular cells, are eliminated.
4. Negative selection:
   - Pre-T lymphocytes, which TCR binds to "self-antigen" presented by the medullar dendritic cells, are eliminated:
     - Pre-T lymphocytes survive if they do not recognize self-antigen.
   - Important step for the development of the immune system's "tolerance to self."
5. Single positive stage:
   - Mature naive T lymphocytes leave the thymic medulla with the blood circulation or efferent lymphatic vessels.
   - The T lymphocytes now:
     - Express:
       - TCR, and
       - Either CD4 or CD8, i.e., are "single positive"
         - CD4 cells are restricted to recognize MHC II molecules
         - CD8 cells are restricted to recognize MHC I molecules
     - Show tolerance towards "self"

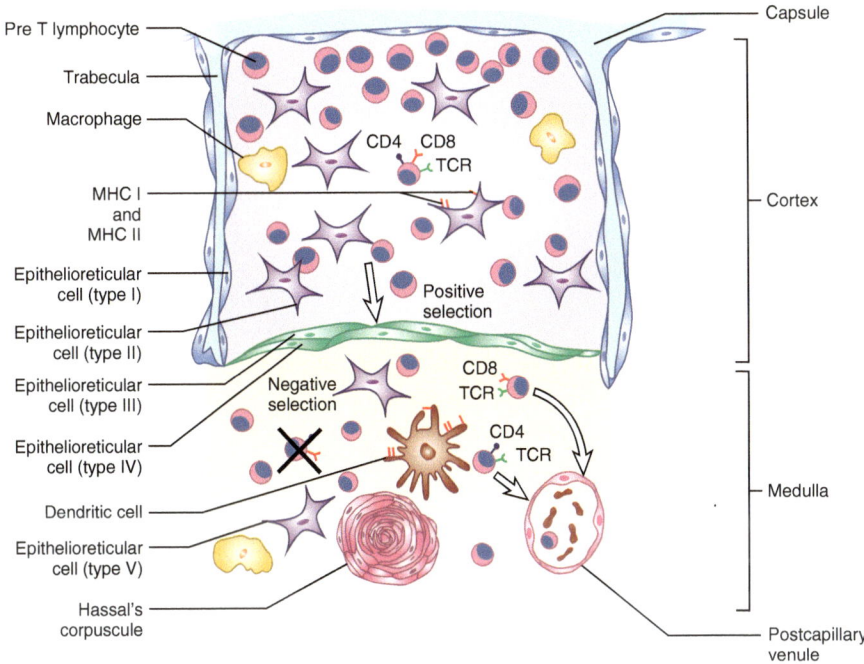

Fig. 19.3 Thymus and the development of T lymphocytes. The positive selection of the developing T lymphocytes takes place in the cortex, and the negative selection takes place in the medulla. The thymic stroma consists of six different epithelioreticular cell types

Blood Supply of the Thymus

Table 19.4 Blood supply of the thymus

	Vessels		Features
Arteries	Thymic arteries (rr. thymici)		
	Arterioles		Run in connective tissue septa to the corticomedullary border
	—	Medullary arterioles	No arterioles in cortex
Capillaries	Cortical capillary loops/networks	Medullar capillary networks	Cortical capillaries are surrounded by epithelioreticular cells, which contribute to a blood–thymus barrier
Veins	Venules at the corticomedullar border	Medullary venules	Postcapillary venules of the corticomedullary border have a specialized cuboidal endothelium, which let the matured T lymphocytes pass into the blood circulation
	Larger veins		

Blood–Thymus Barrier

General

Barrier between cortical pre-T lymphocytes and the lumen of cortical blood vessels

Function

Protection of the microenvironment where the development and maturation of T lymphocytes takes place.

Consists of

- Endothelium of cortical blood vessels
  - Tight junctions between endothelial cells
  - Thick basal membrane
- Macrophages
  - In perivascular connective tissue
- Type I epithelioreticular cells on a basal lamina
  - Surrounding the blood vessels

LYMPH NODE

General

- Small secondary lymphatic organs interposed along the lymphatic vessels.
- Regional lymph nodes form groups as they drain different regions, e.g.:
  - Cervical lymph nodes
  - Axillary lymph nodes
  - Inguinal lymph nodes
  - Lymph nodes associated with:
    - Large blood vessels in mediastinum
    - Large blood vessels in abdomen

Structure

- 1–20 mm long
- Flat, kidney bean shaped
- Surrounded by a thin capsule of dense connective tissue:
  - Trabeculae extend from the capsule into the lymph node.
- Hilum at the concave border
  - Blood vessels enter/exit
  - One efferent lymphatic vessel exits

Function

- Filtration of the lymph on its way back to the blood circulation
- Secondary lymphatic organs, i.e., site for activation of immunocompetent T and B lymphocytes:

- ○ Cell-mediated immune response.
  - ▪ T lymphocytes encounter antigens presented by antigen-presenting cells.
  - ▪ In the paracortex activated cytotoxic T cells proliferate with the assistance of Th1 lymphocytes.
- ○ Humoral (antibody-mediated) immune response.
  - ▪ B lymphocytes encounter antigens presented by follicular dendritic cells or other antigen-presenting cells.
  - ▪ In the lymphatic follicles of the superficial cortex, activated B lymphocytes proliferate with the assistance of Th2 lymphocytes.
  - ▪ B lymphocytes differentiate into plasma cells and migrate towards the medullary cords where they produce antibodies.
- ○ Activated T lymphocytes and B lymphocytes (plasma cells) leave the lymph node in the efferent lymphatic vessel and via the blood recirculate to the target tissue

Consists of (Fig. 19.4)
- • Cortex
  - ○ Superficial cortex (nodular cortex)
  - ○ Deep cortex (paracortex)
  - ○ Subcapsular, cortical, and trabecular lymphatic sinuses
- • Medulla
  - ○ Medullary cords
  - ○ Medullary sinuses

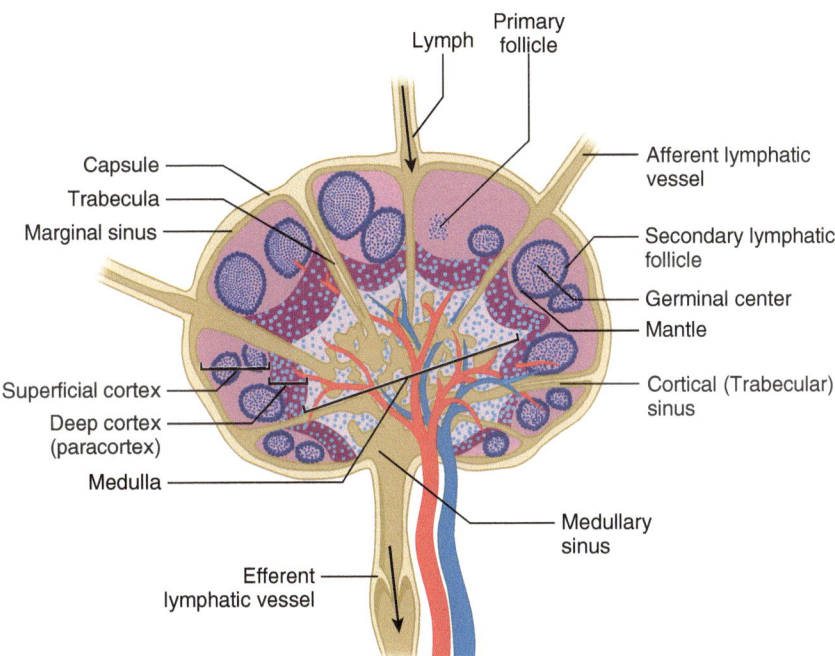

Fig. 19.4 Lymph node. The superficial cortex constitutes a bone marrow-dependent zone, with follicular lymphatic tissue. The deep cortex (paracortex) constitutes a thymus-dependent zone, with diffuse lymphatic tissue. The medulla contains numerous lymphatic sinuses

Light microscopy
See Table 19.5.

High Endothelial Venules

Structure
- Venules with cuboidal endothelium
- Located in the deep cortex (paracortex) of the lymph node

Function
Site where the recirculating immune cells migrate from blood into the lymph node parenchyma (homing)

Table 19.5 Lymph node

	Subdivision	Function	Light microscopy
Cortex			Dark, due to abundant basophilic lymphocytes
• Parenchyma	Superficial cortex	Bone marrow-dependent zone	Follicular lymphatic tissue with primary and secondary lymphatic follicles
	Deep cortex (paracortex)	Thymus-dependent zone	• Diffuse lymphatic tissue • High endothelial venules (HEVs)
	Subcapsular, cortical, and trabecular lymphatic sinuses	Filtration of lymph	See next page
• Stroma			Reticular connective tissue: Meshwork of reticular fibers, covered by reticular cells
Medulla			Light, due to fewer cells and abundant lymphatic sinuses
• Parenchyma	Medullary cords	Site of antibody production	Plasma cells, B lymphocytes, and macrophages
	Medullary sinuses	Filtration of lymph	See next page
• Stroma			Reticular connective tissue: Meshwork of reticular fibers, covered by reticular cells

Lymphatic Sinuses

Structure
- Spaces within the lymph node where the lymph passes on its way through the node.
- Valves in the lymphatic vessels ensure that the flow is one-directional.

Function
Filtration of the lymph:
- The lymph flows through sinuses and is filtered into the surrounding lymphoid tissue by the meshwork of reticular connective tissue and macrophage processes
- Filtered from the lymph are:
  ○ Immune cells, e.g., lymphocytes, dendritic cells, macrophages
  ○ Immune reactive substances, e.g., antigens, pathogens, and tumor cells

Divided into
- Subcapsular sinuses
- Cortical (trabecular) sinuses
- Medullary sinuses

Light Microscopy
- The wall of the sinus is a discontinuous layer of flattened endothelial-like cells
- The lumen of the sinuses is traversed by
  ○ Reticular fibers, surrounded by reticular cell processes (visible in silver staining)
  ○ Processes from macrophages
- Sinuses contain
  ○ Abundant, large macrophages

The pathway of the lymph
1. Lymph capillaries
2. Afferent lymphatic vessels
3. Subcapsular sinuses ⎤
4. Cortical sinuses |
5. Trabecular sinuses ⎬ Within a lymph node
6. Medullar sinuses   ⎦
7. Efferent lymphatic vessel
8. The thoracic duct (ductus thoracicus) or right lymphatic duct (ductus lymphaticus dexter)
9. Large veins at the base of the neck

Blood Supply of the Lymph Node

General
- One or more arteries enter the lymph node at the hilum and branch within the medulla.
- Capillary networks form in the cortex and the medulla.
- High endothelial venules (HEVs) are seen in the paracortex.
- Veins run from cortex, in medullary cords, towards the hilum where they exit the lymph node

SPLEEN

General
- Secondary lymphatic organ located in the left upper quadrant of the abdomen.
- The spleen is, despite its important functions, not necessary for human life.

Structure
- $4 \times 8 \times 12$ cm, 150–200 g
- Capsule of dense connective tissue and strands of smooth muscle tissue
  - Trabeculae of connective tissue from the inner part of the capsule run down into the parenchyma.
  - Medial thickening of the capsule at the hilum.

Function
- Immunological function:
  - In the spleen pathogens/antigens carried by the blood come in contact with the cells of the immune system leading to:
    - Cell-mediated immune response ⎱ Against
    - Humoral (antibody-mediated) immune response ⎰ blood-borne antigens
  - Removal of blood-borne macromolecular pathogens/antigens:
    - Phagocytosed by macrophages in the sheathed capillaries
- Filtration of the blood and thereby removal of old and worn out erythrocytes
- Hematopoiesis, only in fetal life

Consists of (Fig. 19.5, Table 19.6)
- Parenchyma
  - Red pulp
    - Splenic cords
    - Splenic sinusoids
- - - - Marginal zone: Zone between red and white pulp - - - - - - -

- ○ White pulp (Splenic nodules)
  - ▪ Diffuse lymphatic tissue (thymus-dependent zone)
    - • Periarterial lymphatic sheath (PALS)
  - ▪ Lymphatic follicles (bone marrow-dependent zone)
    - • Primary and secondary lymphatic follicles
- • Stroma
  - ○ Reticular connective tissue

Light Microscopy
See Table 19.6.

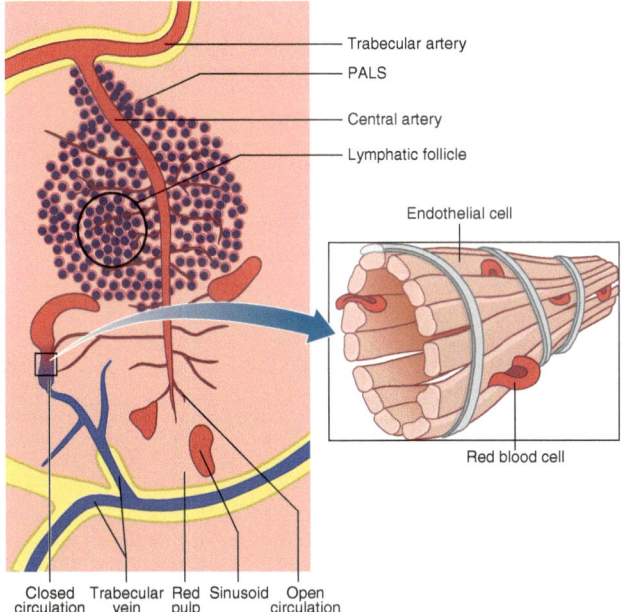

Fig. 19.5 Spleen. The parenchyma of the spleen consists of red and white pulp. Central arteries give off branches as they pass through the white pulp. After passing the white pulp, the central artery branches into penicillary arteries, which either continue into the closed circulation (splenic sinusoids) or empty into the open circulation (splenic cords). Blood cells are filtrated from the splenic cords into the closed circulation of the splenic sinusoids

Table 19.6 The spleen

	Subdivision	Function	Light microscopy
Parenchyma			
• Red pulp	80 %		Eosinophilic
	Splenic cords	Filtration of blood	Reticular connective tissue network filled with: • Blood cells • Macrophages, which phagocyte dead erythrocytes
	Splenic sinusoids	Filtration of blood	Modified capillaries: • ⊘ up to 40–50 μm • Wall consists of characteristic endothelial cells: ○ Fusiform, parallel to the blood flow, cuboidal on cross section ○ The cells are connected only by small contact complexes at each end → gaps between the cells ○ Surrounded by an incomplete basement membrane, resembling the bands of a barrel
• Marginal zone		Zone between red and white pulp	Less heavily packed lymphocytes and dendritic cells
• White pulp	20 %		Intensely basophilic
	Periarterial lymphatic sheath (PALS)	Thymus-dependent zone	• Cylinder of diffuse lymphatic tissue, surrounding the central arteries • With T lymphocytes, macrophages, dendritic cells, and plasma cells
	Lymphatic follicles	Bone marrow-dependent zone	Primary and secondary lymphatic follicles, similar to those of a lymph node
Stroma			Reticular connective tissue • Reticular fibers • Reticular cells

Blood Supply of the Spleen

Structure (Fig. 19.5)

Due to the properties of the vessels, the circulation is divided into:

• Closed circulation
• Open circulation

Function
- Nutrition
- Filtration of the blood
  - Closed circulation:
    - The blood remains intravascular (in the sinusoid lumen)
- Open circulation:
  - The blood empties into the splenic cords and is filtered on its way back into the blood circulation (i.e. into the closed circulation).
  - Old and worn erythrocytes are fragile and end up stuck in the splenic cords, where they are phagocytized by macrophages.

Consists of
See Table 19.7.

Marginal sinus

General
It is debated whether or not the human spleen has well-defined marginal sinuses, as seen in, e.g., rodents.

Structure
5–10 μm wide spaces, located between white pulp and the marginal zone (the zone between white and red pulp)

Function
- Recirculating immune cells enter the white pulp through the marginal sinus and the blood vessels of the marginal zone, i.e., they have a function similar to that of the HEVs of the lymph node.
- Pathogens enter the white pulp of the spleen from the blood vessels of the marginal zone.

MUCOSA-ASSOCIATED LYMPHATIC TISSUE (MALT)

General
- Located in mucous membranes (lamina propria) throughout the body.
- Pathogens reach MALT through the overlying epithelium.

Function
- Secondary lymphatic organs, where immunocompetent lymphocytes are activated.
- Larger accumulations of MALT function as lymph nodes, giving rise to:

Table 19.7 Blood supply of the spleen

	Vessels			Special features
Arteries	The splenic artery (a. splenica) ↓			
	Rr. splenici (end arteries) ↓			
	Trabecular arteries ↓			
	Central arteries			• Embedded in PALS • Actually an arteriole, but called a central artery
	Radiating branches (in white pulp) ↓	Penicillary arteries (in red pulp) ↓		After passing PALS the central arteries branch into penicillary arteries, which radiate out from one shared branching point
Microcirculation	Capillary networks in: • The marginal zone • The white pulp ↓ Marginal sinus ↓	Red pulp capillaries ↓		Some of the red pulp capillaries are sheathed capillaries, i.e., surrounded by a sheath of macrophages
	Splenic cords of the red pulp ↓	Splenic cords of the red pulp ↓		Open circulation, i.e., blood cells are extravascular
	Splenic sinusoids	Splenic sinusoids		Closed circulation, i.e., blood cells are intravascular
Veins	Small red pulp veins ↓			
	Trabecular veins ↓			
	Splenic vein (v. splenica)			

  ○ Cell-mediated immune response
  ○ Humoral (antibody-mediated) immune response
    ▪ IgA are secreted into exocrine discharges or directly onto the luminal surface.
    ▪ IgG and IgM are secreted into the lamina propria.

Consists of
- Diffuse lymphatic tissue
  ○ Abundant IgA-secreting plasma cells
- Dispersed lymphatic follicles (follicular lymphatic tissue)
- Intraepithelial T lymphocytes

Divided into
- Gut-associated lymphatic tissue (GALT)
  ○ Tonsils (Waldeyer's ring) (Chap. 21)
    ▪ Pharyngeal tonsil
    ▪ Palatine tonsils (paired)
    ▪ Lingual tonsils
  ○ Peyer's patches (Fig. 19.6, Table 19.8)
    ▪ Accumulations of diffuse lymphatic tissue and lymphatic follicles
    ▪ Located in the small intestine, most abundant in ileum
  ○ Appendix vermiformis
  ○ Solitary lymphatic follicles
- Bronchus-associated lymphoid tissue (BALT)
- Urinary-mucosa associated lymphoid tissue (UALT)

M cells of GALT

General
Specialized antigen-transporting cells located in the gut epithelium overlying the Peyer's patches.

Function
M cells in the overlying epithelium bring antigens into contact with the lymphatic tissue of the Peyer's patches:
1. Endocytosis of antigens from the gut lumen.
2. Transport of the antigens by transcytosis through epithelium, to the intercellular space/underlying connective tissue.
3. Antigens encounter underlying diffuse and follicular lymphatic tissue of the Peyer's patches.

Light Microscopy
- Cuboidal epithelial cells
- Abundant luminal microfolds (not microvilli)

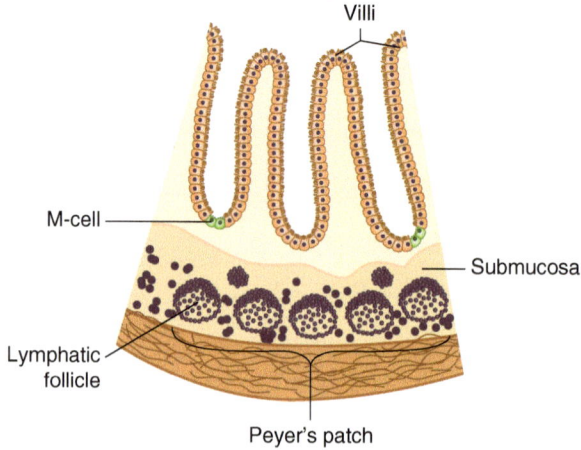

Fig. 19.6 Peyer's patch. In the space between villi of the distal small intestine, M cells appear in the epithelium. Underneath the M cells, both follicular and diffuse lymphatic tissue is seen in the lamina propria

Table 19.8 Overview over the major secondary lymphatic organs

| | Lymphatic vessels | | Antigen reach organ through | Bone marrow-dependent zone (lymphatic follicles) | Thymus-dependent zone | Site of immune cell migration |
	Afferent	Efferent				
Lymph node	+	+	Afferent lymphatic vessels	Superficial cortex	Paracortex	High endothelial venules in the paracortex
Spleen	−	+	The blood → filtrated in the marginal zone and the splenic cords	Follicular lymphatic tissue in relation to PALS	PALS	• Blood vessels of the marginal zone • The marginal sinus
Peyer's patches	−	+	Transcytosis through the overlying epithelium (M cells)	Follicular lymphatic tissue in lamina propria of the small intestine	Diffuse lymphatic tissue in lamina propria of the small intestine	Venules of the diffuse lymphatic tissue in lamina propria

Guide to Practical Histology: The Immune System and the Lymphatic Organs

General
- Lymphocytes:
  - Small, spherical cells
  - Basophilic cytoplasm surrounding a large, intensely basophilic nucleus
- Lymphatic tissues and lymphatic infiltrations:
  - Densely basophilic due to a high density of lymphocytes.
  - In follicular lymphatic tissue, the cells are arranged in rounded aggregations (follicles).

Special staining
Silver:
- Reticular fibers of the stroma of all secondary lymphatic organs and tissues are stained black/brown.

Thymus

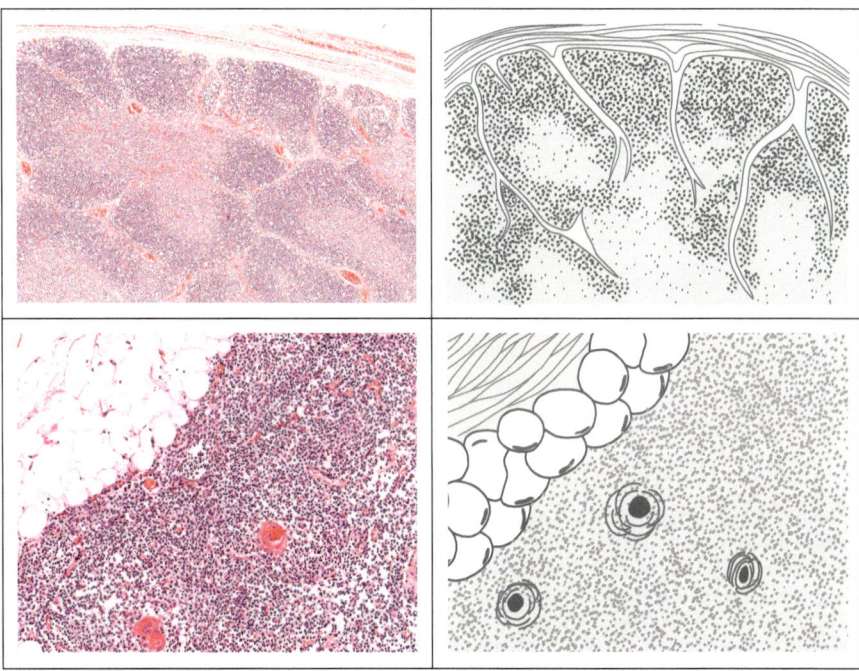

Top panel, left: photomicrograph of the thymus. Magnification: low. Stain: HE (Courtesy of associate professor Steen Seier Poulsen, University of Copenhagen). *Top panel, right*: simplified illustration of the thymus. *Bottom panel, left*: photomicrograph of the thymus: fat infiltrations indicate that the thymus is from an old individual. Magnification: high. Stain: HE (Courtesy of associate professor Steen Seier Poulsen, University of Copenhagen). *Bottom panel, right*: simplified illustration of the thymus

Characteristics

- Low magnification:
  - A dark, basophilic cortex surrounds a lighter, eosinophilic medulla.
  - The parenchyma is incompletely divided into lobules, by trabeculae of dense connective tissue.
  - Capsule of dense connective tissue.
- Higher magnification:
  - Hassall's bodies are seen in the thymic medulla.
- As the individual grows older, the thymic tissue is replaced by adipose tissue, which is why some specimens contain numerous adipocytes.

Can be mistaken for

The parathyroid glands:

- Are not divided into a cortex and a medulla
- Do not contain any Hassall's bodies.

Lymph Node

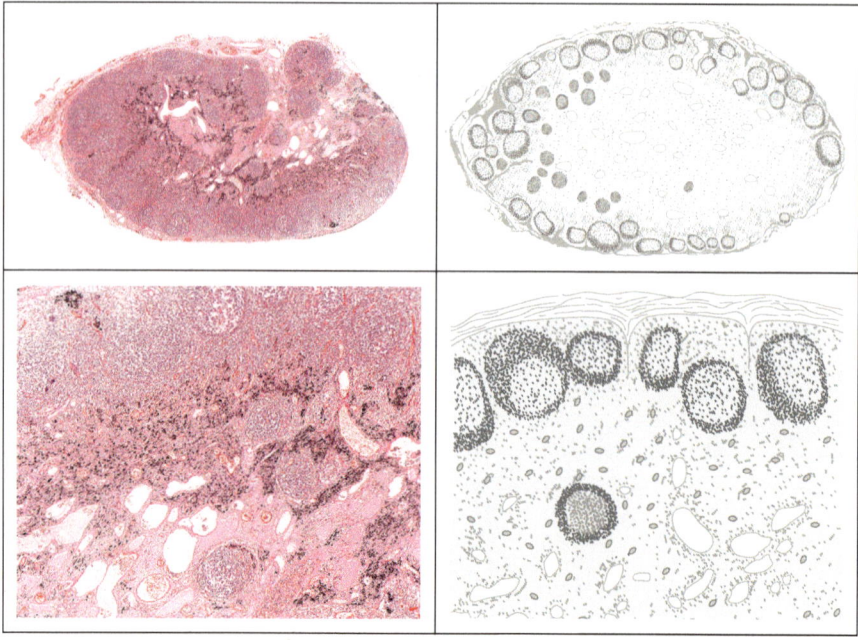

Top panel, *left*: photomicrograph of a lymph node: the lymphatic tissue is black due to accumulated carbon (anthracotic lymphatic tissue). Magnification: low. Stain: HE (Courtesy of associate professor Steen Seier Poulsen, University of Copenhagen). *Top panel*, *right*: simplified illustration of a lymph node. *Bottom panel*, *left*: photomicrograph of a lymph node. Magnification: high. Stain: HE (Courtesy of associate professor Steen Seier Poulsen, University of Copenhagen). *Bottom panel*, *right*: simplified illustration of a lymph node

Characteristics

- Macroscopic:
  - A round or bean-shaped structure surrounded by a connective tissue capsule
- Microscopic:
  - Low magnification:
    - A central light eosinophilic medulla:
      - Contains medullary lymphatic sinuses converging at the hilum
    - A peripheral darker cortex:
      - Lymphatic follicles are seen in the superficial cortex.
      - Diffuse lymphatic tissue is seen in the deeper cortex.

Can be mistaken for

Tonsils (pharyngeal, lingual, and palatine):

- An epithelium covers some part of their surface.
- Do not have a medulla with lymphatic sinuses.

Spleen

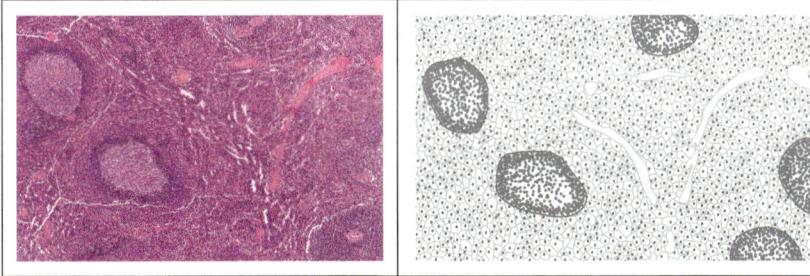

Left: photomicrograph of the spleen with central arteries in PALS. Magnification: low. Stain: HE (Courtesy of associate professor Steen Seier Poulsen, University of Copenhagen). *Right*: simplified illustration of the spleen

Characteristics

- Low magnification:
  - An eosinophilic "ocean" of red pulp, with scattered basophilic "islets" of white pulp
- Higher magnification:
  - The white pulp is seen as basophilic diffuse lymphatic tissue (PALS) surrounding a central artery. Lymphatic follicles are seen associated with the PALS.
  - The central arteries are often located in the periphery of the white pulp.

References

5, 25, 33, 34, 45.

Chapter 20
The Integumentary System

Contents

General
- The skin is a large organ covering the external surface of the body.
  - Continuous with mucosal membranes at all body openings
- Skin thickness (epidermis plus dermis) varies between body regions, e.g.:
  - Thick skin on the back
  - Thin skin on the eyelid

Function
- Barrier, protecting against, e.g.:
  - UV-radiation
  - Mechanical tear
  - Chemical agents
  - Microorganisms, as part of the innate immune system
  - Evaporation → maintenance of the body's fluid balance
  - Heat and cold

© Springer International Publishing Switzerland 2017
A. Rehfeld et al., *Compendium of Histology*, DOI 10.1007/978-3-319-41873-5_20

- Regulation of temperature:
  - Cooling down by
    - Directing the blood through the superficial blood vessels
    - Sweating
  - Keeping warm by
    - Directing the blood away from the superficial blood vessels
    - Rising the hairs as "goose bumps" → keeps warm air trapped on the skin surface (insulation)
- Secretion
  - Endocrine: e.g., inactive vitamin D (cholecalciferol)
  - Exocrine: e.g., sebum
- Absorption, e.g., drugs from drug patches
- Sensory organ

Consists of
- The skin
  - Epidermis:
    - Most superficial layer
    - Epithelium
    - Forms a barrier
  - Dermis:
    - Layer profound to the epidermis
    - Connective tissue
    - Gives strength and elasticity to the skin
  - Hypodermis:
    - Technically not a layer of the skin
    - Traditionally described along with the skin as it binds the skin to deeper structures
    - Adipose tissue and connective tissue
- Epidermal derivatives
  - Hair and hair follicles
  - Nails
  - Glands
- Sensory organs of the skin

Epidermis

General
- The most superficial layer of the skin
- Avascular and nourished by diffusion from capillaries in the underlying stratum papillare of dermis

Structure

- 0.1–1.5 mm thick.
  - The histological terms thick and thin skin relates to the thickness of the epidermis.
    - Thick epidermis is hairless and only seen in the palm and foot sole.
    - Thin epidermis is seen in all other areas.
- The external surface is divided into polygonal areas.
- Parallel ridges are seen in the palm and foot sole.

Consists of (Fig. 20.1)

Keratinized, stratified, squamous epithelium:
- Five defined layers in thin epidermis (no stratum lucidum)
- Six defined layers in thick epidermis (from surface to basement membrane):

6. Stratum disjunctum: cornified keratinized cells, desquamating
5. Stratum corneum: several layers of cornified keratinized cells
4. Stratum lucidum: only seen in thick skin
3. Stratum granulosum: three to five layers of granular cells
2. Stratum spinosum: several layers of spinous cells (prickle cells)
1. Stratum basale: a single layer of basal cells
0. Basement membrane

Growth and differentiation

MEMO-BOX

The layers of epidermis can be remembered by "**D**id **C**inderella **l**eave **g**lass **s**hoe **b**ehind?"

Stratum **d**isjunctum
Stratum **c**orneum
Stratum **l**ucidum
Stratum **g**ranulosum
Stratum **s**pinosum
Stratum **b**asale

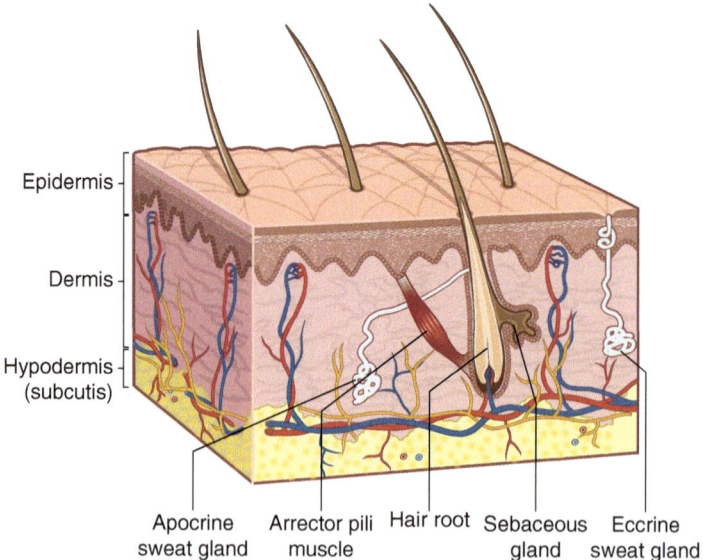

Epidermis

Dermis

Hypodermis
(subcutis)

Apocrine   Arrector pili   Hair root   Sebaceous   Eccrine
sweat gland   muscle   gland   sweat gland

Fig. 20.1 Skin and epidermal derivates

THE CELLS OF EPIDERMIS

Divided into
- Keratinocytes, specialized epithelial cells
- Non-keratinocytes

Keratinocytes

General
- It takes approximately four weeks for a keratinocyte to proliferate, differentiate, and "travel" from stratum basale to stratum corneum, i.e., the skin regenerates in four weeks.
- Keratinocytes are of ectodermal origin.

Structure
- Adjacent keratinocytes are connected through desmosomes, and the basal cells are attached to the basement membrane with focal adhesions and hemi-desmosomes (Chap. 5).
- Keratinocytes of the basal layer are separated from dermis by a basement membrane.

Divided into
From surface to basement membrane:
- Cornified cells, in stratum corneum and disjunctum
- Granular cells, in stratum granulosum
- Spinous cells, in stratum spinosum
- Basal cells, in stratum basale

Light Microscopy
See Table 20.1.

Keratinization

1. Keratinocytes continuously produce keratin filaments as they move up through the stratum basale, spinosum, and granulosum.
2. In the stratum granulosum, keratohyalin granules appear, and their protein content is released into the cytoplasm.
   - The released proteins promote aggregation of keratin filaments into tonofibrils within the cytoplasm of the keratinocytes, i.e., stimulates keratinization.
3. Granular cells become cornified cells as:
   - The cytoplasm fills up with keratin filaments (seen in bundles, tonofibrils).
   - The cells lose their nuclei and organelles.
   - The process is called keratinization and is a kind of apoptosis.
4. Stratum corneum consists of keratinized, dead cells.

Formation of the epidermal fluid barrier

General
1. Membrane-bounded lamellar bodies, containing glycolipids, appear in the stratum spinosum.
2. The glycolipids are exocytosed in stratum granulosum.
3. The lipids form the mortar between the cornified cells (dead keratinocytes) in the stratum corneum and make up a part of the epidermal fluid barrier.

Function
The epidermal fluid barrier prevents loss and absorption of fluid through the skin → assists in maintaining body fluid homeostasis.

Table 20.1 Light microscopy of keratinocytes

Layer	Cell	Nucleus	Ultrastructure	Event in cells	Growth and differentiation ←
6. Stratum disjunctum and 5. Stratum corneum	Cornified cells • Flattened dead eosinophilic cells	No nuclei	• No organelles • Completely filled up with keratin (eosinophilic)	Cells shed off as stratum disjunctum	
4. Stratum lucidum (in thick epidermis)	Cornified cells • Flattened dead eosinophilic cells • Seen as a translucent, light eosinophilic rim	No nuclei	• No organelles • Completely filled up with keratin (eosinophilic)		
3. Stratum granulosum	Granular cells • Steadily more flattened towards the surface of the skin • Contain numerous intensely basophilic keratohyalin granules containing precursor proteins for keratin aggregation	Elongated	• Lamellar bodies are in the peripheral part of the cells • Abundant keratin filaments	Exocytosis of the lamellar bodies in the outer part of stratum granulosum → the lipids form the mortar between the dead keratinocytes of stratum corneum, an important part of the epidermal fluid barrier	
2. Stratum spinosum	Spinous cells • Polygonal • Intercellular bridges: Spinous processes of neighboring cells, connected by desmosomes	Round → ovoid	• Abundant keratin filaments • Membrane-bounded lamellar bodies, (150 nm) containing glycolipids		
1. Stratum basale	Basal cells • Small • Cuboidal • Basophilic	Round	• Abundant free ribosomes • Keratin filaments	Stem cells • Divide frequently • Give rise to new keratinocytes	

Non-keratinocytes

Consist of
- Melanocytes
- Langerhans cells (dendritic cells of the skin)
- Merkel's cells
- Intraepithelial T lymphocytes

Melanocytes

General
- Derived from the neural crest.
- All individuals have the same density of melanocytes.
- Individuals that originate from close to the equator have faster melanin production and greater melanin accumulation in the keratinocytes → more pigment in epidermis and hair

Structure
- Melanocytes are not connected with desmosomes to neighboring keratinocytes, but attached to the basement membrane.
- Epidermal-melanin unit: a melanocyte and the keratinocytes to which it secretes melanin.

Function
- Protection of the DNA of the keratinocytes from UV-radiation, through production of melanin granules (melanosomes).
- Melanin granules are, via a special form of secretion (cytocrine secretion), directly transferred to the cytoplasm of the keratinocytes of the stratum basale.
  - The melanocytes have long cell extensions, which enter the cytoplasm of the surrounding basal cells to deposit melanin granules.
  - The granules are placed on the "sunny side" of the basal cells' nuclei.
  - The melanin granules remain in the keratinocyte as it moves towards the surface of the skin.
- Melanin synthesis is stimulated by paracrine factors secreted by keratinocytes in response to UV-radiation.

Light Microscopy
See Table 20.2.

Langerhans cells

General
Not connected with desmosomes to neighboring keratinocytes

Function
- Antigen-presenting cells (part of the immune system)
- Ingest, process, and transport antigens to regional lymph nodes, where the Langerhans cell presents antigens to lymphocytes (Chap. 19).

Light Microscopy
See Table 20.2.

Merkel's cells

General
- Mechanoreceptor
- Located in relation to the terminal bulb of an afferent nerve fiber, which penetrates the basement membrane
- Attached by desmosomes to keratinocytes in the stratum basale

Function
Slowly adapting mechanoreceptors, detecting light touch

Light Microscopy
See Table 20.2.

Intraepithelial T lymphocytes

General
Part of the immune system: skin-associated lymphoid tissue (SALT) (Chap. 19)

Light microscopy
See Table 20.2.

Table 20.2 Light microscopy of non-keratinocytes

	Cell	Nucleus	Ultrastructure	Location
Melanocytes	• Rounded • Pale • Long cell extensions containing melanin granules	Elongated	• Melanosomes (melanin granules) approximately 1 μm ⊘ • Numerous mitochondria, rER, and well-developed Golgi apparatus	Stratum basale
Langerhans cells	• Weakly stained • Branched cytoplasmic processes form a 3D network in epidermis, able to encounter invading antigens	Dark basophilic	Birbeck granules: striated racquet-shaped granules, with no known function	All of the epidermal layers, most abundantly in stratum spinosum
Intraepithelial T lymphocytes	• Round cell • Thin rim of basophilic cytoplasm	Large, round, dark	Abundant free ribosomes	All of the epidermal layers, most abundantly in the basal layers
Merkel's cells	• Small oval • Dark cytoplasm	Lobulated	Small dense-core granules with neurosecretory material	Stratum basale, especially in areas with great sensibility, e.g., fingertips

Dermis

General
- Dermal thickness varies throughout the body, thickest on the back (4–5 mm).
- Clear border towards the epidermis, not as distinct border towards the hypodermis.

Function
- Mechanical support:
  - Binding epidermis tightly to the subcutaneous tissue.
- Nutritive:
  - Diffusion of nutrients and gasses between the capillaries in dermis' stratum papillare and the cells of epidermis.
- Thermoregulatory:
  - Arteriovenous anastomoses (Chap. 17) in dermis regulate the body temperature through controlled loss of heat.

Consists of
- Stratum papillare (papillary layer)
- Stratum reticulare (reticular layer)
  - In some parts of the body stratum reticulare (and hypodermis) contains muscle tissue.
    - Smooth muscle tissue: areolae, penis, labia majora, scrotum, and the arrector pili muscles (mm. arrector pili).
    - Skeletal muscle tissue: facial muscles and m. platysma.

Light Microscopy
- Stratum papillare
  - Relatively thin layer of well-vascularized loose connective tissue
  - Cells:
    - Macrophages
    - Fibroblasts
    - Mast cells
  - Meissner's corpuscles and associated nerve fibers
  - Well-developed network of blood and lymphatic vessels
- Stratum reticulare
  - Dense irregular connective tissue with collagen and elastic fibers
  - Fewer cells and more fibers than the stratum papillare
  - Cells:
    - Macrophages
    - Fibroblasts
    - Mast cells
  - Pacinian and Ruffini's corpuscles and associated nerve fibers
  - Well-developed network of blood and lymphatic vessels

Dermo-epidermal junction

Structure
- Fingerlike dermal papillae from stratum papillare protrude into the epidermis
  - Interdigitate with ridges from the basal portion of epidermis
- Seen as "waves" on a perpendicular section
- Most noticeable in (histologically) thick skin
- Creates an increased interface between the two layers

Hypodermis (Subcutis)

Structure
- Divided into lobules by septae of connective tissue:
  - Septae are adherent to the dense connective tissue of dermis and of underlying fascia/periosteum.
- Well vascularized

Function
- Energy reserve
- Isolation

Consists of
White adipose tissue (Chap. 11) and loose connective tissue

Epidermal Derivatives

Consist of
- Hair and hair follicle
- Nail
- Glands:
  - Sebaceous glands
  - Eccrine sweat glands
  - Apocrine sweat glands

HAIR AND HAIR FOLLICLES

General
Hair grows all over the body, except on the lips, palms, foot soles, glans penis, clitoris, and labia minora.

Structure
- Hairs are elongated keratinized structures.
- The hair is produced in hair follicles (invaginations of the epidermis).
- A pilosebaceous unit consists of:
  - A hair
  - A hair follicle
  - Associated sebaceous glands and m. arrector pili

Function
- Regulation of body temperature
  - Contraction of the arrector pili muscles → the hair rises to capture warm air close to the skin surface, seen as "goose bumps."
- Tactile sensation

Divided into
- Vellus hairs
  - Thin, "invisible" hairs, e.g., hair on the ventral part of the forearm
- Terminal hairs
  - Coarse "visible" hairs, e.g., on the scalp, in armpits, and around the genitals

Consist of (Fig. 20.1)
- Hair
  - Hair shaft
  - Hair root: anchored in the hair follicle
- Hair follicle
  - Sheaths: run diagonally through dermis, enclosing the hair shaft
    - Epidermal sheaths
      - Internal root sheath
      - External root sheath
    - Glassy membrane
    - Dermal sheath
  - Hair bulb: expanded proximal part of the hair follicle

Light Microscopy
- Hair
  - Medulla (only in terminal hairs): large, vacuolated cells
  - Cortex: keratinized, cuboidal, densely packed cells
  - Cuticle: squamous keratinized cells
- Hair follicle
  - Sheaths:
    - Epidermal sheaths
      - Internal root sheath: surrounds the profound part of the hair root, ends at the level of the sebaceous gland.
      - External root sheath: surrounds the hair, all the way to the epidermis where it is continuous with stratum basale and stratum spinosum.
    - Glassy membrane
      - Avascular, thick basement membrane.
      - Separates the hair follicle from the dermal root sheath.
    - Dermal root sheath
      - Connective tissue sheath
      - The arrector pili muscles run from the middle of the dermal root sheath to the stratum papillare of dermis.
  - Hair bulb:
    - A dermal papilla of well-vascularized connective tissue from the stratum papillare of dermis bulges into the base of the bulb.
    - The area adjacent to the dermal papilla is called matrix, where proliferation and differentiation of keratinocytes lead to formation of the hair.
    - Melanocytes in the matrix are responsible for the pigmentation of the hair.

Hair growth
- The hair is produced through proliferation and differentiation of the cells in the matrix of the hair bulb.
- The hair grows discontinuously and asynchronously, in three phases:
  - Anagen phase:
    - A long period where cells in matrix proliferate and the hair grows
  - Catagen phase:
    - Short period where the hair bulb degenerates and hair growth stops
  - Telogen phase:
    - A long period with inactivity and shedding of the hair

NAIL

Consists of (Fig. 20.2)
- Nail plate
  - Several layers of densely packed, flattened keratinized cells
  - Special areas of nail plate:
    - Lunula
      - A light crescent in the proximal part of the nail
      - Partly covered by the cuticle
    - Nail root
      - Most proximal part
      - Buried in an epidermal fold
- Underlying structures:
  - Nail bed
    - The major (distal) part of the nail lays on the nail bed.
    - Here the epidermis consists of only two layers:
      - Stratum basale
      - Stratum spinosum
  - Matrix
    - A thick epithelium underneath the nail root and lunula
    - Stem cells here:
      1. Proliferate
      2. Move towards the nail root as they differentiate to keratinocytes and produce the keratin of the nail
- Surroundings:
  - Eponychium: epidermal fold covering the nail root
  - Hyponychium: epidermal thickening beneath the free distal end of the nail

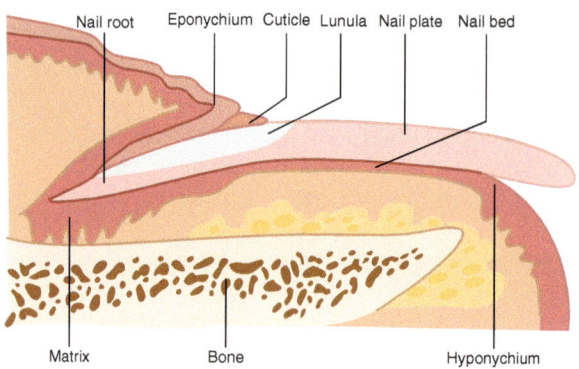

Fig. 20.2 Sagittal section of the distal part of a finger shows a nail plate on a nail bed

GLANDS OF THE SKIN

Consist of (Fig. 20.1, Table 20.3)
- Sebaceous glands
- Sweat glands:
    - Eccrine sweat glands
    - Apocrine sweat glands
- Mammary glands (Chap. 27)

Function
See Table 20.3.

Light Microscopy
See Table 20.3.

Table 20.3 Glands of the skin

	Sebaceous gland	Eccrine sweat gland	Apocrine sweat gland
Type	Simple or branched acinar	Simple coiled tubular	Simple coiled tubular (sometimes branched)

Cells in secretory end piece	• Basophilic, flattened basal cells
	• Cells fill up with lipid droplets, and the nuclei shrink as cells move towards the (non-visible) lumen
	• Connected by desmosomes
		• Stratified cuboidal epithelium:
		  ○ Clear cells (pale in HE, stains pink with PAS)
		  ○ Dark cells (darker due to abundant rER and granules for exocytosis)
		• Contractile myoepithelial cells on the basement membrane
			• Eosinophilic columnar cells:
			  ○ Secretory granules
			  ○ Apical protrusion
			• Contractile myoepithelial cells on the basement membrane

Lumen	Filled up with secretory material	Small lumen	Large lumen

Duct	• Short
	• Opens:
	  ○ Into the superficial portion of a hair follicle (most common)
	  ○ Directly onto skin or mucosal surface
		• Coiled
		• Two layers of densely eosinophilic cuboidal epithelial cells
		• Tonofilaments in apical cytoplasm
		• Opens directly onto skin surface
			• Straight
			• Two layers of eosinophilic cuboidal epithelial cells
			• Tonofilaments in apical cytoplasm
			• Opens into the superficial part of a hair follicle

Location of secretory end piece	Dermis	Deep dermis/superficial hypodermis	Deep dermis/superficial hypodermis
Development	• Outgrowth of the external root sheath of the hair follicle (most commonly) • Develops in puberty	• Invaginates from epidermis, during fetal development	• Invaginates from epidermis, during fetal development • Develops in puberty
Innervation/stimulus	• No innervation • Is stimulated by testosterone	• Autonomous nerve system • Cholinergic neurotransmitters (heat and psychological stress)	• Autonomous nerve system • Adrenergic neurotransmitters (emotional stress)
Distribution	• All over the body, except in palms and foot soles • Abundant in sebaceous areas: face, chest, and back	All over the body, except the lips and the external genitals	• The axilla, areola, nipple, and anogenital area • Ceruminous glands of the ear and the glands of Moll (associated to the eyelashes) are also modified apocrine glands
Product	Sebum	Salty sweat	Milky sweat
Function	Not known	Regulation of body temperature	• Regulation of body temperature • Secretion of pheromones
Secretion (Chap. 6)	Holocrine • The basal cells are filled up with lipids and undergo apoptosis • Cell debris and lipids are discharged as oily sebum	Merocrine • Exocytosis	Merocrine ○ Exocytosis • Apocrine (debated)

Sensory Organs of the Skin

General
Free nerve endings or specialized structures

Function
Convert stimuli into afferent nerve impulses

Divided into
- Free nerve endings (Table 20.4)
  - Free (end freely within the epidermis)
  - Associated with hair follicles
  - Associated with Merkel's cells
- Encapsulated nerve endings (surrounded by a connective tissue capsule)
  - Mechanoreceptors (Table 20.5)
  - Thermoreceptors

Table 20.4 Free nerve endings of the skin

	Location	Function	Sensitive to	Adaptation
Free (most abundant type)	End freely within the epidermis	• Nociception • Thermoreception • Mechanoreception	• Pain • Temperature • Mechanical stimuli	Fast
Associated with hair follicles	Surround bulb of hair follicles	Mechanoreceptor	Mechanical stimuli of hair	Fast
Associated with Merkel's cells	End in a disc-shaped contact with a Merkel's cell in the stratum basale of epidermis	Mechanoreceptor	Mechanical stimuli	Slow

Thermoreceptors (Krause's end bulbs)
Structure
- Small ovoid element
- Located in, e.g., oral mucosa and the skin of genitals

Function
Responsive to low temperature

Consist of
- Thin connective tissue capsule
- An unmyelinated axon ending of a myelinated axon, which branches within the capsule

Table 20.5 Encapsulated mechanoreceptors of the skin

	Meissner's corpuscles	Ruffini's corpuscles	Pacinian corpuscles
Size	150 µm long	1–2 µm long	⊘ > 1 mm in largest dimension
Structure	• Cylindrical element • One to two unmyelinated endings of myelinated axons spiral within the capsule	• Elongated fusiform element • Collagen fibers of dermis pass through the capsule • An unmyelinated ending of a myelinated axon branches between the encapsulated collagen fibers	• Large ovoid element • An unmyelinated ending of a myelinated axon is enclosed by the multilayered capsule
Capsule	• Thin • Flattened Schwann cells	• Thin • Connective issue	• Thick, multilayered • Flattened Schwann cells • Collagen fibers
Function	Sensitive to light touch	Sensitive to stretching of the skin (stimulated by displacement of collagen fibers within the capsule)	Sensitive to pressure and vibration
Adaption	Fast	Slow	Fast
Location	In stratum papillare of dermis	In deep part of dermis	In deep dermis and hypodermis

Guide to Practical Histology: The Integumentary System

Skin (Epidermis + Dermis)

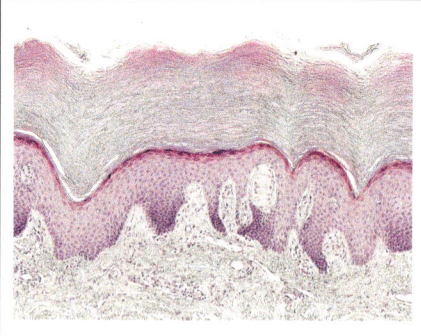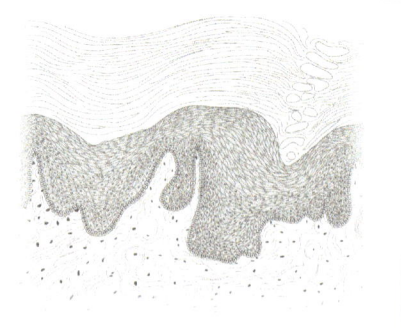

Left: photomicrograph of the skin. Magnification: low. Stain: HE (Courtesy of associate professor Steen Seier Poulsen, University of Copenhagen). *Right*: simplified illustration of the skin

Characteristics
- Epidermis
  - Keratinized stratified squamous epithelium
    - Superficial: mass of pale, flattened eosinophilic lamella (cells, lacking nuclei).
    - Middle layers: cells get gradually flattened towards the surface.
    - Basal: a layer of basophilic cells.
  - The dermo-epidermal border is well defined, and wavy.
- Dermis
  - Superficial: loose connective tissue and capillary loops form papillae, which interdigitate with the epidermis.
  - Profound: dense irregular connective tissue.
  - With hair follicles, sebaceous gland, and sweat glands.

Can be mistaken for
- Esophagus
  - The lumen is lined with nonkeratinized stratified epithelium.
    - Superficial cells have nuclei.
- Vagina
  - The lumen is lined with nonkeratinized stratified epithelium.
    - Superficial cells have nuclei.

Hair Follicle

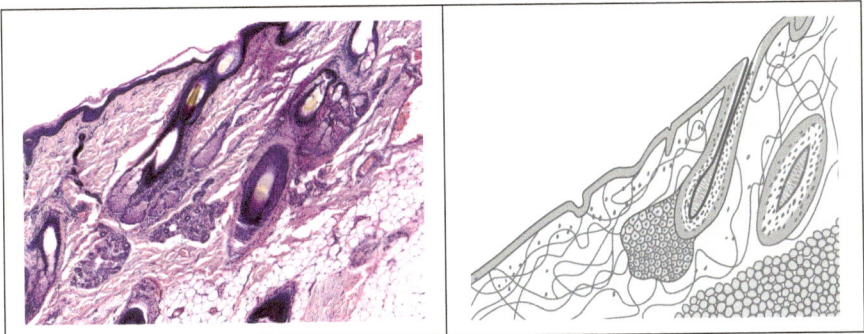

Left: photomicrograph of skin from the scalp with hair follicles, sebaceous glands, and eccrine sweat glands in dermis. There are several tangential sections of each hair follicle (seen in a row), and the superficial part of the duct of the eccrine sweat gland (upper left). Magnification: low. Stain: HE (Courtesy of associate professor Steen Seier Poulsen, University of Copenhagen). *Right*: simplified illustration of skin from the scalp

Characteristics

- An epidermal invagination into the dermis.
  - Dark chords of cells surrounding a lighter channel holding the hair shaft.
- In relation the hair follicle is a sebaceous gland (looks like a "grape cluster").

Sweat Glands

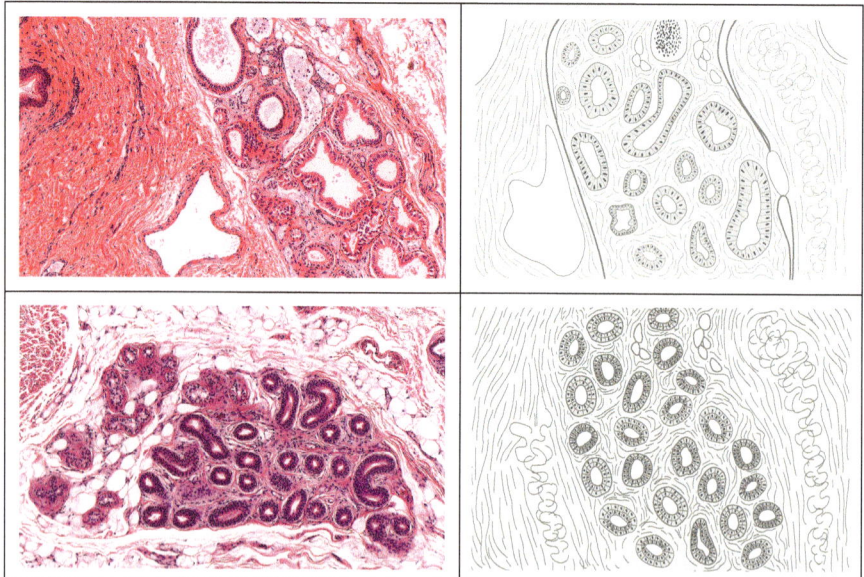

Top left: photomicrograph of the secretory part of an apocrine sweat gland. Magnification: low. Stain: HE (Courtesy of associate professor Steen Seier Poulsen, University of Copenhagen.) *Top right*: simplified illustration of apocrine sweat gland. *Bottom left*: photomicrograph of the secretory part of an eccrine sweat gland. Magnification: low. Stain: HE (Courtesy of associate professor Steen Seier Poulsen, University of Copenhagen). *Bottom right*: simplified illustration of eccrine sweat gland

Characteristics

Groups of cross sections of the tubules are seen in the deep dermis/subcutis.

- Eccrine sweat glands:
  - Thin tubules with a small lumen.
  - The epidermal part of the duct is corkscrew-shaped, seen as multiple cross sections of the duct "on a row."
- Apocrine sweat glands:
  - Thick tubules with a large lumen.
  - The apical part of the gland cells of the secretory end piece bulges into the lumen.

Pacinian Corpuscles

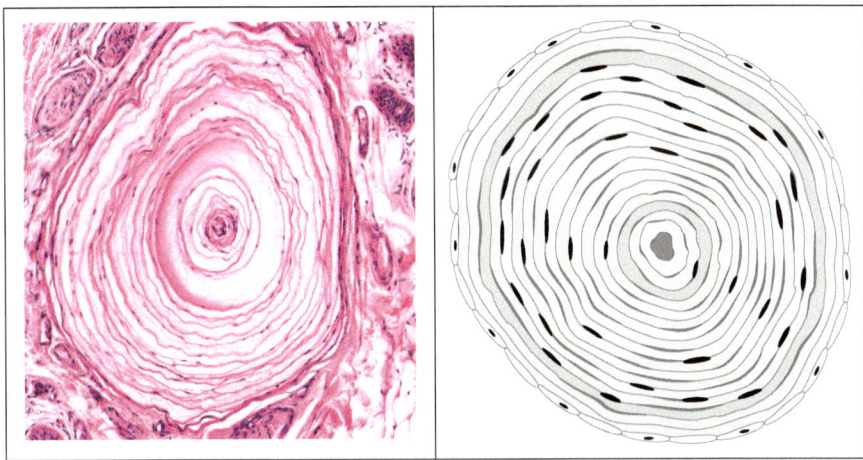

Left: photomicrograph of a Pacinian corpuscle. Magnification: low. Stain: HE (Courtesy of associate professor Steen Seier Poulsen, University of Copenhagen). *Right*: simplified illustration of a Pacinian corpuscle

Characteristics
- Ovoid structures found in the deep dermis and hypodermis
- Concentric lamellae, resembles an onion

Meissner's Corpuscle

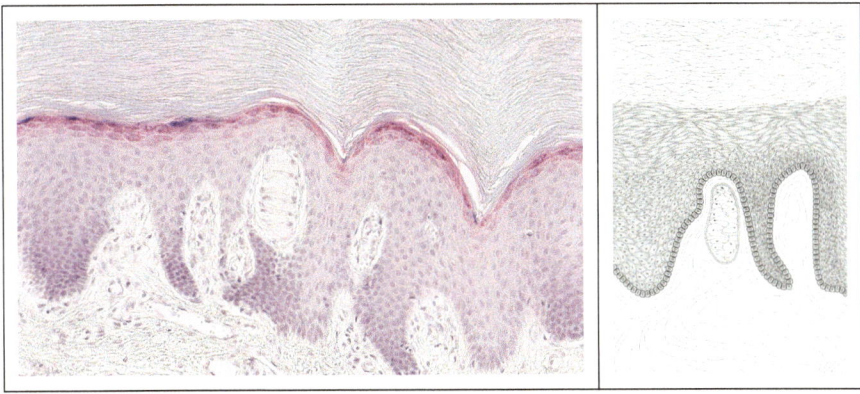

Left: photomicrograph of skin with Meissner's corpuscles (centrally in photo). Magnification: high. Stain: HE (Courtesy of associate professor Steen Seier Poulsen, University of Copenhagen). *Right*: simplified illustration of a Meissner's corpuscle

Characteristics
- Cylinder-shaped structures arranged perpendicular to the skin surface
- With irregular lamellae parallel to the skin surface
- Seen in the papillary layer of the dermis

References

5, 25, 33, 34, 45.

Chapter 21
The Digestive System I: The Alimentary Canal

Contents

Introduction to the Digestive System

General
- A group of organs that work together to digest food and liquids.
- The process of digestion takes place in several stages.

Consists of
- The alimentary canal (canalis alimentarius)
- Associated organs (Chap. 22)
  - Salivary glands (glandulae salivaria)
  - Liver (hepar)
  - Gallbladder (vesica biliaris)
  - Pancreas

© Springer International Publishing Switzerland 2017
A. Rehfeld et al., *Compendium of Histology*, DOI 10.1007/978-3-319-41873-5_21

The Alimentary Canal

General
- A muscular tube that runs between the mouth and the anus
- Lined with a mucous membrane (mucosa)

Function
- Ingestion of food and liquid
- Digestion of food and liquid
- Transportation of food, liquid, chyme, and feces
- Absorption of nutrients
- Excretion of feces

Consists of
- Mouth
  - Oral cavity (cavum oris)
  - Tongue (lingua)
  - Teeth (dentes)
  - Lips (labia oris)
  - Salivary glands (Chap. 22)
- Pharynx
  - Nasopharynx
  - Oropharynx
  - Laryngopharynx
- Esophagus
- Gastrointestinal tract
  - Stomach (ventricle, ventriculus)
  - Small intestine (intestinum tenue)
    - Duodenum
    - Jejunum
    - Ileum
  - Large intestine (intestinum crassum)
    - Colon
    - Rectum
    - Anal canal (canalis analis)

The Mouth and Pharynx

THE MOUTH

General
- First part of the alimentary canal.
- The lips constitute the external boundary.
- Communicates posterior with the oropharynx.

Consists of
- Lips
- Teeth
- Oral cavity
- Tongue
- Salivary glands (Chap. 22)

Lips (Labia oris)

General (Fig. 21.1)
- Paired structure (superior and inferior lip).
- Shape changes with the contraction of the orbicularis oris muscle.

Consists of
- External surface
- Core of skeletal muscle tissue (orbicularis oris muscle)
- Internal surface

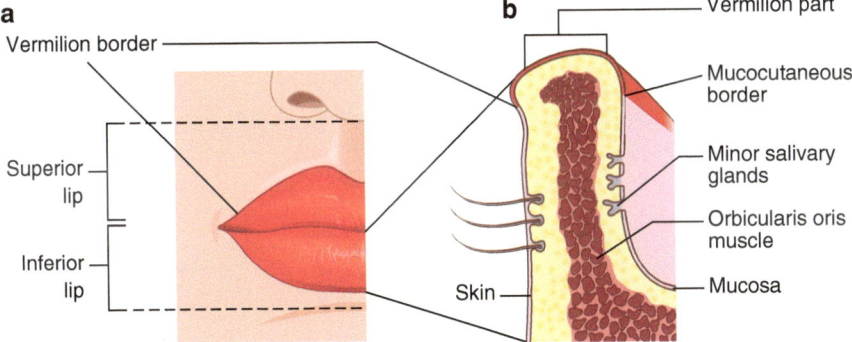

Fig. 21.1 Lips. (**a**) Showing the superior and inferior lip. (**b**) A section of the inferior lip with the external surface and the internal mucosal surface

Light Microscopy (Fig. 21.1, Table 21.1)
- The external surface:
  - Cutaneous part
    - Thin skin with:
      - Hair follicles
      - Sebaceous glands
      - Sweat glands
  - Vermilion part (red area)
    - Thin skin with:
      - Sparse sebaceous glands
      - No hair follicles
      - High dermal papillae, well vascularized → red color
- Core:
  - Skeletal muscle arranged circularly, forming the orbicularis oris muscle
- The internal surface:
  - Lined by mucous membrane (mucosa)
    - Epithelium: nonkeratinized stratified squamous
    - Lamina propria:
      - Loose connective tissue
      - Labial minor salivary glands (mucoserous with mixed end pieces)
      - Nerves

Table 21.1 External surface of the lips

	Part	*Borders*
Superior lip	• Cutaneous part	• Base of the nose
		• Vermilion border (red border)
	• Vermilion part (red area)	• Vermilion border (red border)
		• Mucocutaneous border
Inferior lip	• Vermilion part (red area)	• Mucocutaneous border
		• Vermilion border (red border)
	• Cutaneous part	• Vermilion border (red border)
		• Labiomental crease

Teeth (Dentes)

General

Humans have two sets of teeth:
- Deciduous teeth: the first, temporary set of teeth
- Permanent teeth

Structure (Fig. 21.2)

Each tooth is divided into:
- Crown
- Neck
- Root

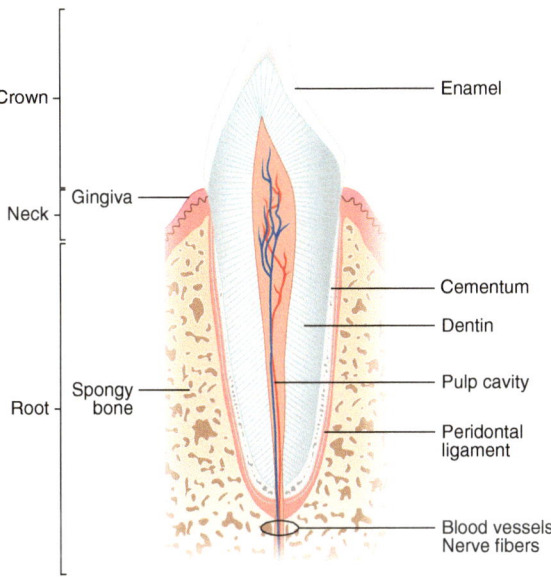

Fig. 21.2 The structure of the crown, the neck, and the root of a tooth

Function
Mastication of food

Consist of (Table 21.2)
- Hard tooth tissue
    - Enamel
    - Cementum
    - Dentin
- Soft tooth tissue
    - Pulp cavity

Table 21.2 Components of the teeth

	Enamel	Cementum	Dentin	Pulp
Structure	White, hard material: • 95 % minerals (hydroxyapatite), as in bone tissue • 5 % water and organic material	Modified bone tissue: • Cementocytes entrapped in a mineralized extracellular matrix	Yellow, hard material: • Type I collagen (90 %) • Dentinal tubules, containing processes of odontoblasts	Loose connective tissue with: • Blood vessels • Nerve fibers
Location	Covers the crown.	Covers the root	Surrounds the pulp cavity	Within the pulp cavity, which spans from the crown to the apex of the root
Function	Protection of the tooth	Attaches the tooth to the surrounding alveolar bone of the jaws	• Forms the pulpo-dentin organ of the tooth • Protection of the pulp	• Nutrition • Sensation
Production	Produced by ameloblasts: • Produced before the tooth erupts from gingiva • Ameloblasts die when the tooth erupts	Produced by modified odontoblasts (cementoblasts)	Produced by odontoblasts, which lie on the inner border of dentin	• Produced in fetal life • With age the amount of cells decreases, and amount of collagen fibers increases

Oral Cavity (Cavum Oris)

General
- A cavity with an irregular shape.
- The teeth divide the oral cavity into:
  - The vestibule
    - The space between lips, cheeks, and teeth
  - The oral cavity proper
    - The cavity posterior to the teeth

Consists of
- Mucosa:
  - Epithelium
    - Masticatory mucosa:
      - Keratinized stratified squamous epithelium
        - Keratinized due to friction from mastication (chewing)
      - Found on the gingiva and the hard palate
    - Lining mucosa:
      - Nonkeratinized stratified squamous epithelium
      - Found in main parts of the oral cavity, e.g., the cheeks and the floor of mouth
    - Specialized mucosa:
      - Contains lingual papillae
      - Can be keratinized or nonkeratinized squamous epithelium
      - Covers the anterior 2/3 part of the dorsal (upper) surface of the tongue
  - Lamina propria
    - Loose connective tissue
- The profound layers
  - Differs, depending of the region of the oral cavity, e.g.:
    - Hard palate, with underlying bone tissue
    - Cheeks with underlying muscle tissue

Tongue (Lingua)

General
- A muscular organ that projects into the oral cavity proper.
- The root of the tongue is attached to several structures, e.g., the hyoid bone.
- Contains several skeletal muscles (the Lingual muscles).

Structure (Fig. 21.3)
The terminal sulcus (sulcus terminalis), a v-shaped groove, divides the dorsal (upper) surface into:
- Anterior 2/3 part
  - Covered with numerous lingual papillae
- Posterior 1/3 part
  - Contains no lingual papillae
  - Contains:
    - Abundant lymphoid follicles
    - Lingual tonsils

Function
- Sensory organ for taste (gustation)
  - Through the taste buds of the lingual papillae
- Grinding of food during mastication
- Takes part in:
  - Articulation (speech)
  - Swallowing

Consists of
- Mucosa
  - Epithelium
    - Specialized mucosa:
      - With lingual papillae
      - Keratinized or nonkeratinized stratified squamous epithelium
      - Covers the anterior 2/3 of the dorsal surface
    - Lining mucosa:
      - Nonkeratinized stratified squamous epithelium
      - Covers the remaining surface of the tongue
  - Lamina propria:
    - Loose connective tissue
    - Serous glands (von Ebner's glands)
- Core of:
  - Skeletal muscle tissue (the lingual muscles)
  - Connective tissue with:
    - Mucous glands
    - Serous glands

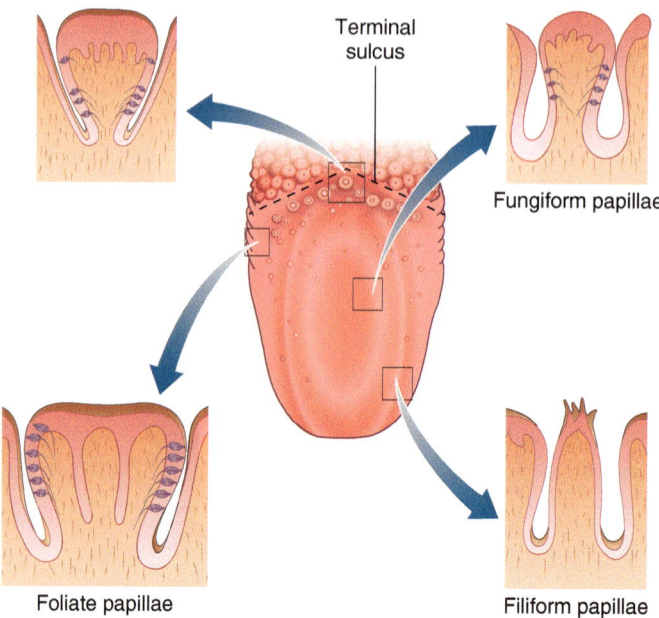

Fig. 21.3 The tongue and the location of the different types of lingual papillae

The lingual papillae

General

- Four types of papillae, scattered with different intensity on the anterior 2/3 of the dorsal upper surface of the tongue:
  - Filiform papillae
  - Fungiform papillae
  - Foliate papillae
  - Circumvallate papillae
- All types except the filiform papillae contain taste buds.

Structure

See Table 21.3.

MEMO-BOX

The name of the papillae can be remembered by:

- Foot, finger, fungus, and cream

Foot: **Fo**liate papillae
Finger: **Fi**liform papillae
Fungus: **Fu**ngiform papillae
Cream: **C**ircumvallate papillae

Table 21.3 Lingual papillae

	Filiform papillae	Fungiform papillae	Foliate papillae	Circumvallate papillae
Shape	Threadlike	Mushroomlike	• Leaflike • Consist of several, parallel ridges	Dome-like
Abundance	Most common type	Second most common type	One on each side of the tongue	8–12
Location	The entire anterior 2/3 dorsal surface of the tongue	• Scattered, solitary among the filiform papillae • Most numerous at the tip of the tongue	Lateral edge of the tongue, just anterior to the palatoglossal arch	• Just anterior to the terminal sulcus • The ducts of the serous glands open into the cleft surrounding the papillae
Taste buds	–	+	+++	+++
Keratinization	++	+	–	–

Taste buds

General (Fig. 21.4)

- Oval clusters of elongated cells found within the epithelia of the oral cavity.
- Apical surface of the cells is in contact with a small opening in the epithelium, the taste pore.
- Located in:
  - Lingual papillae
    - Fungiform papillae
    - Circumvallate papillae
    - Foliate papillae
  - Other locations:
    - The palate
    - Palatoglossal arch
    - Palatopharyngeal arch
    - Oropharynx
    - Larynx

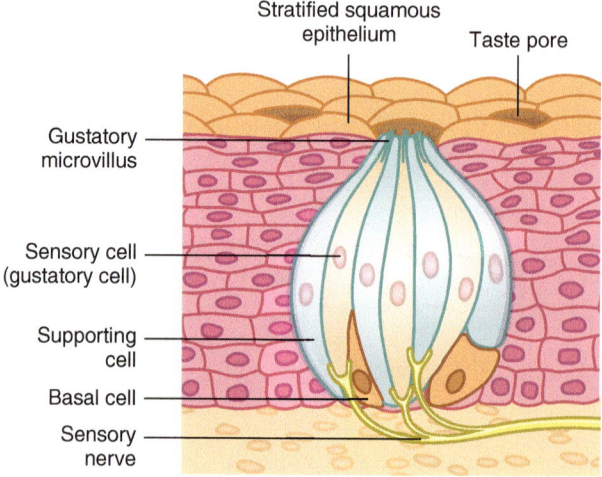

Fig. 21.4 A taste bud and the three cell types, constituting it

Function

Gustation (sense of taste):

- Certain molecules stimulate the taste receptors of the sensory cells, initiating nerve impulses in the afferent nerve fibers
- Taste is divided into:
  - Salty taste, e.g., stimulated by NaCl
  - Sour taste, e.g., stimulated by HCl
  - Sweet taste, e.g., stimulated by sucrose
  - Bitter taste, e.g., stimulated by quinine
  - Umami taste, e.g., stimulated by glutamate

Consist of

Three cell types (Table 21.4 and Fig. 21.4):
- Sensory (gustatory, neuroepithelial) cells
- Supporting (sustentacular) cells
- Basal cells

The lingual muscles

Structure
- Bundles of skeletal muscle cells
- Organized in three planes → precise movement and flexibility of the tongue

Function

Movement of the tongue, which participate in:
- Articulation (speech)
- Mastication
- Swallowing

Table 21.4 Cells of the taste buds

	Sensory cells	Supporting cells	Basal cells
Structure	• Modified elongated columnar epithelial cells • Apical microvilli with taste receptors	• Elongated epithelial cells • Apical microvilli	• Short epithelial cells • Do not reach the apical taste pore
Location	• Most numerous cells • Forms the core of the taste bud	Form the outer wall of the taste bud	At the base of the taste bud
Function	Chemoreceptor cells	Mechanical support for sensory cells	Stem cell for the other two cell types

Divided into
- Extrinsic lingual muscles:
  ○ External origin
  ○ Insertion in the tongue
- Intrinsic lingual muscles:
  ○ Origin and insertion within the tongue

Light Microscopy

Skeletal muscle cells, arranged in various directions

Innervation of the tongue

General

- Motor innervation:
  - Hypoglossal nerve.
  - Except for the palatoglossus muscle, which is innervated by the vagus nerve (cranial nerve X).
- Sensory innervation differs anterior and posterior to the terminal sulcus (Table 21.5 and Fig. 21.3).

Table 21.5   The sensory innervation of the tongue

	Posterior 1/3 part	Anterior 2/3 part
Sensibility	Glossopharyngeal nerve (cranial nerve IX)	Lingual nerve • A branch from the trigeminal nerve (cranial nerve V)
Taste (gustation)	Glossopharyngeal nerve (cranial nerve IX)	Corda tympani • A branch from the facial nerve (cranial nerve VII)

Divided into

- Sensory nerve fibers
  - General: sensibility
  - Special: taste
- Motor nerve fibers
  - Innervation of skeletal muscle cells

PHARYNX

General

- A tube connecting:
  - The nasal cavity with the larynx.
  - The oral cavity with the esophagus.
- A part of:
  - The alimentary canal.
  - The respiratory system (Chap. 18).
- Muscularis mucosae and the submucosa are both lacking in pharynx.

Divided into (Fig. 21.5)

- Nasopharynx (Chap. 18)
  - Superior part
  - Communicates with:

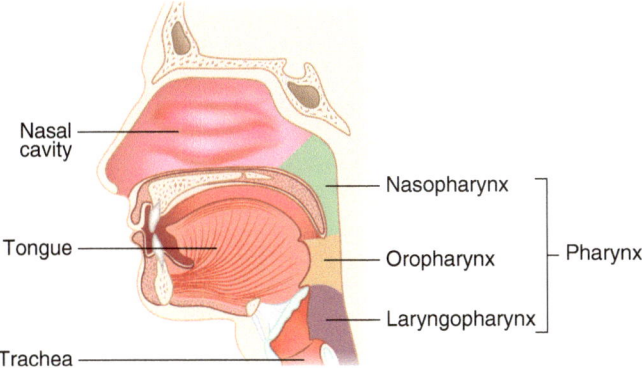

Fig. 21.5 The different parts of pharynx

- Anterior: the nasal cavities
- Lateral: the auditory tubes (Eustachian tubes, tubae auditivae) (Chap. 29)
- Inferior: the oropharynx
    - Contains the pharyngeal tonsil (tonsilla pharyngea)
- Oropharynx:
    - Middle part
    - Communicates with:
        - Superior: nasopharynx
        - Anterior: oral cavity
        - Inferior: laryngopharynx
    - Contains:
        - The most posterior, basal part of the tongue
        - Palatine tonsils
- Laryngopharynx:
    - Inferior part
    - Communicates with:
        - Superior: oropharynx
        - Anterior: larynx
        - Inferior: esophagus

Structure
- Nasopharynx (Chap. 18)
    - Mainly lined with respiratory epithelium
- Oro- and laryngopharynx
    - Mucosa
        - Epithelium
            - Nonkeratinized stratified squamous epithelium
        - Lamina propria
            - Loose connective tissue
            - A thick layer of elastic fibers oriented longitudinally

- External muscular layer (muscularis externa)
  - Skeletal muscle cells arranged in various directions
- Adventitia
  - Dense connective tissue

Tonsils

General
- Secondary lymphatic organs
- Located in the mucosa of:
  - The tongue
  - Nasopharynx
  - Oropharynx
- Constitute the tonsillar ring (Waldeyer's ring)

Structure
Aggregations of diffuse and follicular lymphatic tissue

Function
A part of the immune system, the mucosa-associated lymphatic tissue (MALT) (Chap. 19)

Consist of
See Table 21.6

Table 21.6 Tonsils

	Palatine tonsils	Lingual tonsils	Pharyngeal tonsil (adenoid)
Abundance	Two (paired)	Several	One
Location	In the oropharynx, between the: • Palatoglossal arch • Palatopharyngeal arch	Base of tongue, on the posterior 1/3 dorsal surface	The roof of nasopharynx (Chap. 18)
Mucosa			
• Epithelium	Nonkeratinized stratified squamous epithelium		Ciliated, pseudostratified columnar epithelium
• Lamina propia	Diffuse and follicular lymphatic tissue (Chap. 19)		
• Crypts in the surface	+	+	−
Capsule of dense connective tissue	Thick	−	Thin

Esophagus and the Gastrointestinal Tract

General
- Esophagus and the gastrointestinal tract have the same basic structure of the wall with four layers (from lumen → periphery):
  1. Mucosa
  2. Submucosa
  3. Muscularis externa
  4. Adventitia or serosa
- The functional differences of the distinctive parts are reflected primarily in the mucosal layer.

Structure (Fig. 21.6)
- Mucosa:
  - Epithelium
  - Lamina propria
    - A thin layer of loose connective tissue
    - Mucosa-associated lymphatic tissue (MALT) (Chap. 19)
  - Muscularis mucosae:
    - A thin layer of smooth muscle tissue
- Submucosa:
  - A thick layer of dense irregular connective tissue
  - Contains:
    - Blood vessels
    - Lymphatic vessels
    - Nerves (Meissner's plexus)
- Muscularis externa (tunica muscularis):
  - Two layers of smooth muscle tissue:
    - An inner circularly arranged layer
    - An outer longitudinally arranged layer
  - Myenteric (Auerbach's) nerve plexus located between the muscles layers
- Adventitia or serosa:
  - Adventitia:
    - Loose connective tissue containing:
      - Blood vessels
      - Lymphatic vessels
      - Nerves
    - Covers:
      - Esophagus
        - The major, proximal part
      - Parts of the gastrointestinal tract
        - Where the wall of the gastrointestinal canal is directly attached to neighboring structures, e.g., retroperitoneal organs
        - The whole surface of retroperitoneal parts

- ○ Serosa:
  - ▪ Consists of:
    - • Mesothelium: simple squamous epithelium
    - • Submesothelial loose connective tissue
  - ▪ Covers:
    - • Esophagus
      - ○ The minor, distal part
    - • Gastrointestinal tract
      - ○ Intraperitoneal parts
      - ○ Anterior surfaces of retroperitoneal parts

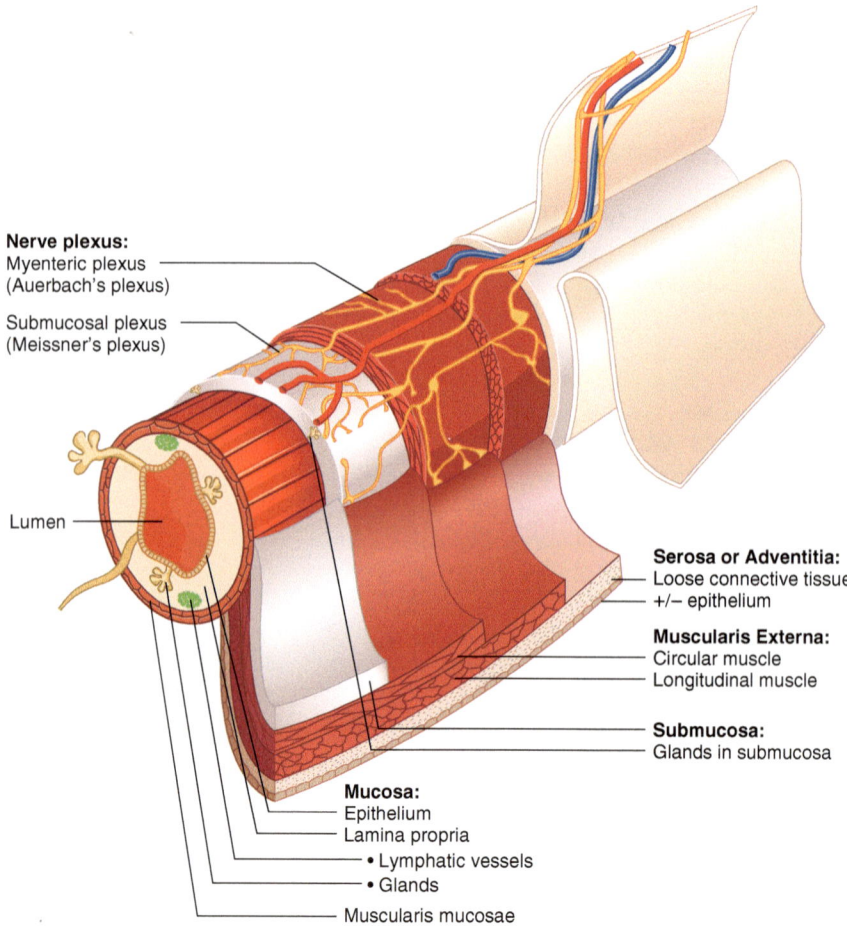

Nerve plexus:
Myenteric plexus
(Auerbach's plexus)

Submucosal plexus
(Meissner's plexus)

Lumen

Serosa or Adventitia:
Loose connective tissue
+/− epithelium

Muscularis Externa:
Circular muscle
Longitudinal muscle

Submucosa:
Glands in submucosa

Mucosa:
Epithelium
Lamina propria
• Lymphatic vessels
• Glands
Muscularis mucosae

Fig. 21.6 The general organization of the wall of the esophagus and gastrointestinal canal

Junctions

General
- The areas where one part of the gastrointestinal tract changes to the next
- Contain transition zones, where the mucosa changes abruptly

Divided into
The name indicates the location, e.g.:
- The gastroduodenal junction, between the stomach and the duodenum
- The ileocecal junction, between the ileum (small intestine) and the cecum (large intestine)
- The recto-anal junction, between the rectum and the anal canal

ESOPHAGUS

General
- A tube from oropharynx to the stomach.
- In close relation to the trachea.
- The lumen is normally collapsed and distends during passage of swallowed food/liquids.
- The epithelium has a rapid turnover.
  - Protects against the abrasive effects of ingested food.

Structure (Table 21.7)
18–25 cm long muscular tube

Function
Transportation of food/liquids from the oropharynx to the stomach

The esophageal wall

Consists of
- Mucosa
  - Epithelium
    - Thick, nonkeratinized stratified squamous epithelium
  - Lamina propria
    - Loose connective tissue
    - Esophageal cardiac glands (Table 21.7)
    - Diffuse lymphatic tissue
  - Muscularis mucosa
    - Thick, longitudinally arranged smooth muscle tissue
    - More extensive in the proximal part of the esophagus

- Submucosa
  - Dense connective tissue
  - Esophageal glands proper (Table 21.7)
  - Submucosal (Meissner's) nerve plexus
- Muscularis externa
  - Layers:
    - Inner circular layer
    - Myenteric (Auerbach's) nerve plexus
    - Outer longitudinal layer
  - Muscle tissue type:
    - The proximal 1/3 part: skeletal muscle tissue
    - The middle 1/3 part: a mixture of smooth and skeletal muscle tissue
    - The distal 1/3 part: smooth muscle tissue
- Adventitia/Serosa:
  - Adventitia
    - Loose connective tissue
    - Covers the major, proximal part
    - Attaches esophagus to surrounding structures
  - Serosa:
    - Consists of:
      - Mesothelium and submestohelial loose connective tissue
    - Covers the most distal part of the esophagus

Table 21.7 Esophageal glands

	Location	End pieces located in	Type	End pieces	Secretion
Esophageal cardiac glands	• Terminal part of esophagus • Similar to the cardiac glands of the stomach	Lamina propria	Branched tubular glands	Mucous end pieces	Neutral mucus
Esophageal glands proper	The entire length of esophagus	Submucosa	Tubuloalveolar glands	Mucous end pieces	Acidic mucus

STOMACH

General
- The widest part of the gastrointestinal tract.
- Shape and size vary with the degree of filling.

Function
- Digestion of food
  - Converts ingested food into chyme by:
    - Mechanic action on food, via contractions/peristaltics
    - Chemical action on food, via secretions (gastric juice)
- Storage of food during digestion

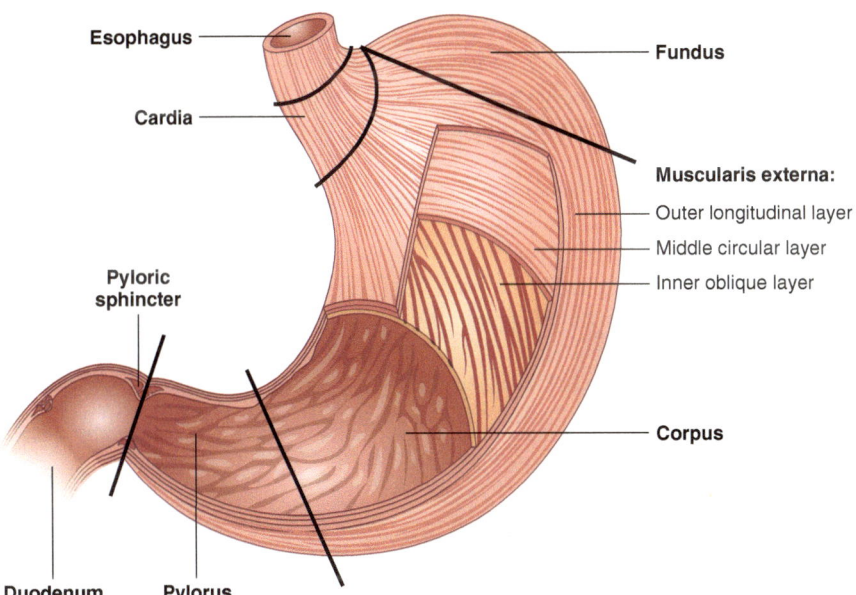

Fig. 21.7 The parts of the stomach

Divided into (Fig. 21.7)
- Cardia
  - Most proximal region
  - Surrounds the esophageal orifice
- Fundus
  - Above a horizontal line intersecting the gastroesophageal junction
- Corpus
  - Central greater part
  - Below a horizontal line intersecting the gastroesophageal junction
- Pylorus
  - Most distal funnel-shaped region
  - Leads to the pyloric sphincter between the stomach and the duodenum

Wall of the stomach

Consists of
- Mucosa
  - Epithelium
    - Simple columnar cells (resemble goblet cells).
      - Mucin granules are located apically, stains pink with PAS.
      - Ovoid, basal nuclei.
    - Secretion of mucus → a protective mucous layer between epithelium and the acidic gastric juice.
  - Lamina propria
    - Loose connective tissue
  - Muscularis mucosa
    - Smooth muscle tissue arranged in two layers:
      - Inner circular layer
      - Outer longitudinal layer
- Submucosa
  - Dense connective tissue with blood and lymphatic vessels
  - Submucosal (Meissner's) nerve plexus
- Muscularis externa (Fig. 21.7)
  - Smooth muscle tissue:
    - Inner oblique layer
    - Middle circular layer
    - Outer longitudinal layer
  - Myenteric (Auerbach's) nerve plexus is located between the muscle layers.
- Serosa
  - Mesothelium and submesothelial loose connective tissue

Inner surface specializations of the stomach

- Rugae
  - Longitudinal mucosal folds
  - Disappears when the stomach is distended
- Mammillated areas
  - Small folds dividing the surface into irregular areas
  - Increase the surface area for secretion
- Gastric pits (foveolae)
  - Millions of small openings.
  - Invaginations of the gastric mucosa.
  - The stomach glands secrete into the bottom of the gastric pits.

Stomach Glands

General
- Named after location of the gland
  - Fundic glands (gastric glands)
  - Cardiac glands
  - Pyloric glands
- Secrete into the bottom of the gastric pits

Structure
Extend from the lamina propria to the bottom of the gastric pits

Fundic glands

General
- Located in the corpus and fundic regions
- Simple, branched tubular glands

Structure (Fig. 21.8)
Each gland is divided into three segments:
- Isthmus segment (luminal part)
- Neck segment
- Fundic segment (deep part)
  - Divides into two to three branches

Function
Production of gastric juice, 2 L per day
- Acidic pH = 1–2
- Takes part in digestion as it contains pepsin, which breaks down proteins

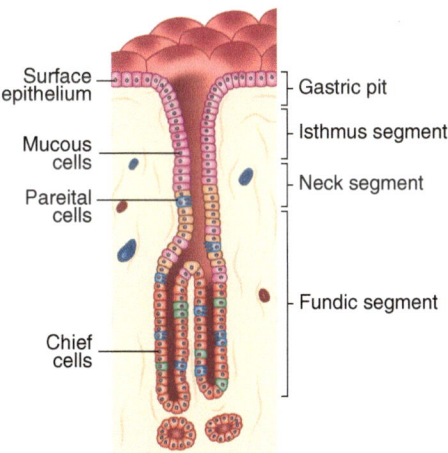

Surface epithelium — Gastric pit
Isthmus segment
Mucous cells
Neck segment
Pareital cells
Fundic segment
Chief cells

Fig. 21.8 The divisions of a fundic gland

Consist of (Table 21.8)

Five different cell types:

1. Mucous neck cells
2. Chief cells
3. Parietal cells
4. Enteroendocrine cells
5. Stem cells:
   - Differentiate into surface epithelial cells and the other cells of the gland

Table 21.8 Cells of a fundic gland

	Mucous neck cells	Chief cells	Parietal cells	Enteroendocrine cells	Stem cells
Location	Neck segment	Fundic segment	Neck segment	Every level of the gland	Isthmus segment (few cells)
Secretion:					None
• Type	Exocrine			Endocrine	
• Product	Mucus	Pepsinogen • Cleaved to pepsin, when in contact with the acidic gastric juice	• Hydrochloric acid (HCl) • Intrinsic factor	Hormones (in response to the luminal content in stomach)	
Life span	6 days	60–90 days	150–200 days	60–90 days	–
Light microscopy	As surface epithelium of the stomach (resemble goblet cells)	Cytoplasm • Basophilic basal part • Acidophilic apical part	• Large triangular cell • Acidophilic cytoplasm • 1–2 spherical nuclei	• Apical microvilli • Basal granules • Varying morphology, depending on type	Columnar cell

MEMO-BOX

The name of cells in the fundic gland can be remembered by:

- **SEC**onds **P**er **M**inute

Stem cells

Enteroendocrine cells

Chief cells

Parietal cells

Mucous neck cells

Cardiac glands

General
- Tubular, coiled, sometimes branched glands
- Located in the cardia region
- Similar to the cardiac glands of the esophagus (Table 21.7)

Function
Secretion of mucus:
- Contributes to the gastric juice
- Contributes to the formation of the protective mucous layer of the surface epithelium

Light Microscopy
Mucous end pieces

Pyloric glands

General
- Branched, coiled tubular glands
- Located in the pyloric region

Consists of
- Simple columnar cells, similar to those of the gastric surface.
  - Cells resemble goblet cells.
    - Mucin granules are located apically (stain pink with PAS).
- Enteroendocrine cells (Table 21.8).

SMALL INTESTINE

General
- The longest component of the gastrointestinal tract
- Suspended in the peritoneal cavity in a sheath of mesothelium, adipose tissue, and connective tissue (the mesentery)
  - Carries blood and lymphatic vessels to the small intestine
- The major site for digestion and absorption
- Receives:
  - Chyme from the stomach
  - Bile from the liver
  - Pancreatic juice from the exocrine pancreas (Chap. 22)

Structure
- Approximately 6 m long tubular structure
- ⊘ 2–3 cm.
- Internal surface area 30 m²

Function
- Digestion
- Absorption of the products of digestion
- Transportation of chyme from the stomach to the large intestine

Divided into (Fig. 21.9, Table 21.9)
Three continuous parts:
- Duodenum
- Jejunum
- Ileum

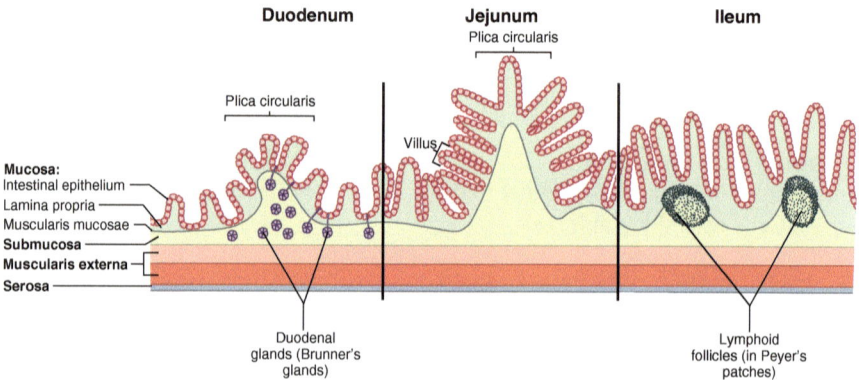

Fig. 21.9 The different parts of the small intestine and how they differ from each other

Table 21.9 The three parts of the small intestine

	Duodenum	Jejunum	Ileum
Level	Proximal (oral) part	Middle part	Distal (anal) part
Approximate length	25 cm	2.5 m	3.5 m
Begins	At the pyloric sphincter, the gastroduodenal junction	Gradually when duodenum changes morphology	Gradually when jejunum changes morphology
Ends	Gradually when duodenum changes morphology	Gradually when jejunum changes morphology	At the ileocecal junction

Wall of the small intestine

Consists of (Tables 21.10 and 21.11, Fig. 21.9)
- Mucosa
- Submucosa
- Muscularis externa
- Serosa

Table 21.10 Layers of the wall of the small intestine

	Duodenum	Jejunum	Ileum
Luminal surface specializations (Table 21.11)			
• Plica circularis	+	+	+
	Except from the first 4–5 cm	Well developed	Gradually disappearing
• Villi (0.5–1.5 mm)	+ Short, thick	+ Longest, thin	+ Long, thin
• Microvilli	+	+	+
Mucosa			
• Epithelium	Simple columnar epithelium, with six cell types • Enterocytes: tall columnar cells with apical brush border (formed by microvilli) • Goblet cells: apical cytoplasm filled with mucin vesicles • Paneth cells • Enteroendocrine cells • M cells (Chap.19) • Stem cells		
• Lamina propria	Loose connective tissue, with • Crypts of Lieberkühn (Table 21.11)		
	• Solitary lymphatic follicles (Chap. 19)		• Aggregated lymphatic follicles (Peyer's patches) (Chap. 19)

• Muscularis mucosae	• Inner layer
	  ○ Circularly arranged smooth muscle tissue
	  ○ Strands extend up into the villi
	• Outer layer
	  ○ Longitudinally arranged smooth muscle tissue		

Submucosa	Loose connective tissue with • Submucosal nerve plexus (Meissner's plexus)		
	• Branched tubular mucous glands (Brunner glands) • Alkaline secretion pH 8.0–9.0	• No glands	
Muscularis externa			
• Inner layer	Circularly arranged smooth muscle tissue		
• Middle layer	Myenteric nerve plexus (Auerbach's plexus)		
• Outer layer	Longitudinally arranged smooth muscle tissue		

Serosa	• Mesothelium and submesothelial connective tissue
	• Covers
	  ○ The entire small intestine
	  ○ The mesentery		

Table 21.11 Luminal surface specializations of the small intestine

	General	Amplification of the surface	Approximate size	Consists of
Plicae circulares	• Transverse folds of mucosa and submucosa • Circularly arranged	3 ×	1 cm	• Mucosa • Submucosa
Villi intestinales	• Projections of the mucosa • Smooth muscle tissue extends from the muscularis mucosae into the core of the villi	10 ×	1 mm	Mucosa
Microvilli	• Projections of the apical cell membrane • Gives the appearance of a striated brush border in the light microscope	20 ×	1 µm	• Apical cell membrane • A core of vertically oriented actin filaments
Crypts of Lieberkühn (intestinal glands)	• Simple tubular glands • Invaginations of the luminal surface epithelium	–	–	Several cell types, e.g.: • Enterocytes • Goblet cells • Intestinal stem cells • Enteroendocrine cells

LARGE INTESTINE

General
- The last part of the gastrointestinal tract
- Receives non-digested chyme from the small intestine

Structure
See Table 21.12.

Function
- Absorption of water and electrolytes
- Transport of feces
- Defecation: elimination of waste products and undigested food as feces

Divided into
Four continuous parts:
- Cecum with vermiform appendix
- Colon
  - Ascending colon
  - Transverse colon
  - Descending colon
  - Sigmoid colon
- Rectum
- Anal canal (canalis analis)

The Wall of the Large Intestine

Consists of (Table 21.12)
- Mucosa
- Submucosa
- Muscularis externa
- Adventitia or serosa

Table 21.12 The layers of the wall of the large intestine

	Vermiform appendix	Colon + cecum	Rectum	Anal canal
Luminal surface specializations				
• Microvilli	+	+	+	+ (disappear distal to the anal transition zone)
Mucosa				

• Epithelium	Simple columnar epithelium with four cell types
	• Enterocytes: tall columnar cells with apical brush border (microvilli)
	• Goblet cells
	  ○ Apical cytoplasm filled with mucin vesicles
	  ○ Secretion of mucin → protection of the surface epithelium and aids the transportation of feces
	• Enteroendocrine cells
	• Stem cells
				Nonkeratinized, stratified squamous epithelium distal to the anal transition zone

• Lamina propria	Loose connective with			
	An almost complete ring of multiple solitary lymphatic follicles penetrating through the muscularis mucosa	• Solitary lymphatic follicles • Crypts of Lieberkühn, similar to those in the small intestine (Table 21.11)		

• Muscularis mucosae	• Inner layer
	  ○ Circularly arranged smooth muscle tissue
	• Outer layer
	  ○ Longitudinally arranged smooth muscle tissue
				Disappears distal to the anal transition zone

Submucosa	Loose connective tissue with • Submucosal nerve plexus (Meissner's plexus)			
	• Without glands			• Anal glands
Muscularis externa				
• Inner layer	Circularly arranged smooth muscle tissue			
	Thin layer	Medium thickness		Thick layer forming the internal anal sphincter

(continued)

Table 21.12 (continued)

	Vermiform appendix	Colon + cecum	Rectum	Anal canal
• Middle layer	Myenteric nerve plexus (Auerbach's plexus)			
• Outer layer	Longitudinally arranged layer of smooth muscle tissue	• Taenia coli: smooth muscle tissue arranged in three longitudinal bands • Haustra coli: sacculations between the taenia coli	Longitudinally arranged layer of smooth muscle tissue	
Adventitia	–	Covers the retroperitoneal parts of the colon	Covers the anal 1/3 of the rectum	Covers the outer surface of the anal canal
Serosa	+	• Covers the intraperitoneal parts of the colon • Have omental appendices: Small projections with abundant adipose tissue	• Covers the anterior surface of the middle 1/3 of the rectum • Covers the proximal 1/3 of the rectum	–

ENTERIC NERVOUS SYSTEM

General
- Intrinsic nervous system of the esophagus and the gastrointestinal tract
- Part of the autonomous nervous system
- Originates from the neural crest (neuroectoderm)

Structure
A nerve plexus consisting of:
- Small ganglion cells (neurons)
- Unmyelinated nerve fibers
- Enteric glial cells

Function
- Control of the esophageal, gastric, and intestinal motility (peristaltics)
- Entero-enteric reflexes, e.g., the gastrocolic reflex
- Defense reactions, e.g., vomiting

Consists of
- Neurons:
  - Efferent neurons
  - Afferent neurons
  - Interneurons
- Enteric glial cells: structurally and functionally similar to astrocytes (Chap. 14)

Divided into
Two nerve plexuses:
- Submucosal (Meissner's) plexus
  - In the submucosal layer
  - Innervates:
    - The muscularis mucosae
    - The vessels of the submucosa
- Myenteric (Auerbach's) plexus
  - Between the two layers of the muscularis externa
  - Innervates:
    - The muscularis externa

ENTERO-ENDOCRINE SYSTEM

General
- A variety of hormone-producing cells
- Located solitary or in groups
- Difficult to identify in routine stains

Function
Secretion of polypeptide hormones
- Control of physiological and homeostatic functions, e.g., peristaltics and gastrointestinal secretions.
- Hormones have auto-, para-, or endocrine actions (Chap. 24).

Structure
Located in:
- The mucosa of the gastrointestinal tract
- The isles of Langerhans in the pancreas (Chap. 22)

Consists of
Multiple cell types, e.g.:
- EC cells:
  - Most common type
  - Located throughout the gastrointestinal tract
  - Secrete serotonin that, e.g., affects intestinal motility and secretions

- D cells:
  - Least common type
  - Located throughout the gastrointestinal tract
  - Secrete somatostatin that, e.g., inhibits intestinal secretions

DIGESTION

General (Table 21.13)
- Physical and chemical breakdown of ingested food and liquids into absorbable substances.
  - Food and liquids need to be broken down into small molecules in order to be absorbed from the intestines into the blood and lymph.
- Takes place in different levels of the alimentary canal.

Table 21.13 Overview of digestion

	Event	Name of digestion product	Secretions aiding digestion	Digestive enzymes break down
Cavum oris proper	Mastication	Food bolus	Saliva, with digestive enzymes	Starches
Esophagus	Transportation	Food bolus	–	–
Stomach	Mixing food bolus and gastric juice	Chyme (semidigested food)	Gastric juice, with digestive enzymes, e.g., pepsin	Proteins
Small intestine	Peristalsis	Chyme (semidigested food)	• Digestive enzymes on intestinal wall • Bile (from the liver) with bile salts • Pancreatic juice (from pancreas via the duct system) with digestive enzymes	• Starches • Proteins • Lipids • Carbohydrates
Large intestine	Peristalsis	Feces	–	–

Divided into
- Mechanical digestion, e.g., mastication
  - Breakdown of food into small pieces
- Chemical digestion
  - Breakdown of small pieces of food into absorbable nutrients

Guide to Practical Histology: The Alimentary Canal

Lip (Labium Oris)

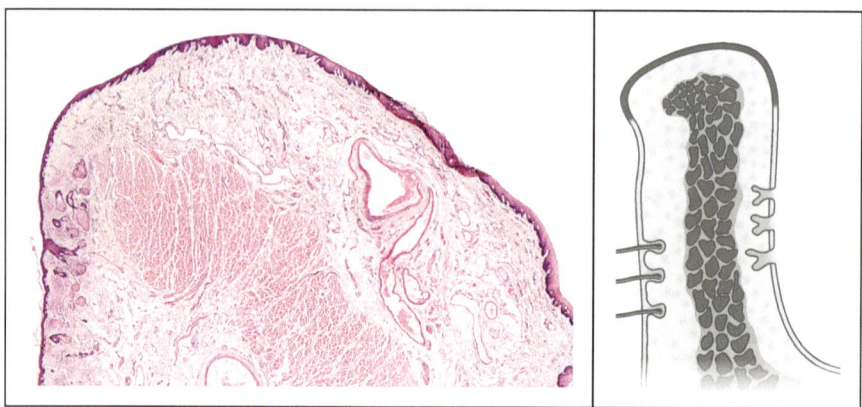

Left: photomicrograph of a lip. Magnification: low. Stain: HE (Courtesy of professor associate professor Steen Seier Poulsen, University of Copenhagen). *Right*: simplified illustration of a lip

Characteristics
- Macroscopic:
  - Shape like a little finger
- Microscopic:
  - Core of skeletal muscle tissue
  - Two surfaces that meet at the apex:
    - Outer surface:
      - Keratinized stratified squamous epithelium
      - With hair follicles
    - Inner surface:
      - Nonkeratinized stratified squamous epithelium
      - Mucoserous and mucous end pieces seen below inner surface

Can be mistaken for

Eyelid:
- Nonkeratinized stratified epithelium contains abundant goblet cells.
- Contains large sebaceous glands below nonkeratinized epithelium.

Tongue

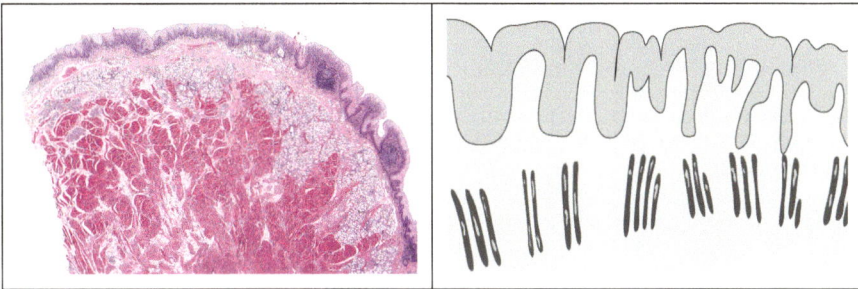

Left: photomicrograph of the tongue. Magnification: low. Stain: HE (Courtesy of professor Jørgen Tranum-Jensen, University of Copenhagen). *Right*: simplified illustration of the tongue

Characteristics

- A core of:
  - Skeletal muscle tissue arranged in unorganized bundles in different directions.
  - Connective tissue:
    - Serous and mucus glands are often seen in the connective tissue.
- The surface is covered with either keratinized or nonkeratinized stratified squamous epithelium.
- The dorsal surface of the tongue is covered with lingual papillae (Table 21.14).

Table 21.14 Lingual papillae

	Filiform papillae	Fungiform papillae	Foliate papillae	Circumvallate papillae
Shape	Threadlike	Mushroomlike	• Leaflike • Consist of several, parallel ridges	Dome-like
Illustration				
Taste buds	−	+	+++	+++
Keratinization	++	+	−	−

Palatine Tonsils

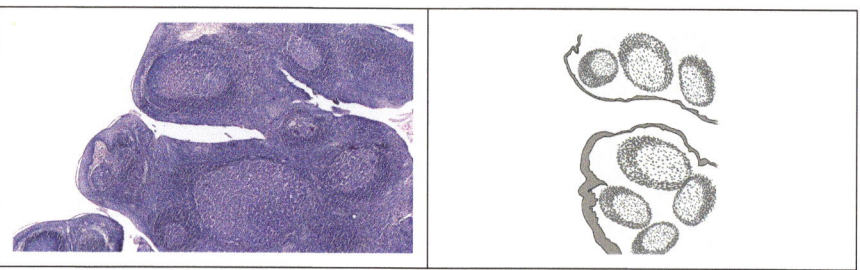

Left: photomicrograph of a palatine tonsil. Magnification: low. Stain: HE (Courtesy of associate professor Steen Seier Poulsen, University of Copenhagen). *Right*: simplified illustration of a palatine tonsils

Characteristics (Table 21.15)
- Partly covered with nonkeratinized stratified squamous epithelium.
- The epithelium invaginates deep into the tonsil (crypts).
- Parenchyma of diffuse and follicular lymphatic tissue.
- Surrounded by a connective tissue capsule.

Can be mistaken for
- Lingual tonsils:
  ○ Smaller
  ○ Without connective tissue capsule
- Pharyngeal tonsil:
  ○ Partly covered with ciliated, pseudostratified columnar epithelium
  ○ Without crypts
- Lymph node:
  ○ Not partly covered with epithelium

Table 21.15   Tonsils

	Palatine tonsils	Lingual tonsils	Pharyngeal tonsil (adenoid)
Mucosa			
• Epithelium	Nonkeratinized stratified squamous epithelium		Ciliated, pseudostratified columnar epithelium
• Lamina propia	Diffuse and follicular lymphatic tissue (Chap. 19)		
• Crypts in the surface	+	+	−
Capsule of dense connective tissue	Thick	−	Thin

Lingual Tonsils

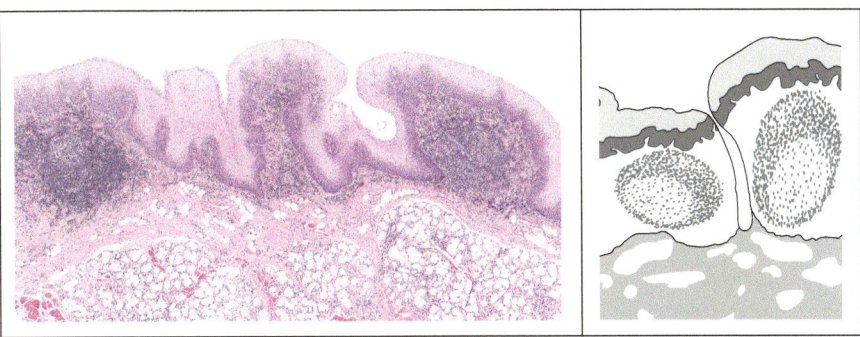

Left: photomicrograph of a lingual tonsil. Magnification: low. Stain: HE (Courtesy of professor Jørgen Tranum-Jensen, University of Copenhagen). *Right*: simplified illustration of a lingual tonsil

Characteristics (Table 21.15)
- Partly covered with nonkeratinized stratified squamous epithelium.
- The epithelium invaginates deep into the tonsil (crypts).
- Parenchyma of diffuse and follicular lymphatic tissue.

Can be mistaken for
- Palatine tonsils:
  - Larger
  - With connective tissue capsule
- Pharyngeal tonsil:
  - Partly covered with ciliated, pseudostratified columnar epithelium
  - Without crypts
- Lymph node:
  - Not partly covered with epithelium

Pharyngeal Tonsil

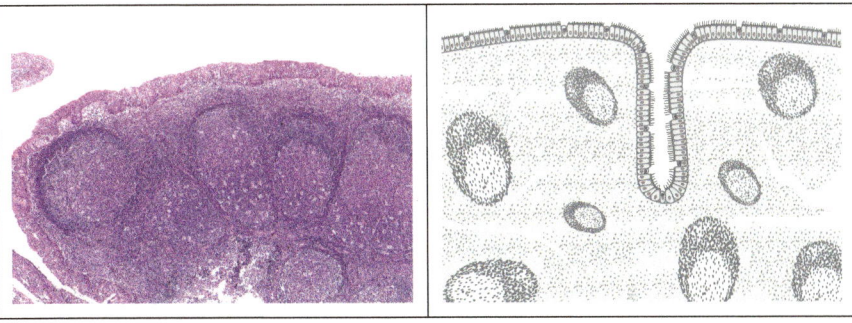

Left: photomicrograph of a pharyngeal tonsil. Magnification: low. Stain: HE (Courtesy of associate professor Steen Seier Poulsen, University of Copenhagen). *Right*: simplified illustration of a pharyngeal tonsil

Characteristics (Table 21.15)
- Partly covered with ciliated, pseudostratified columnar epithelium
- Parenchyma of diffuse and follicular lymphatic tissue
- Surrounded by a connective tissue capsule

Can be mistaken for
- Palatine tonsils:
  - Partly covered with nonkeratinized stratified squamous epithelium
  - With invaginations of epithelium into parenchyma (crypts)
- Lingual tonsils:
  - Smaller
  - Partly covered with nonkeratinized stratified squamous epithelium
  - With invaginations of epithelium into parenchyma (crypts)
  - Without connective tissue capsule
- Lymph node:
  - Not partly covered with epithelium

Soft Palate (Palatum Molle)

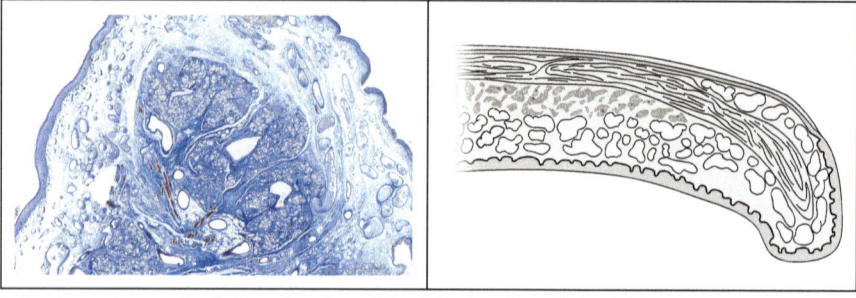

Left: photomicrograph of the soft palate. Magnification: low. Stain: Mallory-Azan (Courtesy of associate professor Steen Seier Poulsen, University of Copenhagen). *Right*: simplified illustration of the soft palate

Characteristics
- Core of skeletal muscle tissue and abundant mucoserous and mucous glands
- Lined with:
  - Nonkeratinized stratified squamous epithelium on one surface
  - Pseudostratified columnar epithelium, with cilia and goblet cells on the other surface

Can be mistaken for
Epiglottis:
  - Contains cores of elastic cartilage

Esophagus

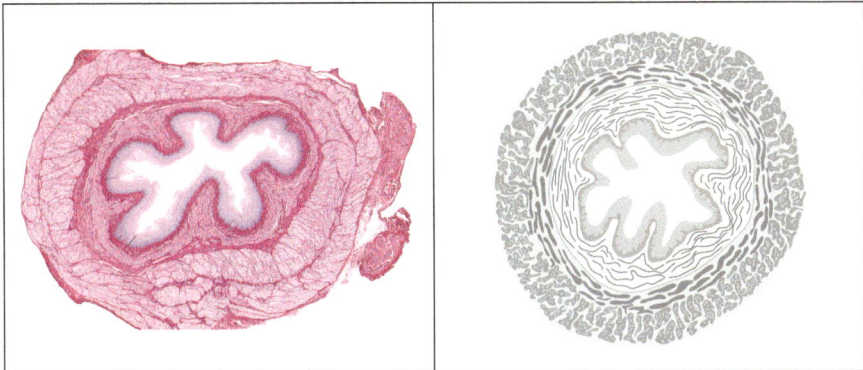

Left: photomicrograph of the esophagus on a cross section. Magnification: low. Stain: HE (Courtesy of associate professor Steen Seier Poulsen, University of Copenhagen). *Right*: simplified illustration of the esophagus

Characteristics
- Cross section: A ring-shaped structure with an irregular/star-shaped lumen.
- Luminal surface is lined with nonkeratinized stratified squamous epithelium.
- Mucous glands (esophageal glands proper) are seen in the submucosa.
- A thick layer of skeletal or smooth muscle tissue is seen profound to the submucosa.

Can be mistaken for
Vagina:
- No mucous glands in the submucosa.
- The luminal epithelial cells are pale, boat shaped, and vacuolated.

GASTROINTESTINAL TRACT

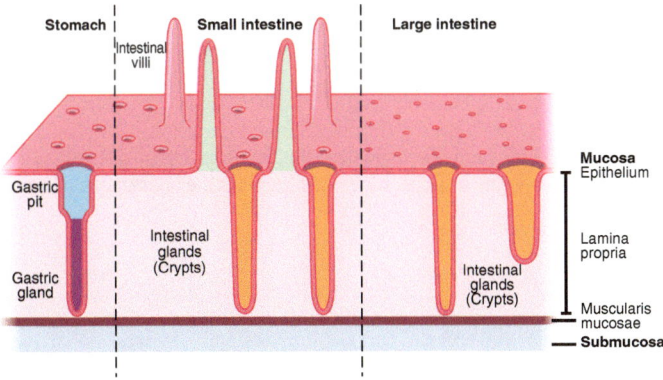

Fig. 21.10 A schematic diagram of the differences in the surface specialization in the different parts of the alimentary canal

Characteristics (Fig. 21.10)

- Villi:
  - ○ Often cut during preparation and appears as isolated islets
  - ○ Seen only in the small intestine
- Crypts/gastric pits:
  - ○ Due to the cut during preparation, they appear as deep holes (small lakes) in the epithelium.
  - ○ Seen in:
    - ▪ Stomach
    - ▪ Small intestine
    - ▪ Appendix
    - ▪ Large intestine

Special Staining

PAS: stains the mucin, mucus glands, and goblet cells dense pink.

Stomach

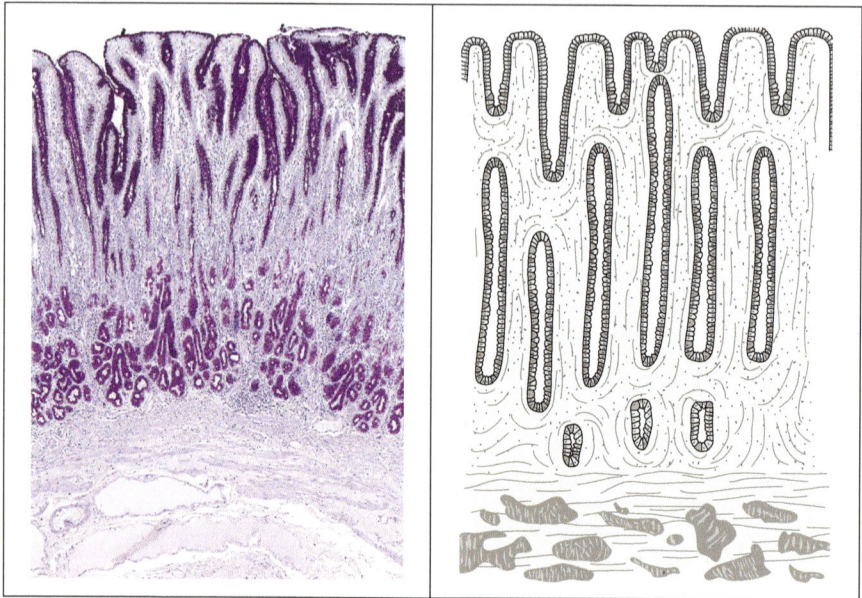

Left: photomicrograph of the stomach. Magnification: low. Stain: HE (Courtesy of associate professor Steen Seier Poulsen, University of Copenhagen). *Right*: simplified illustration of the stomach

Characteristics

- Gastric pits:
  - ○ Funnel-shaped recesses.
  - ○ Ends in the glands, which appear as small lakes.
- The pale surface epithelium resembles an epithelium of goblet cells only.
- Abundant glands in the lamina propria.

Can be mistaken for
- Large intestine:
  - Epithelium with apical brush border (microvilli).
  - Goblet cells are scattered.
- Gallbladder:
  - Epithelium with apical brush border (microvilli).
  - No goblet cells.

Small Intestine

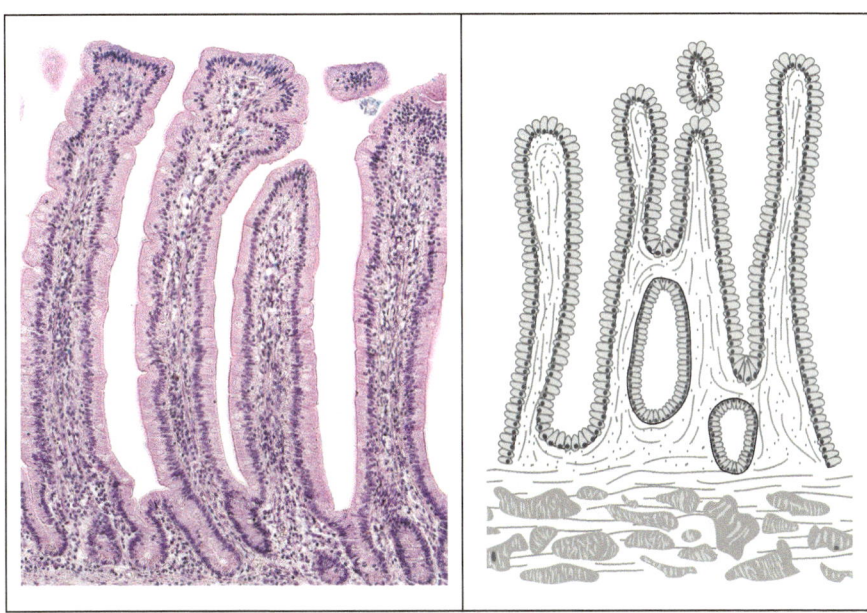

Left: photomicrograph of the small intestine. Magnification: low. Stain: HE (Courtesy of associate professor Steen Seier Poulsen, University of Copenhagen). *Right*: simplified illustration of the small intestine

Characteristics
- Macroscopic
  - Resembles seaweed
- Microscopic
  - Contains villi that offten appear as isolated islets
  - Epithelium with apical brush border (microvilli)
- The different parts can be distinguished from each other (Fig. 21.9, Table 21.16)

Can be mistaken for
- Large intestine:
  - Does not contain villi
- Gallbladder:
  - Does not contain villi
  - Without goblet cells

Table 21.16 How to distinguish the parts of the small intestine

	Duodenum	Jejunum	Ileum
Mucous glands in submucosa	+	–	–
Lymphatic follicles	Solitary	Solitary	Multiple, forming aggregations

Vermiform Appendix

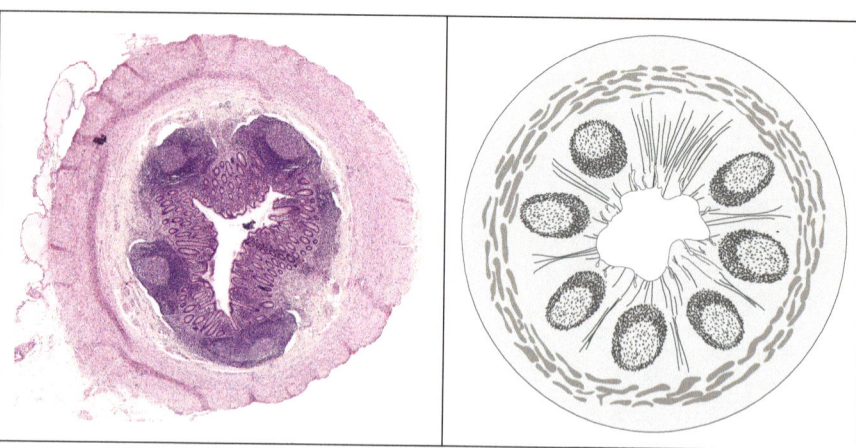

Left: photomicrograph of the vermiform appendix. Magnification: low. Stain: HE (Courtesy of associate professor Steen Seier Poulsen, University of Copenhagen). *Right*: simplified illustration of vermiform appendix

Characteristics
Cross section:
- A ring-shaped structure with a small lumen
- Abundant solitary lymphatic follicles underneath the epithelium
- Crypts

Can be mistaken for
Large intestine:
- Less or no lymphatic follicles

Large Intestine

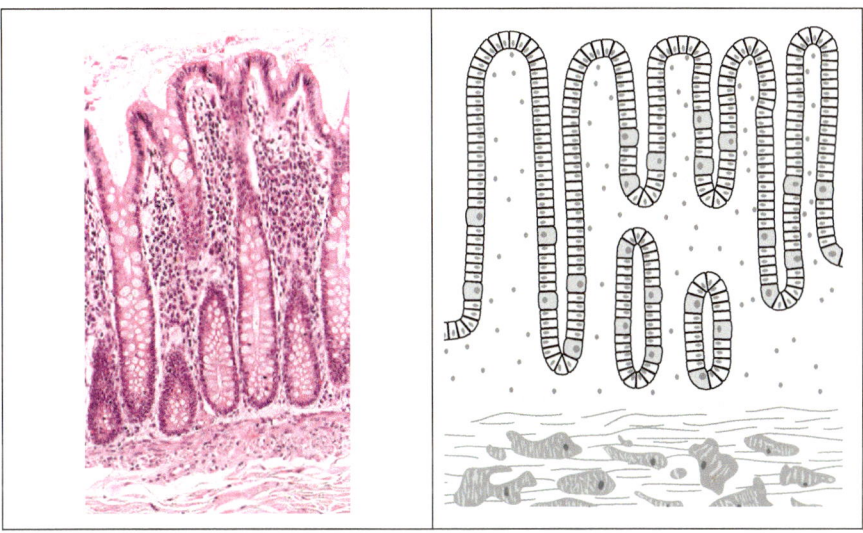

Left: photomicrograph of the large intestine. Magnification: low. Stain: HE (Courtesy of associate professor Steen Seier Poulsen, University of Copenhagen). *Right*: simplified illustration of the large intestine

Characteristics
- Epithelium with apical brush border (microvilli)
- Multiple scattered goblet cells
- Crypts that appear as small lakes

Can be mistaken for
- Stomach:
  - Surface epithelium of mucin secreting cells only (resembles an epithelium of goblet cells only)
  - Abundant glands in the lamina propria
- Small intestine:
  - Contains villi
- Vermiform appendix:
  - Abundant solitary lymphatic follicles underneath the epithelium

References
5, 16, 25, 29, 33, 34.

Chapter 22
The Digestive System II: The Associated Organs

Contents

General
For an introduction to the digestive system, see Chap. 21.

The Associated Organs of the Digestive System

General
- A group of organs located in relation to the alimentary canal
- A part of the digestive system

Consist of
- Salivary glands (glandulae salivaria)
- Pancreas
- Liver (hepar)
- Gallbladder (vesica biliaris)

© Springer International Publishing Switzerland 2017
A. Rehfeld et al., *Compendium of Histology*, DOI 10.1007/978-3-319-41873-5_22

Function
- Facilitation of the digestion of food and absorption of nutrients
- Regulation of, e.g., peristaltics and blood glucose levels

SALIVARY GLANDS

General
Several exocrine glands, located in relation to the oral cavity

Structure
See Table 22.1.

Function
Secretion of saliva
- The secretions differ between the salivary glands.

Divided into
- Three major, paired salivary glands
  - Parotid gland (largest)
  - Submandibular gland
  - Sublingual gland
- Small salivary glands

Consist of
All salivary glands consist of
- Parenchyma
  - Glandular epithelium in secretory end pieces (Chap. 6)
  - Myoepithelial cells
    - Flat cells with long cell extensions
    - Located between the glandular epithelial cells and their basal lamina
    - Contractile cells: contraction aids discharge of secretions from gland
  - Duct system
- Stroma
  - Loose and dense connective tissue

Table 22.1 Overview of the salivary glands

	Location	Capsule of dense connective tissue	Type of secretion	End pieces	Myoepi-thelial cells	Duct
Parotid glands	Infratemporal region	+	Serous	Serous only	+	Parotid (Stensen) duct
Submandibular glands	Submandibular triangle of the neck	+	Mixed seromucous	Serous > mucous	+	Submandibular (Wharton) duct
Sublingual glands	Inferior to the tongue	Not well developed	Mixed mucoserous	Mucous > serous	+	10–12 ducts
Small salivary glands	Throughout the oral cavity	−	Differs between glands	Differs between glands	+	+

Saliva

General
- Fluid with pH 7, composed of the combined secretions of the various salivary glands
- The production is approximately 1000 ml per day.

Function
- Aids digestion, e.g., of starches
- Lubrication
- Antibacterial → e.g., protection of the teeth

Consists of
- Water (99 %)
- Solutes (1 %)
  ○ Proteins, e.g., IgA antibodies
  ○ Enzymes, e.g., lysozyme

PANCREAS

General
- 15 × 20 cm, 100 g
- Elongated exocrine gland, with endocrine islets
- Located retropetrioneally, in close relation to the duodenum

Structure
- No capsule
- Surrounded by a thin layer of connective tissue that extends through the parenchyma as septa, dividing the gland into lobules

Function
- Exocrine secretion:
  - Digestive enzymes
- Endocrine secretion:
  - Hormones, e.g., insulin and glucagon

Divided into
- Head
- Body
- Tail

Consists of (Fig. 22.1)
- Parenchyma
  - Endocrine glandular tissue (the endocrine pancreas)
  - Exocrine glandular tissue (the exocrine pancreas)
  - Duct system
- Stroma of connective tissue

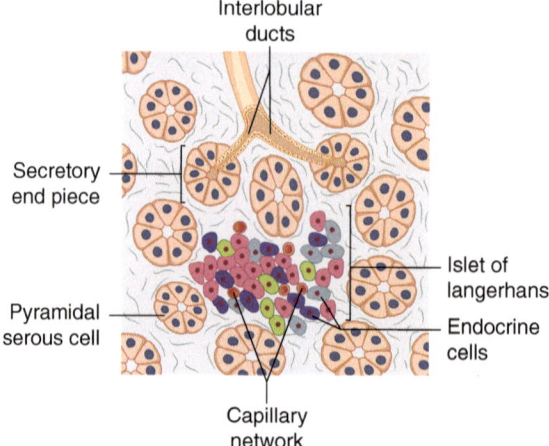

Fig. 22.1 Pancreas. The endocrine cells form aggregations called "islets of Langerhans", which are clearly visible within the exocrine tissue

The Exocrine Pancreas

Structure (Fig. 22.1)
- Tubuloacinar exocrine gland
  - End pieces with simple glandular epithelium of pyramidal serous cells
- Duct system
  - Secretions reach the duodenum through both:
    - The main pancreatic duct
    - The accessory pancreatic duct

Function
- Production of pancreatic juice, containing digestive enzymes
- Secretion of 1500 ml pancreatic fluid per day

Consists of
See Table 22.2.

Table 22.2 The exocrine pancreas

	Epithelium	Light microscopy

End pieces	Simple glandular epithelium of pyramidal serous cells	• Pyramid-shaped cell with apex pointing towards the lumen
		• Cytoplasm
		  ○ Basophilic basally due to abundant rER
		  ○ Acidophilic apically due to zymogen granules
		• Nucleus is large and round, located basally

Intralobular ducts • Intraacinar ducts	Centroacinar cell • Initial part of the duct system	• Small cells with flattened nucleus • Located centrally in the acinar end pieces
• Intercalated ducts	Simple cuboidal/ columnar epithelium	• Low cuboidal/columnar cells with flattened, elongated nuclei
Interlobular ducts	Simple columnar epithelium	Low columnar cells
Main pancreatic duct + accessory pancreatic duct	Simple columnar epithelium	High columnar cells

Regulation of the exocrine secretion

Divided into
- Hormonal control
  - The primary form of regulation.
  - Hormones secreted by enteroendocrine cells in the small intestine stimulate or inhibit the exocrine secretion.
- Neural control
  - Through autonomic innervation.

Endocrine Pancreas

General
- Constitutes 1 % of the pancreatic volume
- A part of the enteroendocrine system

Structure (Fig. 22.1)
- The endocrine cells form aggregations called "islets of Langerhans"
  - The islets of Langerhans vary in size (few cells – hundreds of cells).
  - Scattered throughout the exocrine tissue.
- As in all endocrine tissues, there is a rich network of fenestrated capillaries between the endocrine cells.

Function
Secretion of hormones, e.g., insulin and glucagon, which regulate the blood glucose level

Consists of (Table 22.3)
- Three main islet cells
  - A (α) cells
  - B (β) cells
  - D (δ) cells
- Minor islet cells

Light Microscopy
The islet of Langerhans
- Clusters of pale cells within the exocrine glandular tissue
- Difficult to distinguish between the different types of endocrine cells in routine stains

Table 22.3 Cells in the islets of Langerhans

	% of cells in islets	Secrete	Location
A-cells	15–20%	Glucagon	Located in the peripheral portions of the islets
B-cells	60–70%	Insulin	Located in the central portions of the islets
D-cell	5–10%	Somatostatin	Located in the peripheral portions of the islets
Minor islet cells	5%	For example: • Pancreatic polypeptide • Secretin • Ghrelin	Scattered throughout the islets

LIVER

General
- The largest gland in the human body
- Located in the upper right quadrant of the abdominal cavity
- Mainly covered by serosa
  - Adventitia covers a small posterior area and the area where it attaches to the gallbladder

Structure
- 15 × 14 × 17 cm
- 1.5 kg in adults
- Macroscopically divided into four lobes
  - Right lobe
  - Left lobe
  - The caudate lobe
  - The quadrate lobe

Function
The liver has multiple functions, e.g.:
- Portal function
  - All blood from the gastrointestinal canal passes through the liver.
  - Potentially toxic substances are removed before they reach the systemic circulation.
- Detoxification
  - Degrades toxins, e.g., alcohol and drugs carried to the liver by the blood

- Storage of vitamins, e.g.:
  - Vitamin D: important for the calcium and phosphate homeostasis
  - Vitamin K: important in the synthesis of coagulation factors
- Iron homeostasis
  - Synthesize proteins, e.g., transferrin, involved in the iron transport
- Breakdown of hormones
  - For example, degradation of insulin and glucagon
- Endocrine function
  - Production of, e.g., insulin-like growth factor-1(IGF-1) and angiotensin
- Exocrine function
  - Production of bile, approximately 1 l per day
- Production of plasma proteins
  - For example, albumin and lipoproteins
- Takes part in metabolism
  - Carbohydrate metabolism
    - Storage of glucose in the form of glycogen.
    - Glycogen in the liver can be broken down to glucose when needed.
  - Lipid metabolism
    - For example, cholesterol synthesis
  - Protein metabolism
    - For example, amino acid synthesis

Consists of (Fig. 22.2)
- Capsule of Glisson
  - Thin layer of dense connective tissue
- Parenchyma
  - Liver cells (hepatocytes) arranged in cords, one cell layer thick.
  - Sinusoids separate the cords of hepatocytes.
- Stroma
  - Loose connective tissue surrounding the hepatocytes
  - Septa of dense connective tissue
    - Continuous with the connective tissue capsule
    - Divide the parenchyma of the liver into lobes and lobules
    - Surround the portal (Glisson's) triads, which consist of:
      - A branch from the portal vein
      - A branch from the hepatic artery
      - A bile duct

Divided into (Table 22.4 and Fig. 22.2)
There are three ways to divide the liver into units:
1. The classical liver lobule
2. The liver acinus
3. The portal lobule

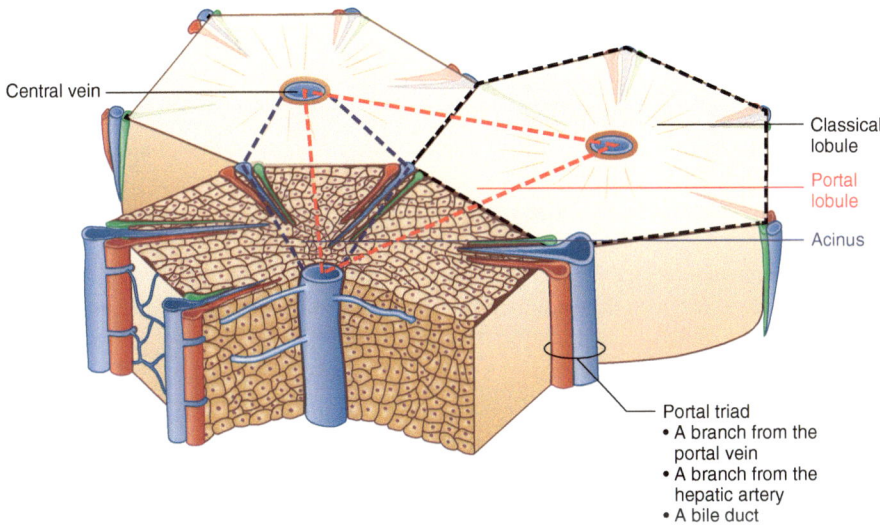

Central vein

Classical lobule

Portal lobule

Acinus

Portal triad
• A branch from the portal vein
• A branch from the hepatic artery
• A bile duct

Fig. 22.2 The general liver organization. The three functional divisions and their relations are shown

Light Microscopy
- Hepatocytes
  - ○ Polygonal cell, often binucleate.
  - ○ ⊘ 20–30 μm
  - ○ Eosinophilic cytoplasm.
  - ○ Abundant mitochondria.
  - ○ Microvilli project into the perisinusoidal space
- Sinusoids
  - ○ Endothelium
  - ○ Discontinuous basement membrane
  - ○ Multiple erythrocytes in the lumen

The Classical Liver Lobule

General (Fig. 22.2)
The smallest structural (anatomical) unit of the liver

Structure
- Hexagonal shaped, 2×1 mm
- Surrounding a central vein
- Separated by sparse interlobular connective tissue septa

Consists of (Fig. 22.3)
- Hepatic cords
  - Formed from one cell layer of hepatocytes
  - Separated by the sinusoids
  - Radiate from the central vein towards the periphery of the lobule
- Sinusoids
  - Irregular-shaped vascular spaces
  - Drains to the central vein
- Perisinusoidal spaces (spaces of Disse)
  - Spaces between the endothelium of the sinusoids and the hepatocytes of the hepatic cords
  - Filled with blood plasma

Table 22.4 Units of the liver

	Type	Shape	Drained by
The classic liver lobule	Smallest structural unit	Hexagon	Central vein
Liver acinus	Smallest functional unit	Rhombus	Terminal branches from portal triads
Portal lobule	Exocrine unit	Triangular	Portal triad

The Liver Acinus

General (Fig. 22.2)
The smallest functional (metabolic) unit of the liver

Structure
- Rhombus shaped
  - The short axis is the border between two classical lobules, where the terminal branches of the portal triad run.
  - The long axis is a direct line between two central veins.
- Consists of tissue from two neighboring classical liver lobules.

The Portal Lobule

General (Fig. 22.2)
- An exocrine unit of the liver.
- An interlobular bile duct of a portal triad is draining bile from the portal lobule.

Structure
- Contains tissue from three neighboring classical liver lobules
- Triangular shape
  - A portal triad in the center
  - A central vein in each corner

The Blood Supply of the Liver

General

- Two afferent (supplying) blood vessels
  - The hepatic artery from the celiac trunk (truncus coeliacus)
  - The hepatic portal vein from the gastrointestinal tract
- One efferent (draining) blood vessel
  - The hepatic vein to the inferior vena cava

Divided into

See Table 22.5.

Table 22.5 Blood supply of the liver

	Venous part	Arterial part
Afferent blood vessels	The hepatic portal vein	The hepatic artery
• % of blood supply	75% of the blood supply to the liver	25% of the blood supply to the liver
• Content of blood	Venous blood from the gastrointestinal tract carrying, e.g.: • Nutrients absorbed in the intestine • Pancreatic hormones	Arterial oxygenated blood
Intrahepatic blood vessels	Interlobular blood vessels ↓	
	Sinusoids ↓	
	Central vein (terminal hepatic venule) ↓	
	Sublobular vein ↓	
Efferent blood vessels	Hepatic veins ↓	
	Inferior vena cava	

Liver sinusoids

General (Fig. 22.3)
- Irregularly shaped vascular spaces between hepatocyte cords
  - Drain into the central vein
  - Radiate from the central vein towards the periphery of the classical liver lobule
- Separated from the hepatocytes by the perisinusoidal space (space of Disse)

Structure

From lumen → periphery
- Kupffer cells (macrophages) on the luminal surface of the endothelium
- Endothelium with fenestrations and gaps between endothelial cells
- Discontinuous basement membrane

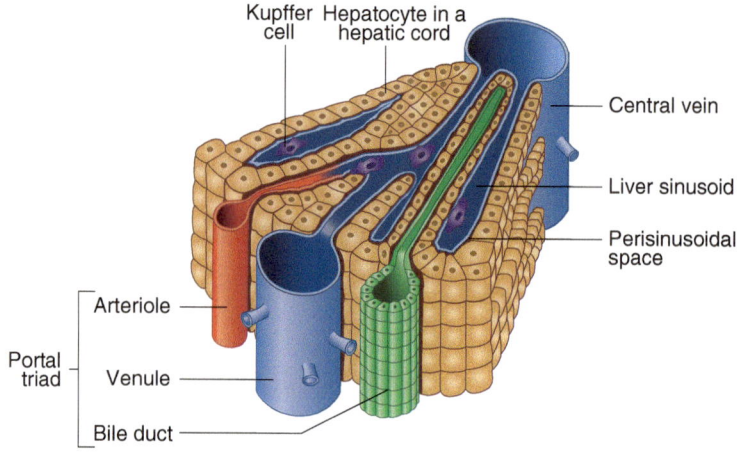

Fig. 22.3 The liver sinusoids and their relation to the hepatocytes in the hepatic cords

Perisinusoidal space (space of Disse)

General
- The space that separates the liver sinusoids from the hepatocytes.
- Microvilli from the hepatocytes project into the perisinusoidal space.
- Filled with blood plasma.
- Contains hepatic stellate cells (Ito cells):
  - Store vitamin A
  - Cytoplasm filled with lipid droplets where vitamin A is stored

The Biliary Tree

General (Fig. 22.3)
- A three-dimensional system of canals, containing bile
- >2 km of interconnected ducts and ductules
- Lined primarily by cholangiocytes

Structure
See Table 22.6.

Function
Transportation of bile
- From hepatocytes → intrahepatic bile ducts → extrahepatic bile ducts → 1 or 2
  1. Cystic duct (ductus cysticus) → gallbladder → cystic duct (ductus cysticus)
     → 2
  2. Common bile duct (ductus choledochus) → duodenum

Table 22.6 Bile ducts

	Luminal ⌀	Location	Lining
Intrahepatic bile ducts			
• Bile canaliculi	0.5 µm	Between adjacent hepatocytes	Two adjacent hepatocytes • Specialized surface • Sealed off from surroundings by tight junctions
• Canals of Hering	1.0 µm	Between cords of hepatocytes	• Hepatocytes • Cholangiocytes ○ Cuboidal cells • Hepatic stem cells
• Intrahepatic bile ductules	1.0–1.5 µm	Between cords of hepatocytes	Cholangiocytes • Cuboidal cells
• Interlobular bile ducts (form part of portal triads)	15–40 µm	In the connective tissue stroma	Cholangiocytes • Cuboidal → columnar cells
Extrahepatic bile ducts	> 40 µm	Outside of the liver	Cholangiocytes • Columnar cells

Divided into
- Intrahepatic bile ducts
  - Bile canaliculi
  - Canals of Hering
  - Intrahepatic bile ductules
  - Interlobular bile ducts
- Extrahepatic bile ducts
  - Right and left hepatic duct
  - Common hepatic duct
  - The cystic duct
  - Common bile duct

Cholangiocytes

Structure
- Epithelial cells
- Cuboidal in the ductules → columnar in the ducts
- Apical microvilli and one primary cilium projecting into the lumen

Function
Monitor and modify bile:
- The primary cilium senses changes in the bile flow, composition, and osmolarity.
- Cholangiocytes modify the bile via secretion and absorption.

Bile

General
- 1 L per day, secreted by the hepatocytes.
- Modified by cholangiocytes.
- Reaches the duodenum through the common bile duct.
- Many of the bile components are recycled via the portal circulation:
  - Hepatocytes → biliary tree → intestine → portal circulation → hepatocytes.

Consists of
- Water
- Bile salts
- Bile pigments
- Lipids
- Electrolytes

Function
- Involved in the absorption of fat
  - Secreted bile salts emulsify lipids → aid absorption of lipids.
- Excretion of:
  - Cholesterol
  - Bilirubin
  - Iron
  - Copper

GALLBLADDER

General
- Pear-shaped distensible pouch.
- Volume of 50 ml.
- Located under the right liver lobule.
- The wall resembles the general structure of wall in the gastrointestinal tract, but lacks the muscularis mucosa and the submucosa.

Function
- Storage of bile
- Concentration of bile
  - Removes 90% of the water content of the bile

Consists of
- Mucosa
- Muscularis externa
- Adventitia/serosa
  - Adventitia where the gallbladder is attached to the liver
  - Serosa on the free inferior surface

Light Microscopy
- Mucosa
  - Simple columnar epithelium
    - Cholangiocytes
      - Apical brush border (formed by microvilli)
      - Ovoid nuclei, basally located
      - Connected to neighbor cells by tight junctions
  - Lamina propria
    - Thick layer of loose connective tissue with mucous glands
    - Abundant fenestrated capillaries and venules
    - Many different cells, e.g.:
      - Lymphocytes
      - Plasma cells
- Muscularis externa
  - Bundles of smooth muscle cells, randomly arranged
  - Abundant collagen and elastic fibers between the cells
- Adventitia/serosa
  - Adventitia
    - Loose connective tissue
  - Serosa
    - Mesothelium and submesothelial loose connective tissue

Secretion of bile

General

Bile secretion is stimulated by ingestion and digestion of food:
1. Fatty chyme in the lumen of the proximal duodenum
2. Secretion of the hormone cholecystokinin by enteroendocrine cells in the small intestine
3. Contraction of the smooth muscle tissue of the gallbladder wall
4. Discharge of bile into the duodenum

Guide to Practical Histology: The Associated Organs of the Digestive System

Parotid Gland

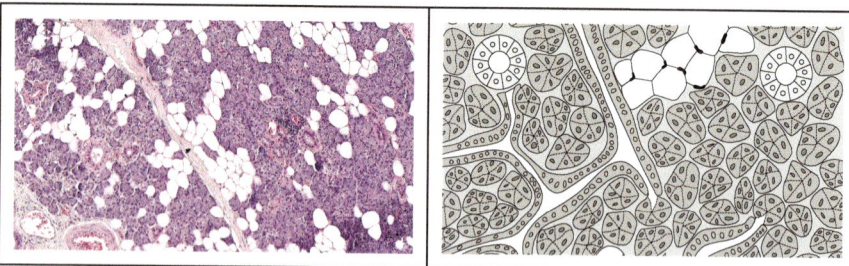

Left: photomicrograph of the parotid gland. Magnification: low. Stain: HE (Courtesy of professor Jørgen Tranum-Jensen, University of Copenhagen). *Right*: simplified illustration of the parotid gland

Characteristics
• Serous end pieces (Chap. 6)
• Often with multiple adipocytes (large white (empty) polyhedral cells) within the exocrine tissue.

Can be mistaken for
The lacrimal gland
• No fat infiltrations.
• The lumen of the serous end pieces is larger and easily recognizable.

Submandibular Gland

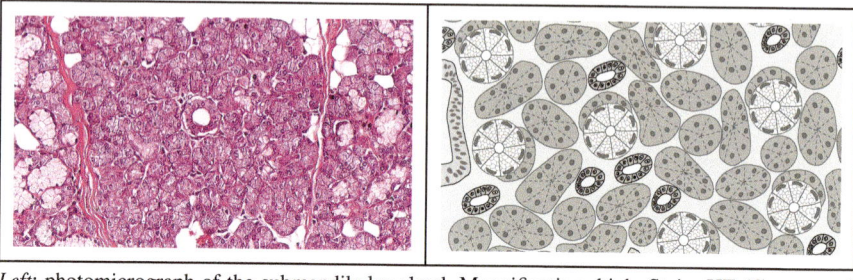

Left: photomicrograph of the submandibular gland. Magnification: high. Stain: HE (Courtesy of associate professor Steen Seier, University of Copenhagen). *Right*: simplified illustration of the submandibular gland

Characteristics
Mixed seromucous gland (Chap. 6)
- Serous end pieces (majority of end pieces in gland)
- Mucous end pieces
- Mixed end pieces

Can be mistaken for
Sublingual gland
- Mucous end pieces make up the majority of the gland.

Sublingual Gland

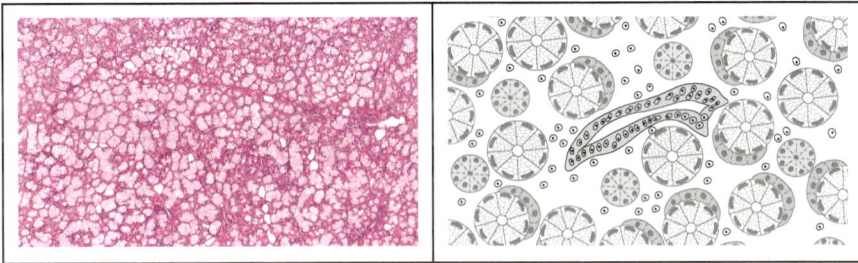

Left: photomicrograph of the sublingual gland. Magnification: low. Stain: HE (Courtesy of associate professor Steen Seier, University of Copenhagen). *Right*: simplified illustration of the sublingual gland

Characteristics
Mixed mucoserous gland (Chap. 6)
- Serous end pieces
- Mucous end pieces (majority of end pieces in gland)
- Mixed end pieces

Can be mistaken for
Submandibular gland
- Serous end pieces make up the majority of the gland.

Pancreas

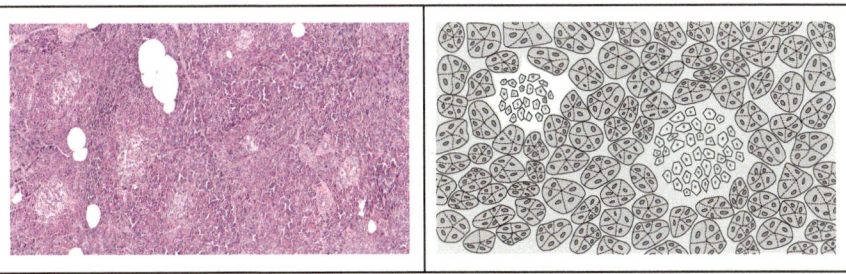

Left: photomicrograph of the pancreas. Magnification: low. Stain: HE (Courtesy of professor Jørgen Tranum-Jensen, University of Copenhagen). *Right*: simplified illustration of the pancreas

Characteristics
- Exocrine tissue
  - Serous end pieces.
  - End pieces have cells located in the center (centroacinar cells).
- Endocrine tissue
  - Islets of pale cells (islets of Langerhans).
  - Islets are scattered throughout the exocrine tissue.

Liver

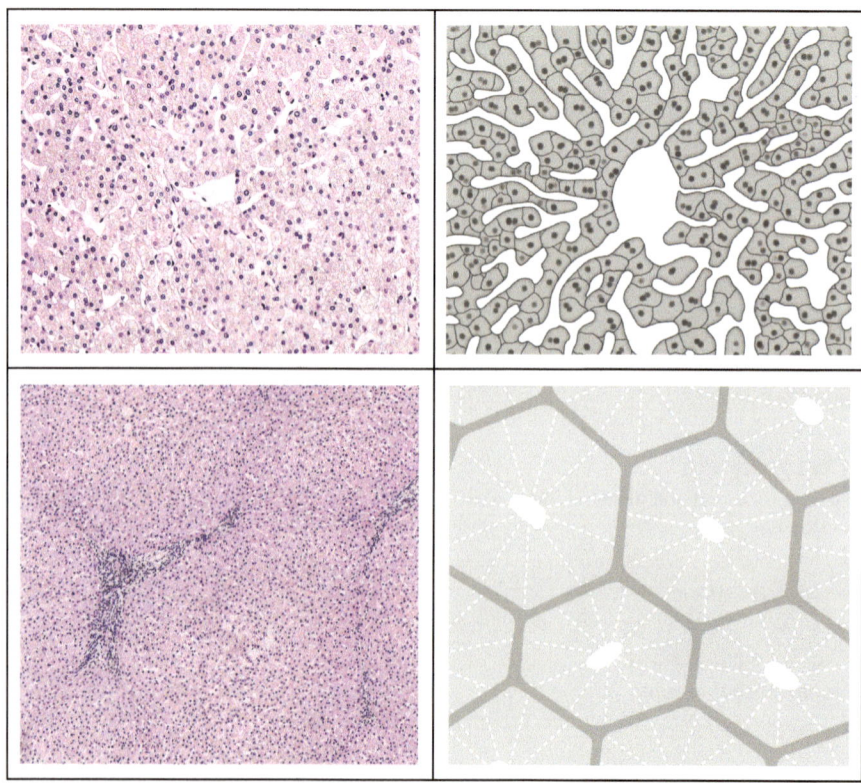

Top left: photomicrograph of the liver. Magnification: low. Stain: HE (Courtesy of associate professor Steen Seier, University of Copenhagen). *Top right*: simplified illustration of the liver. *Bottom left*: photomicrograph of the liver. Magnification: high. Stain: HE (Courtesy of associate professor Steen Seier, University of Copenhagen). *Bottom right*: simplified illustration of liver lobuli

Characteristics
Homogenous, cellular parenchyma with irregular, hexagonal structures and systematically scattered white holes:
- Two types of rounded holes:
  - Central veins (larger)
  - Venules of portal triads

- Sinusoids
  - Irregularly shaped white spaces between the cell strands
  - Contain acidophilic erythrocytes

Gallbladder

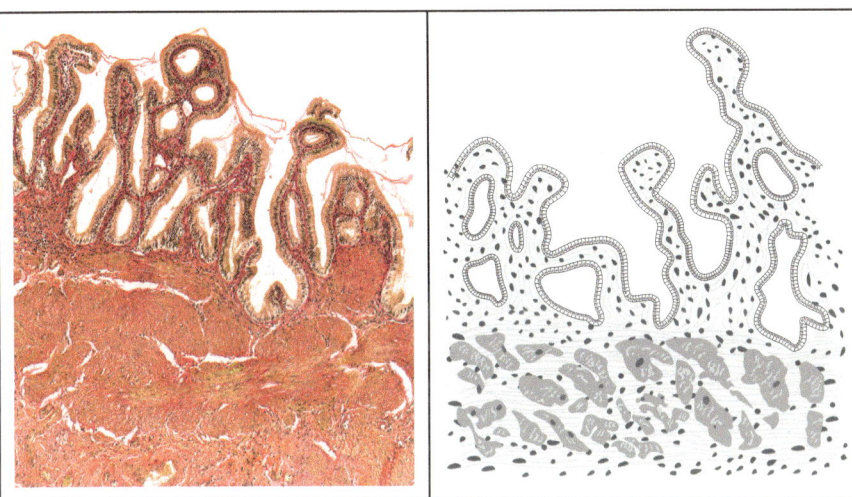

Left: photomicrograph of the gall bladder. Magnification: low. Stain: Sirius red (Courtesy of professor Jørgen Tranum-Jensen, University of Copenhagen). *Right*: simplified illustration of the gallbladder

Characteristics
- Luminal surface lined with regular high columnar epithelium
  - Apical brush border (microvilli)
  - Without goblet cells
- The muscle layer (muscularis externa) contains bundles of smooth muscle cells, collagen and elastic fibers.

Can be mistaken for
- Stomach
  - Surface epithelium of mucin-secreting cells only (resemble an epithelium of goblet cells only)
    - Without apical brush border
  - Abundant glands in the lamina propria
- Small intestine
  - Abundant goblet cells in epithelium

References
5, 25, 33, 34, 41.

Chapter 23
The Urinary System

General

The urinary system (the renal system) eliminates wastes from the human body and maintains homeostasis of, e.g., electrolyte levels and blood volume.

Consists of

- Kidneys
- Urinary tract
  - Renal pelvises
    - Minor calyces
    - Major calyces
  - Ureters
  - Bladder
  - Urethra

© Springer International Publishing Switzerland 2017

A. Rehfeld et al., *Compendium of Histology*, DOI 10.1007/978-3-319-41873-5_23

The Kidney (Ren, Nephros)

General
Paired organ, located retroperitoneally, on the posterior abdominal wall

Structure
- $3 \times 6 \times 12$ cm, 150 g
- Bean-shaped organ, convex laterally and concave medially

Function
- Excretion of metabolic waste products and foreign substances
- Maintenance of homeostasis of:
  - Blood pressure
  - Body fluid volume and osmolality
  - Electrolyte concentration
  - pH (acid–base balance)
    - Maintenance of the pH homeostasis, together with buffering agents, e.g. the bicarbonate buffer system, and the respiratory system
    - Reabsorbs filtered bicarbonate from urine and excretes acids into urine
- Endocrine function
  - Secretion of:
    - Erythropoietin (EPO), crucial for erythropoiesis
    - Renin
  - Conversion of 25(OH)-vitamin D into the active form, 1,25(OH)-vitamin D

Consists of (Fig. 23.1)
- Capsule
  - Thin layer of dense connective tissue
  - Forms a hilum on the concave medial border, where vessels, nerves, and the ureter enter/exit the kidney
- Tissue
  - Stroma: sparse interstitial connective tissue
  - Parenchyma
    - Cortex
    - Medulla
- Sinus, with:
  - Minor calyces, 8 per kidney
  - Major calyces, 2–3 per kidney
  - Renal pelvis
  - Adipose tissue and vessels

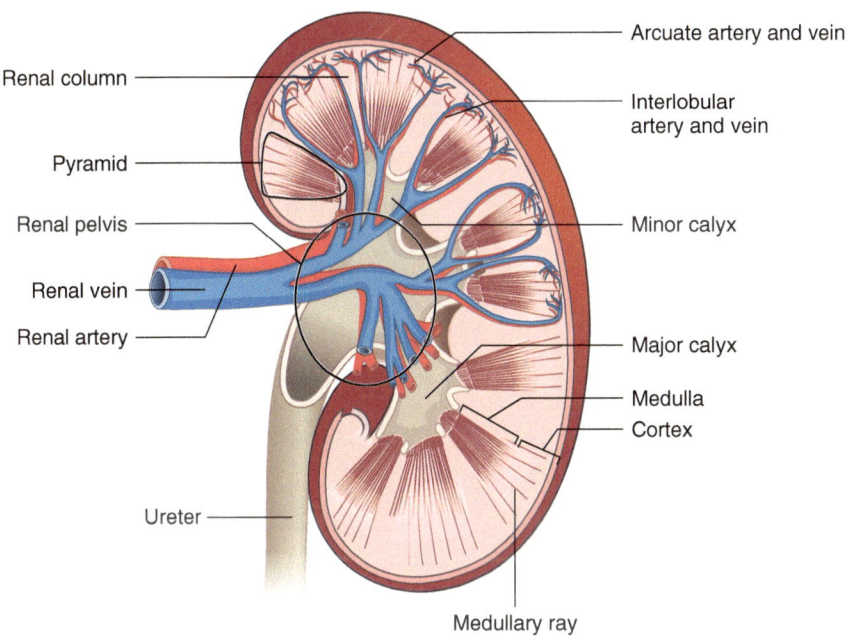

Fig. 23.1 The kidney

Divided into

- Lobes
  - A lobe consists of:
    - A pyramid
    - The surrounding cortex
  - Lobes are further divided into lobules.
- Lobules
  - A lobule consists of:
    - A central medullary ray
    - The surrounding cortex, i.e., the nephrons emptying into the collecting ducts of the medullary ray
  - Lobules are further divided into functional units.
- Functional units
  - A nephron
  - The smallest functional unit of the kidney

Parenchyma of the Kidney

General
The parenchyma consists of nephrons and collecting ducts (Fig. 23.2).

Divided into
- The cortex: outer darker part (1/3), which contains:
  - Renal corpuscles
  - Proximal convoluted tubules
  - Distal convoluted tubules
  - Collecting tubules
  - Collecting ducts
  - Capillary net
- The medulla: inner lighter part (2/3), which contains:
  - Straight tubules
  - Collecting ducts
  - Vasa recta

Structure
- The cortex consists of:
  - Medullary rays
    - Straight tubules and collecting ducts that project into the cortex from the medulla
    - Regarded as a part of the cortex
  - Cortical labyrinth
    - Cortical tissue surrounding the medullary rays
- The medulla consists of:
  - Pyramids
    - 8–12 pyramids per kidney
    - The pyramid's apex (papilla) points into a minor calyx, where collecting ducts empties into a minor calyx, at area cribrosa
  - Renal columns
    - Cortical tissue projects into the medulla, surrounding the medullary pyramids.
    - Regarded as a part of medulla.

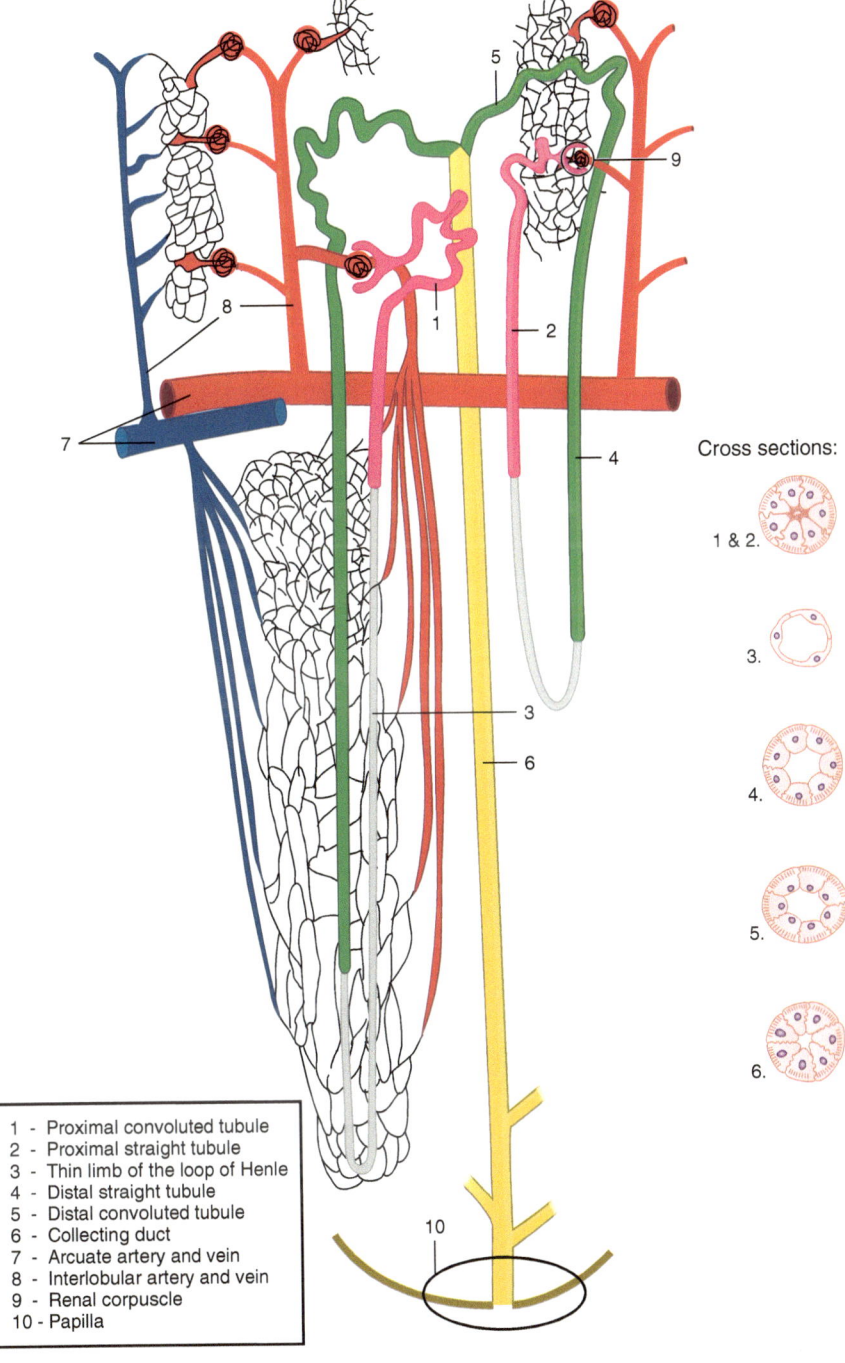

Cross sections:

1 & 2.

3.

4.

5.

6.

1 - Proximal convoluted tubule
2 - Proximal straight tubule
3 - Thin limb of the loop of Henle
4 - Distal straight tubule
5 - Distal convoluted tubule
6 - Collecting duct
7 - Arcuate artery and vein
8 - Interlobular artery and vein
9 - Renal corpuscle
10 - Papilla

Fig. 23.2 Nephrons, collecting ducts, and associated blood supply. Cross sections show the characteristics in the different parts of the tubule and the collecting duct

Interstitial Tissue of the Kidney

General
- Connective tissue surrounding nephrons, collecting ducts and vessels
- Sparse in the cortex, more abundant in the medulla

Consists of
- Cortex
  - Macrophages and other antigen-presenting cells
  - Fibroblasts
    - Erythropoietin (EPO) is secreted by some of the cortical fibroblast in response to hypoxia.
- Medulla
  - Myofibroblasts-like cells containing lipid droplets

NEPHRON

General
There are two million nephrons per kidney.

Function
Excretion of metabolic waste products and foreign substances
- Excretion = glomerular filtration − tubular selective reabsorption + tubular specific secretion

Consists of (Figs. 23.2 and 23.3)
- Renal corpuscule
  - Glomerulus
  - Mesangium
  - Bowman's capsule
- Tubule
  - Proximal convoluted tubule
  - Proximal straight tubule ⎤
  - Thin segment   ⎬ Constitutes the loop of Henle
  - Distal straight tubule   ⎦
  - Distal convoluted tubule

Divided into
Based on location of their renal corpuscle, nephrons are divided into:
- Juxtamedullary nephrons
  - Relatively few
  - Renal corpuscles located in the deeper part of the cortex, close to the base of the medullary pyramid
    - Long loops of Henle
- Cortical/subcapsulary nephrons
  - Renal corpuscles located in the superficial part of the cortex
  - Short loops of Henle
- Intermediate nephrons

MEMO-BOX
- Juxtamedullary nephrons: "juxta" is latin for "near" → located within the cortex, near the medulla.
- Subcapsulary nephrons: "sub" is latin for "below" → located within the cortex, below the capsule.

Renal Corpuscle

Structure
⊘ 200 µm

Function
Filtration of the blood, producing primary urine (glomerular ultrafiltrate)
- 180 L per 24 h.
- Substances are filtrated according to size, shape, and electrical charge.

Consists of
- Glomerulus
- Mesangium
- Bowman's capsule
  - Parietal layer
    ---Urinary space: space formed between the two layers----
  - Visceral layer

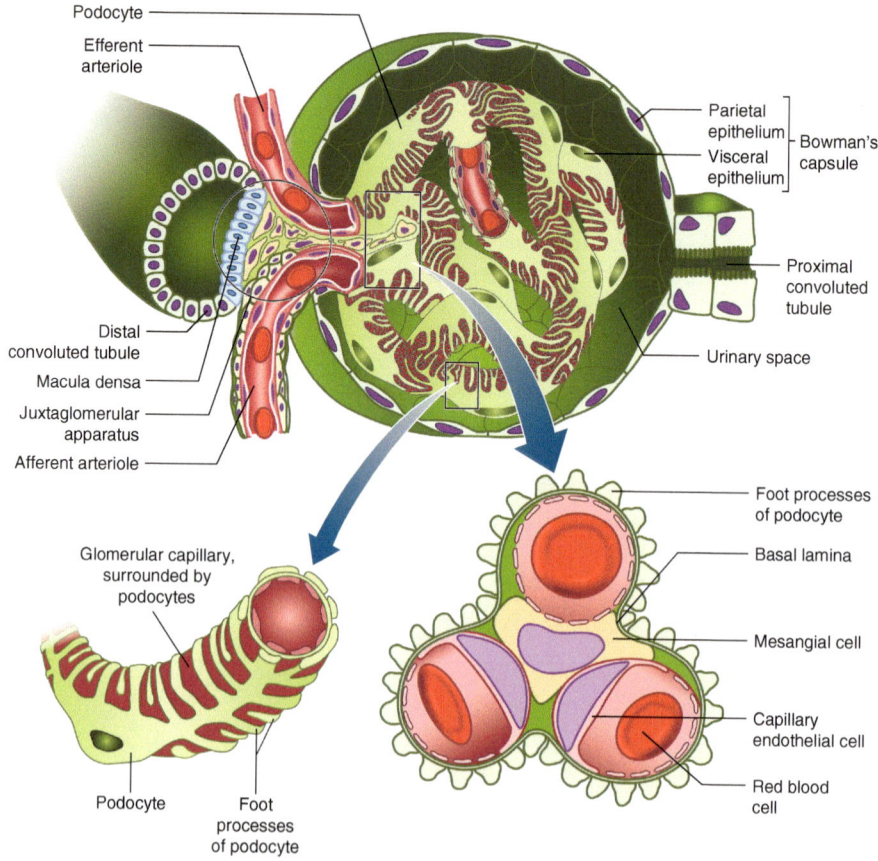

Fig. 23.3 Renal corpuscle. Glomerulus surrounded by the Bowman's capsule

Light Microscopy (Fig. 23.3)

- Glomerulus
  - Tuft of fenestrated capillaries, invaginated by the Bowman's capsule
    - Endothelium with fenestrations, 70–90 nm, without diaphragms
  - Thick (300 nm) negatively charged basement membrane, consisting of a fusion of the basal membranes of the glomerular endothelium and the podocytes
    - Stains pink with PAS
- Mesangium
  - Mesangial cells
  - Matrix (stains pink with PAS)
- Bowman's capsule
  - An epithelial cup, with two layers
    - Partial layer:
      - Simple cell layer continuous with the epithelium of the proximal tubule

- Visceral layer
  - Simple cell layer surrounding the capillaries of the glomerulus.
  - The cells are called podocytes.
    - Their cell body is placed some distance from the capillary wall.
    - Podocytes have primary processes, branching into
      - Secondary processes, further branching into
        - Foot processes (pedicles).
        - Pedicles interdigitate with pedicles from neighboring podocytes, like a zipper, almost entirely covering the basal lamina of the endothelium.

The glomerular filtration barrier

General
A physiological and anatomical barrier that limits the passage of small molecules from the blood of the glomerular capillaries to the urinary space of the Bowman's capsule

Consists of
- Endothelium (glomerular capillaries)
- Glomerular basal lamina
  - Lamina rara externa
  - Lamina densa
  - Lamina rara interna
- Filtration slits of the visceral layer of Bowman's capsule
  - 40 nm wide
  - Space between interdigitating pedicles of neighboring podocytes
  - Covered by an ultrathin diaphragm

Mesangial cells

General
- A part of the mesangium of the renal corpuscle
- Located both within and outside the glomerulus
  - Intraglomerular mesangial cells
  - Extraglomerular mesangial cells (Lacis cells)

Function
- Secretion of mesangial matrix
- Phagocytosis
- Mechanical support
  - Cytoplasmic processes with contractile elements extend around the endothelial cells of the glomerulus
- Extraglomerular mesangial cells form a part of the juxtaglomerular apparatus (JGA)

Light Microscopy
- Difficult to distinguish from neighboring podocytes and endothelial cells, in routine sections.
- Mesangial cells stain darker and have darker and larger nuclei than neighboring endothelial cells

Renal Tubule

General
- Continuous tube from the urinary pole of the Bowman's capsule to the collecting duct
- Lined with simple epithelium, which varies in the various parts (Fig. 23.2)

Function
Modulates the primary urine (glomerular ultrafiltrate) through:
- Reabsorption
- Secretion

Consists of
From the urinary pole of the Bowman's capsule → the collecting duct (Fig. 23.2)
- Proximal thick segment
  - Proximal convoluted tubule
  - Proximal straight tubule
- Thin segment
- Distal thick segment
  - Distal straight tubule
  - Distal convoluted tubule

Tubule epithelium
General
- The epithelium varies in the different parts of the tubule.
- The standard tubule cell:
  - Single-layered cuboidal/columnar epithelium.
  - Nucleus: centrally placed.
  - Cytoplasm: light acidophilic.
  - Apical surface: few, short microvilli.

- ○ Basal surface: basal striations due to abundant elongated mitochondria.
- ○ Lateral surface:
  - ▪ Well-developed tight junctions.
  - ▪ Lateral folds/interdigitations interacting with similar processes of neighboring cells.
- Special features of the "standard" cell in different part of the renal tubule are described below

Light Microscopy
- Proximal convoluted tubule
  - ○ Strongly acidophilic
  - ○ Well-developed basolateral interdigitations
  - ○ Brush border (microvilli) on apical surface, stained pink with PAS
  - ○ Active endocytosis apparatus:
    - ▪ Deep invaginations between the microvilli
    - ▪ Multiple vesicles and lysosomes
  - ○ Collapsed lumen in routine section
- Proximal straight tubule
  - ○ As the proximal convoluted tubule, but less developed
- Thin segment
  - ○ Squamous cell with flattened nuclei:
    - ▪ In cortical nephrons:
      - • Type I: flattened cell with few lateral interdigitations and organelles
    - ▪ In juxtamedullary nephrons:
      - • Type II: Taller cell, with plentiful organelles and small microvilli
      - • Type III: Simpler cell, few microvilli
      - • Type IV: Simpler cell, no microvilli
- Distal straight tubule
  - ○ Appearance close to standard tubule cell, but with:
    - ▪ Apical nuclei
    - ▪ Apical surface may bulge into the lumen
    - ▪ Macula densa: Cells in the last part of the distal straight tubule, which are thinner and more densely packed (see below)
- Distal convoluted tubule
  - ○ Appearance close to standard tubule cell, but with:
    - ▪ Less eosinophilic cytoplasm
    - ▪ Often apical nuclei
  - ○ Often open lumen in routine section

Macula Densa

General
- Located in the last part of the distal straight tubule
- Part of the juxtaglomerular apparatus (JGA)

Structure
- Tubule cells are thinner and more densely packed.
- The cells come in close apposition with the afferent and efferent arterioles at the renal corpuscle's vascular pole.
- The cells are in close relation to the extraglomerular mesangial cells and juxtaglomerular (JG) cells, through an incomplete basal lamina.

COLLECTING DUCT

Structure
- Runs from the cortex (in a medullary ray) through medulla and ends in area cribrosa at the papilla (apex of the medullary pyramid).
- The distal convoluted tubules of the nephrons empty into the collecting duct via:
  - A shorter connecting tubule or
  - An arched, longer collecting tubule

Function
- Concentrate the urine, due to regulation of excretion of Na^+, K^+, H^+, and H_2O
- Transport the urine from several nephrons to a minor calyx

Light Microscopy
Simple cuboidal epithelium, with two cell types
- Light cells (principal cells, collecting ducts (CD) cells)
  - Most numerous cell type
  - Central, round nuclei
  - Pale staining
  - Apical surface bulges into the lumen
- Dark cells (intercalated (IC) cells)
  - Central, round nuclei
  - Rich in mitochondria → densely stained
  - Apical surface bulges into the lumen
  - Not present in the deepest part of the collecting duct

JUXTAGLOMERULAR APPARATUS

General
Structure located where the afferent arteriole of the glomerulus comes in close contact with the macula densa of the distal straight tubule

Function
- Regulation of blood pressure through activation of the Renin–Angiotensin–Aldosterone system
- The secretion of renin is regulated by
  - Macula densa: monitors the Na^+ concentration of the urine
  - The juxtaglomerular (JG) cells: senses the blood pressure in the afferent arteriole of the glomerulus

Consists of
- JG cells
  - Modified smooth muscle cells in the wall of the afferent arteriole
  - Rounded cells with spherical nuclei
  - Secretory granules containing renin
- Macula densa
- Extraglomerular mesangial cells (Lacis cells)

BLOOD SUPPLY OF THE KIDNEY

Structure (Figs. 23.1 and 23.2)

Renal artery (a. renalis) from the aorta
↓
4–5 segment arteries: functional end arteries, i.e., not anastomosing
↓
Interlobar arteries (aa. interlobares) run between pyramids
↓
Arcuate arteries (aa. arcuatae): run in the corticomedullary border, at the base of the pyramids
↓
Interlobular arteries (aa. interlobulares) run in the cortical labyrinth, between the medullary rays, straight to the subcapsular area
↓
Afferent arterioles
↓
Glomerular capillaries (glomerulus)
↓
Efferent arterioles
↓

In cortical nephrons:	In juxtamedullary nephrons:
Peritubular capillary network (fenestrated)	Approximately 25 descending vasa recta
↓	↓
Interlobular veins (vv. interlobulares)	Medullary capillary network (fenestrated)
	↓
	Approximately 25 ascending vasa recta

Arcuate veins (vv. arcuate)
↓
Interlobar veins (vv. interlobares)
↓
Renal vein (v. renalis)

The Route of the Urine

General

Renal corpuscles → tubules → collecting/connecting tubules → collecting ducts → minor calyces → major calyces → pelvis → ureter → urinary bladder → urethra

Urinary Tract

General
- The structure of the wall is the similar through the whole proximal part of the urinary tract, but differs in the urethra.
- The thickness of the wall increases towards the urinary bladder.
- The thickness of the urinary bladder wall differs with the degree of distention.
  - It is more constant in the trigone area (between the two ureteric orifices and the internal urethral orifice) in the posterior part of the bladder.

Function
- Transport of the urine from the kidneys to the exterior.
- The urinary bladder is a reservoir for the urine.

Consists of
- Minor calyces (8 per kidney) ⎤
- Major calyces (2–3 per kidney) ⎥ ⎬ Paired
- Pelvis ⎥
- Ureter ⎦
- Urinary bladder (vesica urinaria)
- Urethra (female/male)

Wall of the Proximal Part of the Urinary Tract
Consists of
- Mucosa
- Muscularis
  - Two layers of smooth muscle cells.
    - Three layers in distal ureters and urinary bladder
  - The urinary bladder muscle is known as m. detrusor vesicae.
- Adventitia/serosa

Light Microscopy
- Mucosa
  - Epithelium
    - Urothelium/transitional epithelium (Chap. 5).
    - 2–3 layers in calyces → 3–7 layers in the bladder.
    - Morphology differs with distension of the bladder wall (Table 23.1).
  - Lamina propria
    - Dense connective tissue
- Muscularis
  - Inner layer
    - Longitudinally arranged smooth muscle cells
  - Outer layer
    - Circularly arranged smooth muscle cells
  - Additional outer layer
    - Only in distal ureters and the bladder
    - Longitudinally arranged smooth muscle cells
  - The internal urethral sphincter is a circular formation of smooth muscle cells around the internal urethral orifice (non-voluntary).
- Adventitia/serosa
  - Serosa: on the anterior part of ureters and superior part of the bladder
    - Submesothelial connective tissue
    - Mesothelium
  - Adventitia: On the posterior part of ureters and inferior part of the bladder
    - Connective tissue

Table 23.1 Light microscopy: mucosa of the urinary bladder

		Contracted bladder	Distended bladder
At low magnification		Mucous membrane folded	Mucous membrane smooth
At high magnification	Basal layer	• Several layers of small basophilic cuboidal/columnar cells • On a thin basement membrane	• Few layers of basophilic cuboidal cells • On a thin basement membrane
	Middle layer	Several layers of pale polyhedral cells	Few/no pale polyhedral cells
	Luminal layer	"Umbrella cells" • Large pale rounded cells • Convex towards lumen • Plaques in apical plasma-lemma = microfolds allowing the epithelium to be stretched when the bladder distend	• "Umbrella cells" are flattened • Each umbrella cell covers several underlying cells
Number of cell layers in the epithelium		Seven cell layers ──────────────→	Three cell layers

Female Urethra

Structure
- 4 cm long
- Luminal ⊘: proximally 9 mm → distally 6 mm
- Runs from the internal urethral orifice in the bladder to the external orifice in the vestibule

Function
Transports urine from bladder to the external environment

Wall of Female Urethra

Consists of
- Mucosa
  - Epithelium
    - Several types
      - Proximal part is primarily lined with urothelium
      - Distal part is primarily lined with stratified squamous epithelium
    - Intraepithelial mucous glands
  - Lamina propria
    - Loose connective tissue
    - Large venous plexuses, resemble the male corpus spongiosum
- Muscularis
  - Continuous with muscle of the urinary bladder.
  - The external urethral sphincter (m. sphincter urethra externus) is a voluntary (skeletal) muscle, located where the urethra crosses the pelvic floor.
- Adventitia
  - Connective tissue continuous with the adventitia of the vagina

Male Urethra

Structure
- 15–20 cm long
- Luminal ⊘: proximally 10 mm → distally 6 mm
- Runs from the internal urethral orifice in the bladder to external orifice on glans penis

Function
- Transports urine from the urinary bladder to the external environment
- Transports semen from the prostate and the ejaculatory ducts (Chap. 26) to the external environment

Divided into
- Prostatic urethra
  - Runs from the inferior part of the urine bladder, through the prostate
- Membranous urethra
  - Runs from prostate gland apex to the bulb of the penis
- Penile/spongy urethra
  - Runs through corpus spongiosum

Light Microscopy
See Table 23.2.

Table 23.2 Male Urethra

	Length	Epithelium	Surrounded by	Shape of lumen	Additional info
Prostatic urethra	3 cm	Urothelium	Prostate, smooth muscle cells	Banana-shaped	Ejaculatory ducts and small prostatic ducts empty into this part of urethra
Membranous urethra	1 cm	Stratified/pseudostratified columnar epithelium	• Skeletal muscle of pelvis floor • The external urethral sphincter (voluntary)	Star-shaped	
Penile urethra	15 cm	• Pseudostratified columnar epithelium → stratified squamous epithelium • With urethral intraepithelial mucous glands	Corpus spongiosum (see Chap. 26)	Transverse ovoid → T shaped → Sagittal ovoid	• Ducts from bulbourethral glands empty into this part of urethra • Ducts of urethral glands (Littre glands)

MEMO-BOX

To remember the parts of the male urethra – **p**rostatic, **m**embranous, and **s**pongy – think of a female problem: **P-M-S** (premenstrual syndrome).

Guide to Practical Histology: The Urinary System

Kidney

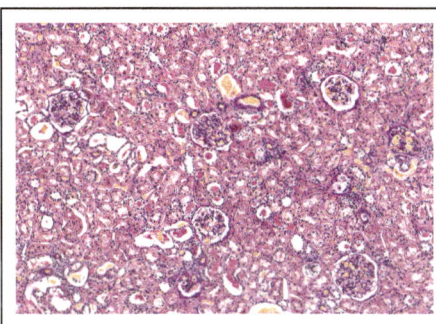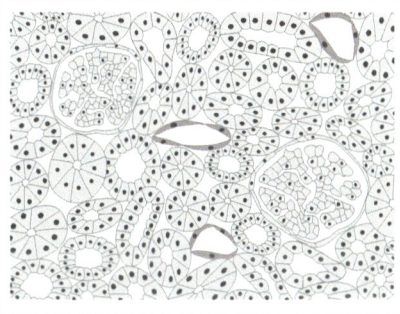

Left: photomicrograph of kidney cortex. Magnification: low. Stain: PAS (Courtesy of associate professor Steen Seier Poulsen, University of Copenhagen). *Right*: simplified illustration of the kidney cortex

Characteristics
- The cortex is granulated, with numerous rounded corpuscles and cross sections of tubules.
  - High magnification: corpuscles are seen as coils of vessels (glomeruli) surrounded by a white thin brim (urinary space of Bowman's capsule).
- Medulla is striated due to numerous parallel tubules, running perpendicular to the cortical surface.
  - There are no corpuscles in the medulla.

Can be mistaken for
The lacrimal gland
- Has no corpuscles

Special staining
PAS: stains certain structures pink
- The glycocalyx of the podocytes of the glomeruli
- The basal lamina of the glomeruli
- The mesangial region of the corpuscles

Ureter

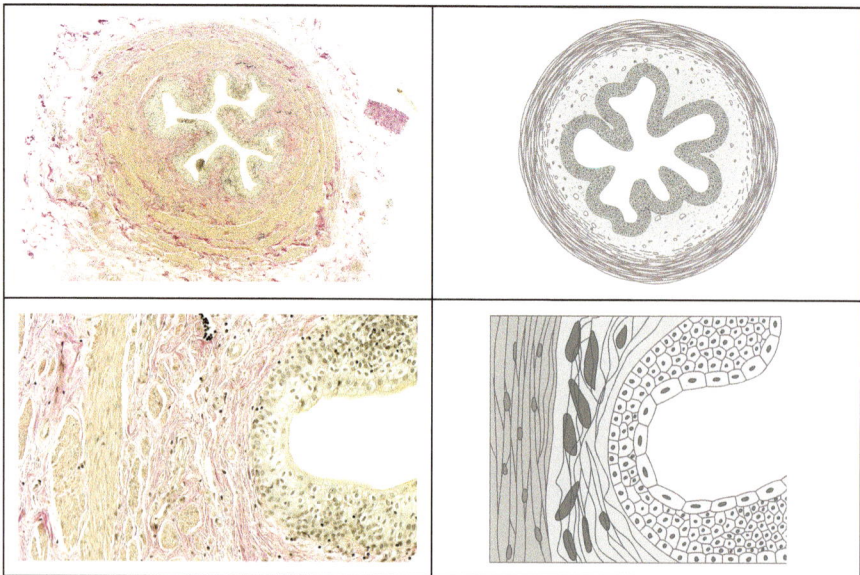

Top panel, left: photomicrograph of a cross section of the ureter. Magnification: low. Stain: Van Gieson (Courtesy of professor Jørgen Tranum Jensen, University of Copenhagen). *Top panel, right*: simplified illustration of a cross section of the ureter. *Bottom panel, left*: Photomicrograph of a cross section of ureter. Magnification: High. Stain: Van Gieson (Courtesy of professor Jørgen Tranum Jensen, University of Copenhagen). *Bottom panel, right*: Simplified illustration of a cross section of the ureter

Characteristics
Cross section
- A ring-shaped structure with a small star-shaped lumen.
- Luminally lined with urothelium.

Can be mistaken for
- Ductus deferens
  - Lined with pseudostratified epithelium.
  - An extremely thick layer of smooth muscle tissue surrounds the mucosa.
- Fallopian tube
  - Lined with simple columnar epithelium
  - Great mucosal folds (looks like curly kale)

Urinary Bladder

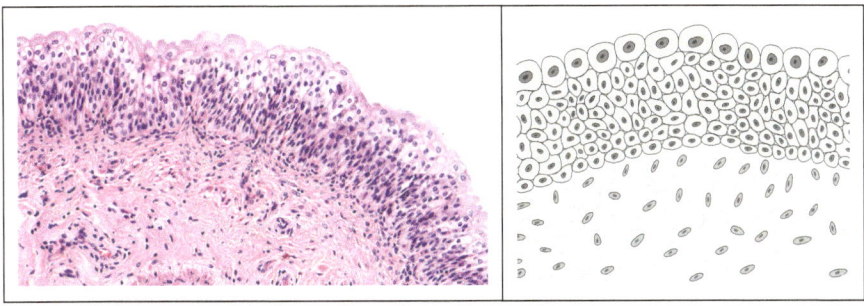

Left: photomicrograph of the urinary bladder wall (urothelium of a contracted (empty) urinary bladder). Magnification: high. Stain: HE (Courtesy of associate professor Steen Seier Poulsen, University of Copenhagen). *Right*: simplified illustration of the urothelium of the urinary bladder wall

Characteristics
- Wall
  - ○ Lumen is lined with urothelium.
  - ○ Thick layer of smooth muscle tissue
    - ▪ The smooth muscle fibers are arranged in three layers, in various directions.
- Appearance depends on the degree of contraction (fullness) of the urinary bladder (Table 23.3).

Table 23.3 Microscopic characteristics of the urinary bladder wall

		Contracted wall (empty bladder)	Distended wall (full bladder)
Low magnification	Mucous membrane (luminal surface)	Folded	Smooth
	Underlying layers of smooth muscle tissue	Thick	Thin
High magnification	Superficial layer of large, pale cells	Rounded cells, convex towards lumen	Cuboidal or flattened cells
	Middle layers of pale polyhedral cells	Several layers	Few/no layers
	Basal layers of basophilic cells	Several layers	Few layers

References

5, 17, 25, 31, 33, 34, 35, 45.

Chapter 24
The Endocrine System

Contents

General

- In this chapter the following discrete endocrine organs are described:
  - Pituitary gland (hypophysis)
  - Pineal gland
  - Thyroid gland
  - Parathyroid glands
  - Adrenal glands

© Springer International Publishing Switzerland 2017
A. Rehfeld et al., *Compendium of Histology*, DOI 10.1007/978-3-319-41873-5_24

- Many other tissues and organs contain cells with endocrine functions. Organs and tissues with this "secondary" endocrine function are described in other chapters:
  - Ovaries (Chap. 25)
  - Placenta (Chap. 25)
  - Testicles (Chap. 26)
  - Pancreas (Chap. 22)
  - Enteroendocrine cells of the gastrointestinal tract (Chap. 21)
  - Liver (Chap. 22)
  - Kidney (Chap. 23)
  - Heart (Chap. 17)
  - Adipose tissue (Chap. 11)

Structure
- Endocrine cells are found
  - Solitary, e.g., enteroendocrine cells
  - In endocrine tissues, e.g., in the pancreas
  - In endocrine organs (glands), e.g., the thyroid gland
- Endocrine tissues are highly vascularized as they:
  - Need materials for hormone production
  - Release their hormones to the blood, which transport the hormones throughout the body

Function
- Regulation of the action of cells, tissues, and organs via secretion of hormones → maintenance of homeostasis and management of multiple physiological processes, including:
  - Growth
  - Development
  - Metabolism
  - Reproduction
- The endocrine system works together with the nervous system:
  - Generally the endocrine system acts slowly, whereas the nervous system acts rapidly.

Light Microscopy
- Endocrine tissues contain many capillaries
- Parenchyma in endocrine glands (Chap. 6) consists of:
  - Trabecular endocrine tissue, or
  - Follicular endocrine tissue (only seen in the thyroid gland)

Hormones

General
A hormone is defined as the secretory product from an endocrine cell, which is transported with the bloodstream to target cells (effector cells).

Function
- Alter actions in target cells.
- Hormones only act in target cells, i.e., cells with the adequate receptors for the specific hormone.

Divided into
- Peptide hormones
  - Fast action
  - Bind to membrane-bound receptors and act via intracellular signaling pathways (second messengers)
- Steroid hormones
  - Slow action
  - Bind to receptors in the nucleus (or in the cytoplasm) and act by altering gene transcription and thereby protein synthesis
- Amine hormones
  - Act like peptide hormones
  - Except the thyroid hormones, which act like steroid hormones

Action of a hormone
Endocrine cell: synthesize and secrete hormones to the blood.
↓
Hormones are carried by the blood to target cells.
↓
In the target cells, the hormones act by binding to specific receptors.

Types of Hormone Receptors
Divided into
- Intracellular receptors
  - Localized in nucleus/cytoplasm
  - Bind:
    - Steroid hormones, which easily diffuse through the cell membrane
    - Thyroid hormones, which are transported across the cell membrane with carrier proteins
  - Have a slow response: affects gene transcription and thereby protein synthesis
  - For example, estrogen receptors
- Cell surface receptors
  - Mainly bind peptide/amine hormones (except the thyroid hormones)
  - Have a fast response: acts via intracellular signaling pathways

- ○ Divided into:
  - ▪ Ion-channel-coupled receptors
  - ▪ G-protein-coupled receptors
    - • For example, adrenergic receptors
  - ▪ Catalytic receptors, e.g., tyrosine kinases
    - • For example, insulin receptors

Types of Hormone Action

Divided into
- Endocrine
  - ○ Hormone is transported by the blood to target cells
  - ○ Hormone acts peripherally, on cells throughout the body
  - ○ Typical mode of action for classical hormones
- Paracrine
  - ○ Hormone diffuses to nearby cells.
  - ○ Hormone acts on neighboring cells.
  - ○ This mode of action is seen for, e.g., growth factors.
- Autocrine
  - ○ Hormone targets the secreting cell itself.
  - ○ The secreting cells express receptors for their secreted hormone.
  - ○ This mode of action is seen for, e.g., cytokines.

Feedback Systems

General
- Secretion of a hormone is often controlled by feedback from the target cells.
- Types of feedback
  - ○ Negative feedback
  - ○ Positive feedback

Negative feedback
- A response attenuates stimulation of hormone secretion (Fig. 24.1).
- Secretion of the hormone is
  - ○ Inhibited by
    - ▪ A high concentration of the hormone or
    - ▪ A high level of "hormone response"
  - ○ Stimulated by
    - ▪ A low concentration of the hormone or
    - ▪ A low level of "hormone response"
- Two examples
  1. $\uparrow$TSH $\rightarrow$ $\uparrow$ T_3 and T_4 $\rightarrow$ $\downarrow$TSH $\rightarrow$ $\downarrow$ T_3 and T_4 $\rightarrow$ $\uparrow$TSH $\rightarrow$ and so on
  2. $\uparrow$Blood glucose $\rightarrow$ $\uparrow$ insulin $\rightarrow$ $\downarrow$ blood glucose $\rightarrow$ $\downarrow$insulin $\rightarrow$ and so on

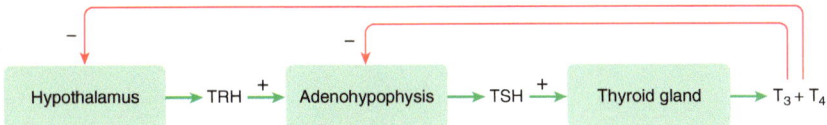

Fig. 24.1 Negative feedback. TRH from the hypothalamus stimulates the thyrotropes of the anterior lobe of the pituitary gland (adenohypophysis) to secrete TSH. TSH stimulates secretion of thyroid hormones (T3 and T4) from the thyroid gland. T3 and T4 inhibit secretion of both TRH and TSH

Positive feedback

- A response amplifies the hormone secretion.
- Not persistent, ends abrupt.
- Rare, e.g., seen prior to ovulation, where high levels of estrogen stimulate a peak of luteinizing hormone (LH) secretion.
  - ↑↑ estrogen → ↑↑ LH → ovulation.
  - Under normal conditions high levels of sex hormones will inhibit secretion of gonadotropins (LH and follicle stimulating hormone (FSH)) from the pituitary.

Pituitary Gland (Hypophysis)

General
- Small gland in close relation to the hypothalamus
- Located in sella turcica, in the sphenoid bone of the cranium
- Surrounded by a venous plexus

Structure
10×12 mm, 0.5 g

Divided into (Fig. 24.2)
- Adenohypophysis, anterior lobe
  - Pars tuberalis
  - Pars intermedia
  - Pars distalis
- Neurohypophysis, posterior lobe
  - Pars nervosa
  - Infundibulum

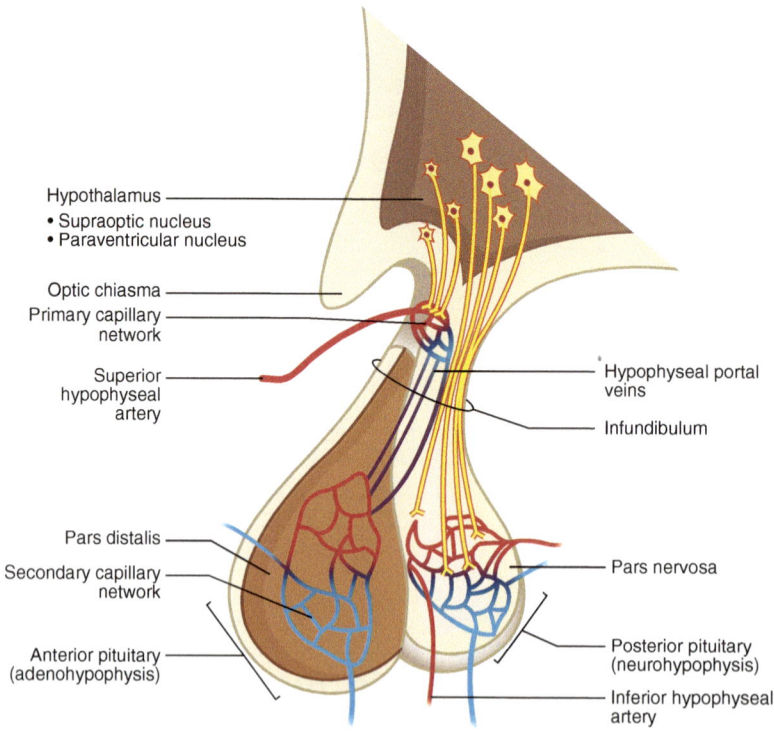

Fig. 24.2 Pituitary gland. Hormones from the hypothalamus reach the adenohypophysis through the hypothalamic-hypophyseal portal system. Axons from the hypothalamic nuclei run in the infundibulum, to the neurohypophysis

Consists of
- Adenohypophysis
  - Glandular epithelium
    - Trabecular endocrine tissue
  - Derived from ectoderm in the oropharynx (Rathke's pouch)
- Neurohypophysis
  - Nerve tissue
  - Derived from neuroectoderm of the diencephalon

ADENOHYPOPHYSIS

Function
- Controls the action of other endocrine tissues and organs, via secretion of regulatory (tropic) hormones
  - Gonadotropins
    - Follicle-stimulating hormone (FSH)
    - Luteinizing hormone (LH)

- ◦ Thyroid-stimulating hormone (TSH)
- ◦ Adrenocorticotropic hormone (ACTH)
- Regulation of non-endocrine tissues, via secretion of hormones
  - ◦ Growth hormone (GH)
  - ◦ Prolactin (PRL)
- All adenohypophyseal hormones are peptide hormones

Consists of
- Pars tuberalis
  - ◦ Sheaths of cells, surrounding the infundibulum of the neurohypophysis
- Pars intermedia
  - ◦ Thin brim of cells
  - ◦ Located between pars distalis of the adenohypophysis and pars nervosa of the neurohypophysis
  - ◦ Remnant of the lumen of Rathke's pouch
- Pars distalis
  - ◦ Main part of the adenohypophysis
  - ◦ Parenchyma
    - ▪ Chromophobes, 50% of cells in pars distalis
      - • Progenitor cells
      - • Chromophils that have emptied their cytoplasmic vesicles through exocytosis
    - ▪ Chromophils, secretory cells with hormones in cytoplasmic vesicles (Table 24.1)
      - • Acidophils, 40% of cells in pars distalis
        - ◦ Lactotropes, producing PRL
        - ◦ Somatotropes, producing GH
      - • Basophils, 10% of cells in pars distalis
        - ◦ Thyrotropes, producing TSH
        - ◦ Gonadotropes, producing gonadotropins: FSH and LH
        - ◦ Corticitropes, producing ACTH
  - ◦ Stroma
    - ▪ Folliculo-stellate cells
      - • Stellate cells with long cellular processes, surrounding the endocrine cells
    - ▪ Reticular fibers

Light Microscopy
- Pars tuberalis: cords of cells, abundant vessels.
- Pars intermedia: basophils and chromophobes, surrounding follicles of colloid.
- Pars distalis.
  - ◦ Cords or clusters of cells in relation to a dense network of fenestrated capillaries
  - ◦ Small amount of stroma
- The hormones (or precursors) synthesized in the basophils are all glycoproteins, which is why the granules are stained pink with PAS.

Table 24.1 Chromophils

	Cell shape	Nucleus	Granules stain with	Product	Target organ	Secretion primarily regulated by
Basophils						
• Thyrotropes	Large, polygonal	Round, eccentric	HE: weakly basophilic PAS: pink	TSH	Thyroid gland	Stimulation • Thyrotropin-releasing hormone (TRH) Inhibition • Thyroid hormones (T$_3$ and T$_4$)
• Gonadotropes	Small, ovoid	Round, eccentric	HE: weakly basophilic PAS: pink	FSH LH	Gonads	Stimulation • Gonadotropin-releasing hormone (GnRH) Inhibition • Estrogen and progesterone • Testosterone • Inhibin
• Corticitropes	Polygonal	Round, eccentric	HE: weakly basophilic PAS: pink	ACTH	Adrenal glands	Stimulation: • Corticotropin-releasing hormone (CRH) Inhibition • Cortisol
Acidophils						
• Lactotropes	Polygonal	Ovoid	HE: acidophilic	PRL	Mammary glands	Inhibition • Dopamine
• Somatotropes	Ovoid	Round, central	HE: acidophilic	GH	Several	Stimulation • Growth hormone-releasing hormone (GHRH) Inhibition • Somatostatin • Insulin-like growth factor 1 (IGF-1)

NEUROHYPOPHYSIS

General
- The hormones of the neurohypophysis are produced in neurosecretory neurons, with cell bodies located in the hypothalamic nuclei:
  - ○ Supraoptic nucleus (nucleus supraopticus)
  - ○ Paraventricular nucleus (nucleus paraventricularis)
- Axons of neurosecretory neurons do not end in a synapse with another neuron or target cell, but in relation to the fenestrated capillaries of pars nervosa of the neurohypophysis.

Function
Storage site for neurohormones that regulate non-endocrine tissues
- Antidiuretic hormone (ADH)
- Oxytocin (OX)

Consists of
- Pars nervosa
  - Pituicytes: specialized glial cells
  - Endings of nonmyelinated nerve fibers from nuclei in hypothalamus
- Infundibulum
  - Hypothalamic-hypophyseal tracts of nerve fibers
  - Connected to the hypothalamus via the median eminence

Light Microscopy
- Pituicytes
  - HE: only round/oval nuclei are visible.
  - Silver stain: abundant cytoplasmic processes are seen.
- Nonmyelinated nerve fibers
- Fenestrated capillaries
- Herring bodies
  - Accumulations of secretory material in the axons
  - Mallory-Azan: stained blue

BLOOD SUPPLY OF THE PITUITARY

Function
Regulatory substances from the hypothalamus reach the endocrine cells of the pars distalis in the adenohypophysis via the hypothalamic-hypophyseal portal system.

Structure
- All capillaries are fenestrated, with a large ⊘.
  - The capillaries are called "sinusoidal" even though they are not true sinusoids.
- Derived from two sets of arteries (Fig. 24.2):
1. Superior hypophyseal arteries → primary capillary network in the upper part of infundibulum → hypophyseal portal veins in the pars tuberalis → secondary capillary network in pars distalis → hypophseal veins → sinus cavernosus.
2. Inferior hypophyseal arteries → capillary plexus in pars nervosa → hypophseal veins → sinus cavernosus.

Pineal Gland

General
Appendix on the roof/posterior wall of the third ventricle

Structure
- 4 × 7 mm, 150 mg
- Flattened, pine cone shaped gland

Function
- Contributes to the regulation of diurnal body rhythms, through circadian secretion of melatonin:
  1. Circadian variation in blood melatonin levels →
  2. Changes in the activity of the hypothalamus, pituitary gland, and other endocrine tissues →
  3. 24-hour rhythm of physiological functions and behavior
- The pineal gland translates neural input, regarding light and darkness into variations in endocrine functions, e.g., secretion of GH, which peaks during sleep.
  ○ Melatonin release from pinealocytes is
    ▪ Inhibited by light
    ▪ Stimulated by darkness

Consists of
- Cells
  ○ Pinealocytes
    ▪ Principal cell type, 95 %
    ▪ Melatonin secreting
    ▪ Cytoplasmic processes, end in relation to surrounding capillaries
  ○ Interstitial cells
    ▪ Supporting glial cells, 5 %
- Acervuli cerebri (corpora arenacea, brain sand)
  ○ Calcified concretions with concentric lamella
- Stroma
  ○ Capsule, consisting of the innermost meninges, pia mater
  ○ Septa from the capsule divide the gland into lobules
  ○ Well-developed network of continuous capillaries

Light Microscopy
- Pinealocytes.
  ○ In cords/clumps.
  ○ Large, weakly basophilic cells.
  ○ Large, round nuclei.
  ○ The cytoplasmic processes are not seen in HE stain.

- Interstitial cells
  - Smaller, darker nuclei
  - Cytoplasmic processes only seen in silver stain
- Acervuli cerebri
  - Large, rounded basophilic structures
- Capillaries
  - Seen as strands of multiple erythrocytes

Thyroid Gland

General
Bilobed gland located in the anterior part of the neck, just inferior to the larynx

Structure
- 25 g
- Butterfly-shaped gland
- Consist of
  - Two lobes, each $5 \times 2.5 \times 2.5$ cm
  - Isthmus, a thin rim of tissue that unites the two lobes
  - Pyramidal lobe, inconsistent, extends upwards from the isthmus
- Surrounded by:
  - Capsule of connective tissue
    - Sends septa into the gland and divides it into irregular lobes
  - An additional thin layer of connective tissue surrounds the gland

Function
Secretion of
- Thyroid hormones: T_3 and T_4 (amine hormones)
- Calcitonin (peptide hormone)

Consists of (Fig. 24.3)
- Parenchyma
  - Follicular endocrine tissue
    - Follicles, the functional unit of the gland
      - Follicular cells
      - C cells
- Stroma (interfollicular space)
  - Loose connective tissue
  - Fenestrated capillaries

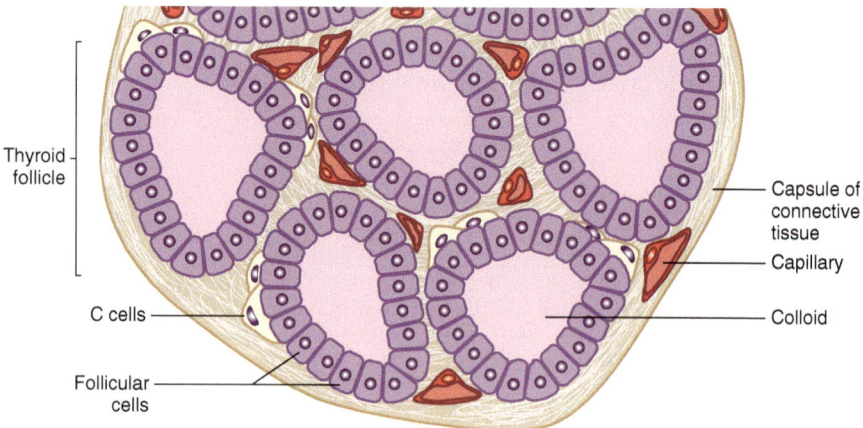

Fig. 24.3 Thyroid gland. The thyroid follicle consists of a brim of simple epithelium (follicular cells) surrounding a central space filled with colloid. Small groups of C cells are located between the follicular cells and their basement membrane. The interfollicular connective tissue has abundant capillaries

Thyroid follicle

Structure
- Spherical structure
- ⊘ 50 μm–1 mm

Consists of
From center → periphery
- Colloid
  - Gelatinous substance
  - Contains extracellular stored secretions, e.g.:
    - Enzymes
    - Thyroglobulin
      - An iodinated glycoprotein
      - The inactive stored precursor of T_3 and T_4
- Follicular cells
  - Participate in the production of T_3 and T_4
- Parafollicular cells (C cells)
  - Produce calcitonin
  - Derived from crista neuralis
- Basal lamina

Light Microscopy

- Colloid
  - HE: acidophilic
  - PAS: heavily pink
- Follicular cells
  - Simple epithelium
    - Epithelial height varies with secretory activity
      - Passive gland: squamous/cuboidal epithelium
      - Active gland: columnar epithelium
    - Microvilli and pseudopodia on apical surface
    - Round, pale nuclei with one to several prominent nucleoli
    - Cytoplasm
      - Weak basophilic, due to rER
      - Vesicles
        - Subapical granules
        - Colloid droplets
        - Lysosomes
- Parafollicular cells (C cells)
  - Fewer than the follicular cells
  - Located between the follicular cells and the basal lamina, never in contact with the colloid
  - Seen solitary or in groups of 3–4 cells
  - Large, pale cells with a large, light nucleus

Production of thyroid hormone

1. Follicular cells concentrate iodide (I⁻) from the blood and pump it into the colloid.
2. Iodide (I⁻) is oxidized to iodine (I) in the colloid.
3. Follicular cells produce uniodinated thyroglobulin, which is secreted to the colloid.
4. In the colloid, in relation to the luminal surface of the follicular cells, the thyroglobulin becomes iodinated.
5. T3 and T4 residues are formed within the iodinated thyroglobulin molecule.
6. Follicular cells endocytose colloid as droplets in endosomes, which fuse with lysosomes → T3 and T4 are liberated from the iodinated thyroglobulin molecule and released to the blood.

Parathyroid Glands

General
Four small glands located in relation to the thyroid gland, often posteriorly, but the location may vary

Structure
- Four ovoid glands (number may vary), arranged in two pairs
- 130 mg in total
- 0.3 × 0.5 cm each
- Thin capsule of connective tissue

Function
Secretion of parathyroid hormone (PTH), a peptide hormone crucial in the regulation of plasma levels of calcium

Consist of
- Parenchyma
  - Principal (chief) cells
    - Secrete PTH
  - Oxyphil cells
    - No known secretory activity
    - Number increases with age
- Stroma
  - Adipocytes
    - Number increases with age → 60–70 % of gland in elderly.
  - Well-developed network of fenestrated capillaries.
  - Connective tissue septa from the capsule divide the parenchyma into diffusely defined lobules.

Light Microscopy
Compactly packed cords of cells
- Principal cells
  - Small, polygonal cells
  - Slightly acidophilic
  - Central nuclei
  - Lipofuscin vesicles, glycogen, and lipid droplets
- Oxyphil cells
  - Large, round
  - Heavily acidophilic
  - Solitary or in clusters
  - Small, basophilic nuclei

- Adipocytes
  - ○ ⊘ 15–150 µm
  - ○ Rounded/polyhedral cells
  - ○ Peripheral, flattened nucleus
  - ○ Contain a single large lipid droplet, which fills up almost all of the cytoplasm
    - ▪ Lipid leaches out during routine preparation → only the nucleus and a thin rim of cytoplasm are left → the cell looks like a hollow circle.

Adrenal Glands

General

Paired glands located retroperitoneally, in relation to the superior poles of the kidneys

Structure

- Paired, flattened, triangular glands.
- 1 × 3 × 5 cm.
- 10 g together.
- Thick capsule of connective tissue.
- Connective tissue trabeculae run from the capsule down into the cortex, carrying vessels and nerves.

Consist of (Fig. 24.4)

- Cortex
- Medulla

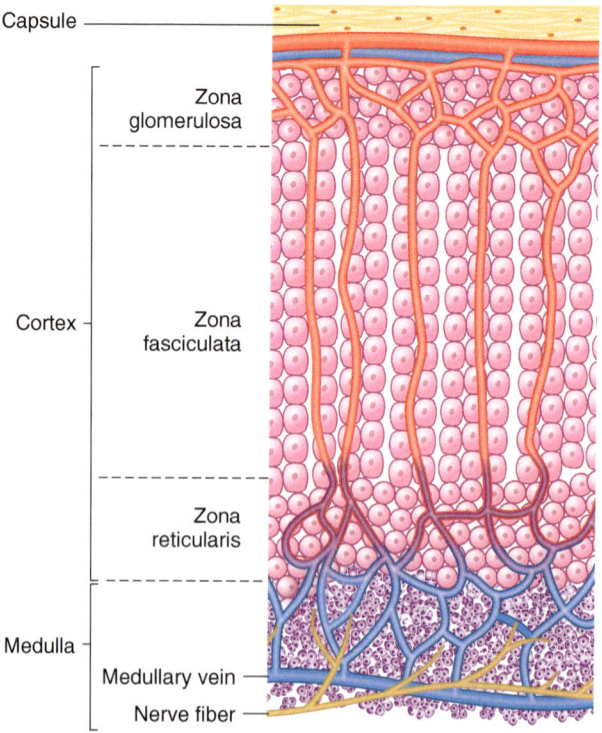

Fig. 24.4 The adrenal gland

ADRENAL CORTEX

General
- 90% of the volume of the gland
- Derived from the urogenital ridge (mesoderm)

Function
Secretion of steroid hormones
- Mineralocorticoids, e.g., aldosterone
- Glucocorticoids, e.g., cortisol
- Gonadocorticoids, e.g., androstenedione (androgen)

Divided into

Three concentric zones
- Zona glomerulosa, 15 % of the volume
- Zona fasciculata, 80 % of the volume
- Zona reticularis, 5 % of the volume

Consists of
- Parenchyma
  ○ Trabecular endocrine tissue with steroid hormone-producing cells
    ▪ Cells generally contain abundant sER, mitochondria, and lipid droplets.
    ▪ Appearance differs in the three zones of cortex (Table 24.2).
- Stroma
  ○ Capsule of dense connective tissue sends trabeculae into the cortex.
  ○ Reticular fibers.
  ○ Fenestrated capillaries.

Light Microscopy

See Table 24.2.

Table 24.2 Adrenal cortex

	Cells arranged in	Cells	Ultrastructure	Nucleus	Capillaries
Zona glomerulosa	Compact arches and clusters	• Small columnar/ pyramidal • Acidophilic cytoplasm, with small basophilic clumps	• sER • Mitochondria with regular, shelflike cristae • Few lipid droplets • rER • Golgi apparatus	• Round • Densely basophilic	Well-developed network of fenestrated capillaries (called sinusoids) run between cells arches
Zona fasciculata	Radiating columns (1–2 cells wide)	• Large, polyhedral • Slightly acidophilic cytoplasm with abundant vacuoles → popcorn-like appearance due to leached out lipids (artifact)	• Highly developed sER • Mitochondria with tubular cristae • Abundant lipid droplets • rER • Golgi apparatus	Pale	Radiating cell columns are separated by fenestrated capillaries (called sinusoids)
Zona reticularis	Anasto- mosing network	• Small, columnar cells • Acidophilic cytoplasm • "Dark cells": containing lipofuscin granules	• sER • Mitochondria with tubular cristae • Few lipid droplets • Little rER • Golgi apparatus	Densely basophilic	Anastomosing cords of cells are separated by fenestrated capillaries (called sinusoids)

ADRENAL MEDULLA

General
- 10% of the volume of the gland
- Derived from the neural crest (ectoderm)

Structure
- Numerous presynaptic sympathetic nerve fibers form synapses with chromaffin cells of the adrenal medulla.
- The chromaffin cells lack axons and release their secretions into the fenestrated capillaries of the medulla.
  - The chromaffin cells can be thought of as altered postsynaptic sympathetic neurons, lacking axons.

Function
Secretion of catecholamines (peptide hormones)
- Epinephrine (adrenaline) 90%
- Norepinephrine (noradrenaline) 10%
- Catecholamines are released in response to an impulse from the presynaptic sympathetic nerve fibers.

Consists of
- Parenchyma
  - Chromaffin cells
- Stroma
  - Ganglion cells
  - Connective tissue
  - Fenestrated capillaries in a well-developed network

Light Microscopy
- Diffuse border between the medulla and zona reticularis of the cortex
- Chromaffin cells
  - In clusters/cords
  - Large, epitheloid
  - Weakly basophilic cytoplasm with fine granules
    - Granules stain brown with chrome salt fixations
- Fenestrated capillaries
- Ganglion cells
  - Rarely seen

Ultrastructure

Chromaffin cells

- rER, mitochondria, and well-developed Golgi apparatus
- Abundant vesicles with secretory material
  - Norepinephrine in large vesicles with dense cores
  - Epinephrine in smaller, homogenous, and less dense vesicles
  - A cell either contains norepinephrine or epinephrine vesicles, not both

BLOOD SUPPLY OF THE ADRENAL GLANDS

Structure

- Both cortical "sinusoids" and medullary capillaries are fenestrated.
- There are no veins in the cortex.
- Cortical hormones reach the medulla with the blood draining from cortical "sinusoids" to medullary capillary network → thus, cortical hormones can influence the production of catecholamines.

Consists of

See Table 24.3 and Fig. 24.4.

Table 24.3 Blood supply of the adrenal glands

	Vessels		Features
Arteries	Superior, middle, and inferior suprarenal arteries ↓		Originate from the phrenic artery, aorta and the renal artery, respectively
	Subcapsular plexus ↙ ↘		Branch just underneath entering the capsule
	Cortical arterioles ↓	Medullary arterioles ↓	Medullary arterioles run in the cortical connective tissue trabeculae
Capillaries	Cortical "sinusoids" ⟶ ↓	Medullary capillary network ↓	The cortical "sinusoids" drain into: • The medullary capillary network • The collecting veins at corticomedullary border
Veins	Collecting veins at corticomedullary border ↓		
	Central adrenomedullary veins ↓		
	Suprarenal vein		

Guide to Practical Histology: The Endocrine System

General
Endocrine glandular tissue is well vascularized.
- Trabecular endocrine tissue
  - Numerous capillaries are seen as white cords filled with red erythrocytes, in between the strands/groups of endocrine cells.
- Follicular endocrine tissue
  - Numerous capillaries are seen as small white spaces filled with red erythrocytes, in the interfollicular connective tissue.

The Pituitary Gland

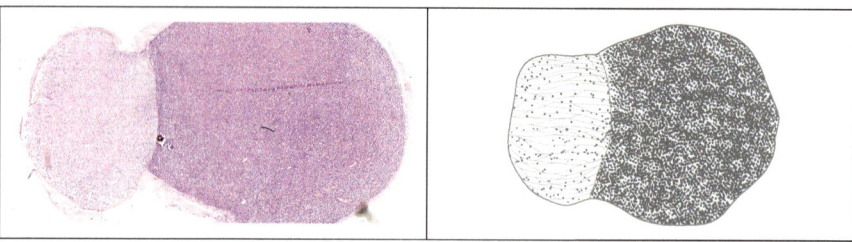

Left: photomicrograph of the pituitary gland. The adenohypophysis to the *right* and the neurohypophysis to the *left*. Magnification: low. Stain: HE (Courtesy of associate professor Steen Seier Poulsen, University of Copenhagen). *Right*: simplified illustration of the pituitary gland

Characteristics
- Macroscopic
  - Two distinct components:
    - A larger, darker adenohypophysis
    - A smaller, lighter neurohypophysis
- Microscopic
  - Two distinct components:
    - A heavily stained adenohypophysis
      - Basophilic, eosinophilic, and pale cells in cords, separated by capillaries
    - A pale neurohypophysis
      - Rich in nerve fibers (fibrillar appearance)
      - Contains rounded eosinophilic bodies (Herring bodies)

The Thyroid Gland

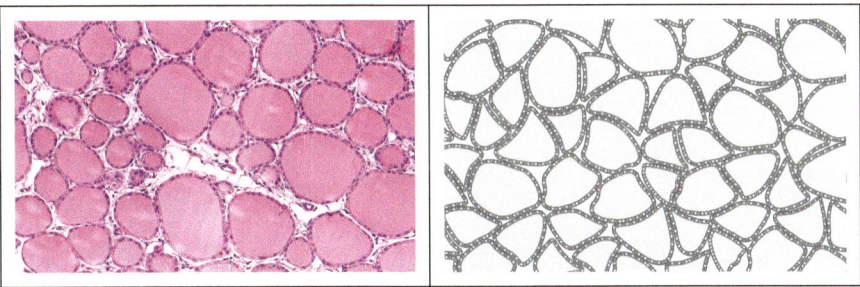

Left: photomicrograph of the thyroid gland. Magnification: low. Stain: HE (Courtesy of professor Jørgen Tranum Jensen, University of Copenhagen). *Right*: simplified illustration of the thyroid gland

Characteristics
- Consists of multiple large follicles:
  - Rings/circles of simple epithelium.
  - Epithelium surrounds a lumen filled with homogenous eosinophilic material (colloid).
- Between follicles there are thin strands of loose connective tissue with capillaries.

The Parathyroid Glands

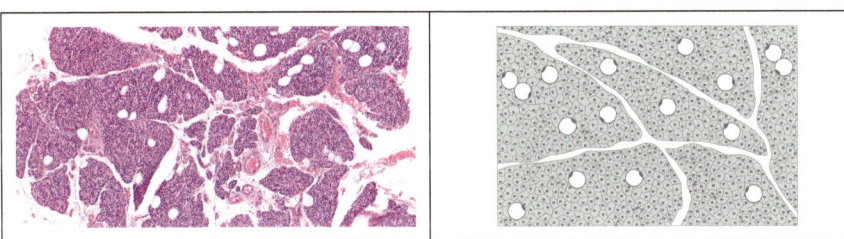

Left: photomicrograph of the parathyroid gland. Magnification: low. Stain: HE (Courtesy of associate professor Steen Seier Poulsen, University of Copenhagen). *Right*: simplified illustration of the parathyroid gland

Characteristics
- An "ocean" of basophilic chief cells.
- Scattered adipocytes are seen as large, white (empty) polyhedral cells in the basophilic "ocean."
- Numerous capillaries are seen between the cells.

Can be mistaken for
Thymus
- Divided into a dark cortex and a light medulla
- Contains eosinophilic lamellar bodies (Hassall's bodies)

The Adrenal Glands

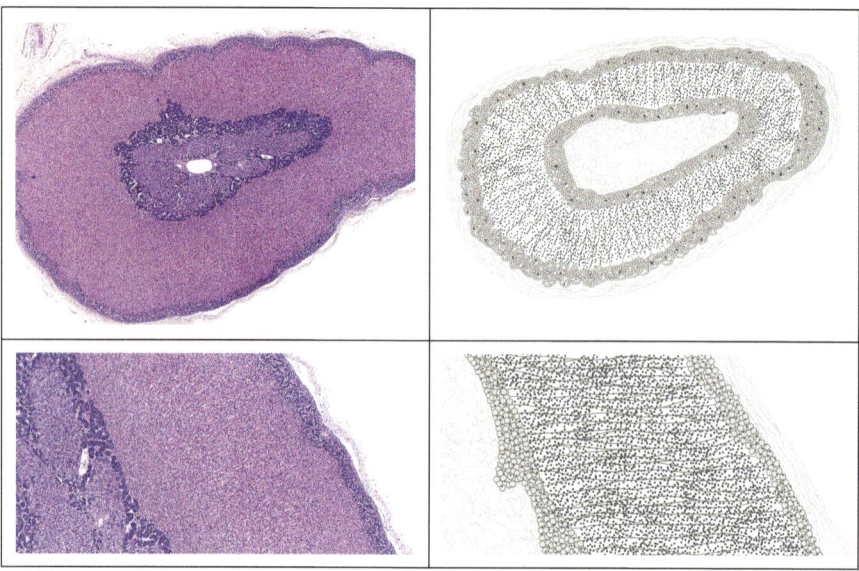

Top panel, left: photomicrograph of the adrenal gland. Magnification: low. Stain: HE (Courtesy of associate professor Steen Seier Poulsen, University of Copenhagen). *Top panel, right*: simplified illustration of the adrenal gland. *Bottom panel, left*: photomicrograph of the adrenal gland. Capsule to the right and medulla to the left. Magnification: high. Stain: HE (Courtesy of associate professor Steen Seier Poulsen, University of Copenhagen). *Bottom panel, right*: simplified illustration of the adrenal gland

Characteristics
- Macroscopic
  - Often seen as a dark tissue brim (cortex) surrounding a lighter center (medulla).
  - Sometimes the difference in color between the two parts is difficult to spot.

- Microscopic
  - Most superficial is a connective tissue capsule.
  - Cells in the most superficial layer of the cortex are arranged in groups.
  - In deeper parts of the cortex, popcorn-like cells are arranged in radiating, parallel strands, perpendicular to the capsule.
  - Most central is an irregular and thin medulla.
  - Numerous capillaries are seen between the cells.

References

5, 15, 25, 33, 34, 45.

Chapter 25
The Female Reproductive System

Contents

General Introduction to the Reproductive Systems

General
Enables human reproduction, through several steps:
- Development of gametes
- Fertilization of the egg
- Development of the embryo → fetus
- Labor
- Nursing of the child (Chap. 27)

© Springer International Publishing Switzerland 2017
A. Rehfeld et al., *Compendium of Histology*, DOI 10.1007/978-3-319-41873-5_25

REPRODUCTIVE ORGANS

Divided into
- Primary (gonads) (Table 25.1)
  - ○ Production/maturation of gametes (oocytes or spermatozoa)
  - ○ Production of sex hormones
- Secondary/accessory
  - ○ Facilitates the fertilization, primary through peristaltic movements and secretions

Table 25.1 Primary reproductive organs (gonads)

	Gonad	Gamete	Epithelial support cell	Stromal support cell
Female	Ovary	Oocyte (egg)	Granulosa cell	Theca cell
Male	Testicle	Spermatozoon (sperm cell)	Sertoli cell	Leydig cell

SEX

General
Humans, and many other species, have sexual specialization, and their population consists of two different individuals:
- Females
- Males

Divided into
- Genetic sex
  - ○ Established at fertilization by presence/absence of a Y chromosome
- Gonadal sex
  - ○ The gonadal sex is determined in 6th–7th week of gestation.
  - ○ Established by the SRY gene (on the Y chromosome):
    - ▪ Expression of the SRY gene → activation of male determining genes → male development from the sexually indifferent stage
    - ▪ No expression of the SRY gene → female development from the sexually indifferent stage
- Biological sex
  - ○ Due to influence of sex hormones, behavior and appearance differ between the female and male phenotype.

The Female Reproductive System

Consists of
- Internal reproductive organs
  - Ovaries
  - Fallopian tubes
  - Uterus
  - Vagina
- External reproductive organs (vulva)
  - Mons pubis
  - Labia majora and minora
  - Erectile bodies: clitoris and vestibular bulbs
  - Vestibule, with minor and major vestibular glands

General
The female reproductive system changes through life.
- Puberty:
  - The female reproductive organs grow and develop
- - - - -Menarche- - - - - -
  - First menstruation
  - Marks the end of puberty and beginning of fertile period
- Fertile period:
  - During the fertile period an ovulation takes place approximately every 28–30 day, causing a menstrual bleeding once a month.
- - - - -Menopause- - - - - -
  - Marks the end of fertile period
  - Ovulations and endocrine function of the ovaries terminates →
    - Infrequent and eventually ceased menstruations
    - Slow atrophy of the female reproductive organs, as estrogen levels drop
- Post-menopausal period

The Internal Reproductive Organs

OVARY

Structure
- Paired, ovoid organs located in the pelvis.
- $1 \times 2 \times 3$ cm, 6–8 g each.
- Size differs with age and pregnancy.
- The ovaries atrophy after menopause.

Function

- Oogenesis: proliferation (in fetal life) and maturation of the female gametes, oocytes
- Production of sex hormones:
  - Estrogens
    - Stimulates growth and development of internal and external reproductive organs
    - Causes female sex characteristics, e.g., breast development
    - Both theca and granulosa cells of the ovaries are important in estrogen production:
      - Estrogen precursor (androstenedione) is produced in theca cells.
      - Androstenedione diffuses to the granulosa cells where it is aromatized to estradiol.
  - Progesterone
    - Causes secretory changes in the endometrium, which prepare uterus for pregnancy
    - Prepares the mammary gland for lactation (during pregnancy)
- The ovary function is controlled by the gonadotropins secreted from the pituitary gland:
  - Follicle-stimulating hormone (FSH)
  - Luteinizing hormone (LH)

Consists of

- Medulla
  - Centrally located loose connective tissue
  - Sex hormone producing ovarian hilar cells
  - Vessels and nerves
- Cortex
  - Stroma
    - Loose, cellular connective tissue
    - Hormone-producing interstitial cells, derived from atretic follicles
  - Parenchyma: Ovarian follicles (Table 25.2, Fig. 25.1):
    - Oocytes
    - Epithelium surrounding oocytes
- Capsule (tunica albuginea)
  - Thin layer of dense connective tissue.
  - The external surface is covered with a simple, cuboidal epithelium, called germinal epithelium.

Light Microscopy

See Table 25.2.

Table 25.2 Ovarian follicles and their development

	Primordial follicle	Primary follicle	Secondary (antral) follicle	Graafian, mature follicle	Corpus luteum	Corpus albicans
Follicle development				→	OVULATION	→
General	Most abundant follicle type			A Single, large follicle Ø >10 mm	Remaining part of an ovulated Graafian follicle	Degenerated corpus luteum
Location	Superficial part of cortex	Superficial part of cortex	Deeper part of cortex	Spanning the cortex	Cortex	Cortex
Oocyte	Primary oocyte: • 30-35 µm • Large, eccentric nucleus with 1 or more nucleoli • Acidophilic cytoplasm	Growing oocyte: Increasing Ø	Growing oocyte: Ø 100-125 µm	Secondary oocyte (at ovulation): Ø150 µm	-	-
Zona pellucida	-	Extracellular glycoprotein layer • Produced by the oocyte • Stains intensely with acidophilic stains and with PAS			-	-
Surrounding epithelium: Central	Single layer of squamous follicle cells	One -> multiple layers of cuboidal granulosa cells derived from the follicle cells • As the follicle grows fluid filled spaces appear between the granulosa cells → Spaces fuse and from an antrum. • The fluid, liquor folliculi, is viscous and highly osmotic.	• Cumulus oophorus:a prominence of granulosa cells, which surround the oocyte and protude into the antrum. • Antrum: a crescent shaped space filled with liquor folliculi	• Corona radiata: granulosa cells surrounding the oocyte. Persist to after ovulation • Antrum grows bigger.	Granulosa lutein cells: • Big, polyhedral cells • Pale cytoplasm • Plentiful sER • Mitochondria with tubular cristae	Cells undergo autolysis, and hyaline material accumulates between them.
Peripheral			• Multiple layers of cuboidal granulosa cells derived from the follicle cells	• Multiple layers of cuboidal granulosa cells derived from the follicle cells		
Basal lamina	+	+	+	+	-	-
Surrounding stroma	-	Stromal cells forms a cover of connective tissue, theca folliculi	Theca folliculi differentiates into: • Theca interna • Highly vascularized • Cuboidal/polyhedral steroid secreting cells with many LH-receptors • Fibroblasts and collagen bundles • Theca externa • Connective tissue and smooth muscle tissue		Theca lutein cells: • Smaller • Darker cytoplasm • Plentiful sER • Mitochondria with tubular cristae	Cells undergo autolysis, and hyaline material accumulates between them.

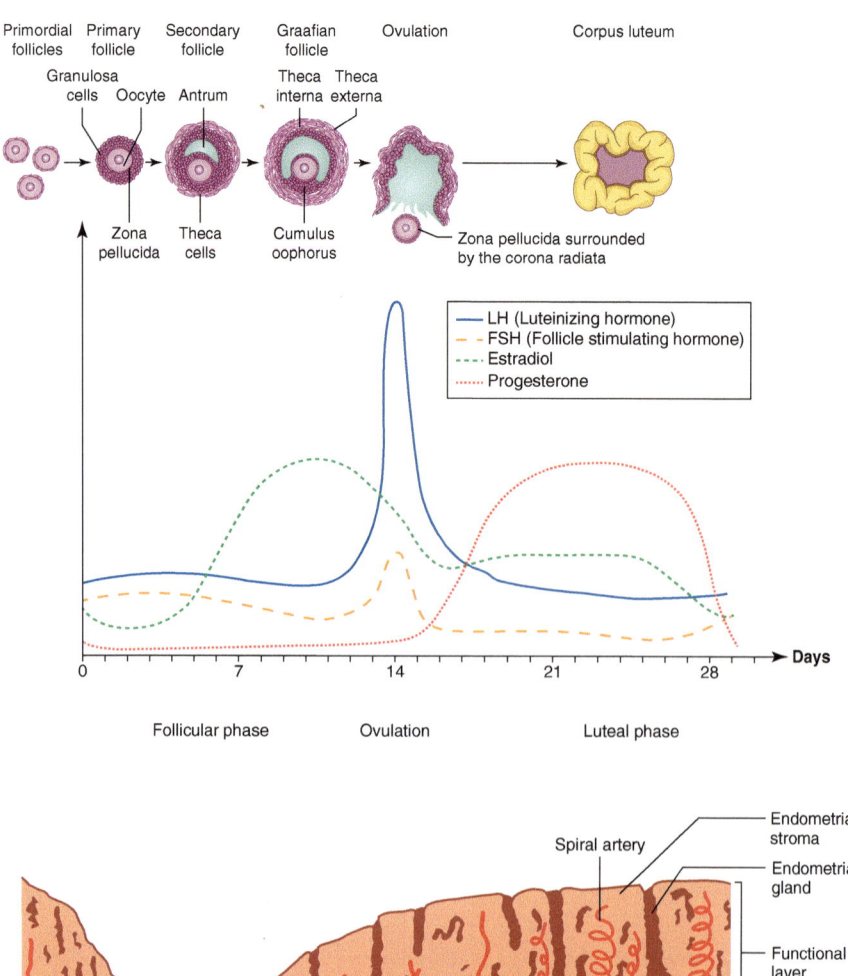

Fig. 25.1 Ovarian follicle development, ovarian, and endometrial cycles. FSH stimulates follicular growth and development. A peak in the level of LH triggers ovulation. Progesterone levels rise when the ovulated follicle turns into a corpus luteum

Follicle Development and Ovulation

Follicle development

General (Fig. 25.1 and Table 25.2).

1. Every day a small cohort of primordial follicles starts growing/maturing, independent of the concentration of follicle-stimulating hormone (FSH) from the pituitary gland

2. At a certain size, the growth becomes FSH-dependent as the granulosa cells develop FSH receptors

3. The follicles with the right size and right amount of FSH receptors continue to grow and mature as the level of FSH rises

4. As the follicles grow, they produce estrogens, causing FSH levels to fall, through negative feedback on the pituitary gland

5. The follicle with the most abundant FSH receptors "survives" the decreased level of FSH and continues to develop into a dominant Graafian follicle, which goes through ovulation

Ovulation

General (Fig. 25.1 and Table 25.2)

- The discharge of a secondary oocyte with surrounding zona pellucida and corona radiata from the Graafian follicle.
- Usually, only one follicle goes through ovulation each month.

Formation

A peak in plasma levels of luteinizing hormone (LH) stimulates the ovulation.

1. Just prior to ovulation, the Graafian follicle protrudes from the ovarian surface.
   - Tunica albuginea, theca interna, theca externa, and the outer layer of granulosa cells are stretched and thinned. The thinned area is called follicular stigma.
2. Three steps occur simultaneously:
   - Enzymatic proteolysis breaks down the wall at the stigma.
   - Smooth muscle cells in theca externa contract.
   - The follicle grows due to increased production of liquor folliculi.
3. The follicle bursts
   - The oocyte and liquor folliculi are expelled into the abdomen.
   - The oocyte is transported via the fallopian tube to the uterine cavity.

Maturation of oocytes

1. Fourth week of gestation: primordial germ cells arise in the embryonic yolk sac.
2. Sixth week of gestation: primordial germ cells invade the gonads (ovaries).
3. In female fetuses the primordial germ cells differentiate into oogonia, which proliferate and differentiate into primary oocytes.
   - Meiosis I is initiated in the fetal life but first completed at ovulation.
     - Primary oocyte (46×2) ⟶ Secondary oocyte (23×2)
       ⟶ First polar body (23×2)
   - Meiosis II is only completed if the oocyte is fertilized.
     - Secondary oocyte (23×2) ⟶ Mature oocyte, ovum (23×1)
       ⟶ Second polar body (23×1)

Corpus Luteum and Corpus Albicans

Corpus Luteum

Formation

1. After ovulation a blood clot fills up the collapsed Graafian follicle.
2. The basal lamina is degraded, and vessels and loose connective tissue from the theca enter the follicle.
3. Granulosa and theca interna cells are "luteinized", i.e., they become steroid producing, and are called:
   - Granulosa lutein cells
   - Theca lutein cells

Function

- In every menstruation cycle, secretion of
  - Progesterone (primarily) ⎱ Prepare the endometrium
  - Estrogen ⎰ for a potential pregnancy
- In first trimester of pregnancy, secretion of e.g.:
  - Progesterone
  - Estradiol
  - Relaxin

Light Microscopy

- Granulosa lutein cells are big, polyhedral, with a pale cytoplasm.
- Theca lutein cells are smaller, with a darker cytoplasm.
- Both have abundant sER and mitochondria with tubular cristae (characteristic for steroid hormone-producing cells).

Divided into

The corpus luteum faces different fates, depending on the presence or absence of hCG from the trophoblast (i.e., presence or absence of fertilization).

- Corpus luteum of pregnancy:
  - If fertilization occurs, hCG from the trophoblast prevents the degradation of the corpus luteum.

- ○ Function depends on a combination of paracrine and endocrine secretions, called luteotropins.
- ○ Increases in size → ⊘ 2–3 cm.
- ○ Persists through the whole pregnancy, although the function decreases gradually after 8 weeks.
- Corpus luteum of menstruation
  - ○ If fertilization does not occur, the absence of hCG leads to degeneration of the corpus luteum 10–12 days after ovulation.

Corpus albicans

- After pregnancy or menstruation, the corpus luteum slowly degenerates to a white scar, the corpus albicans, which slowly disappears from the ovarian cortex.
- Has no endocrine function.

Ovarian Cycle

Function
- The ovarian cycle controls the endometrial cycle.
- FSH and LH from the pituitary gland stimulate the ovaries to produce estrogens and progesterone during the development of follicles. Estrogens and progesterone in turn affect the endometrium and the mucous membranes in fallopian tube and cervix.

Divided into (Fig. 25.1)
1. Follicular phase:
   - FSH from the pituitary gland stimulates follicle growth and maturation.
   - Growing follicles produce estrogens.
   - Duration approximately 14 days.
- - - - Ovulation - - - -
2. Luteal phase:
   - Corpus luteum produces progesterone (primarily) and estrogen.
   - Duration approximately 14 days.

Atresia

- Degeneration of oocyte (apoptosis) and follicle, without ovulation.
- Approximately 400 follicles go through ovulation during a woman's fertile period.
- The rest (>99 %) of all oocytes/follicles goes through atresia.
- The process starts in fetal life.

FALLOPIAN TUBE (UTERINE TUBE)

Structure
- Paired tubular organ
- 10–12 cm long, muscular tube
- Outer ⌀: 8 mm (infundibulum) → 2 mm (uterine/intramural part)

Function
- Transports the oocyte from the ovary to the uterine cavity.
- Fertilization and initial embryonic development (zygote → morula) habitually take place in the fallopian tube.

Consists of (Table 25.3)
Lateral → medial (from ovary to uterus):
- Infundibulum
    - Funnel shaped, most lateral part of the fallopian tube
    - With fimbriae, fringe, that helps sweeping the ovulated oocyte into the fallopian tube
- Ampulla
    - Widest and longest part.
    - Here fertilization habitually takes place.
- Isthmus
    - Narrow part close to the uterus
- Uterine part
    - Passes through the uterine wall, opens into the uterine cavity

Wall of fallopian tube

Consists of
- Mucosa
    - Thin longitudinal folds, well developed in ampulla, smaller in isthmus
- Tunica muscularis
    - Smooth muscular tissue
- Tunica serosa (peritoneum)

Light Microscopy
See Table 25.3.

Table 25.3 The wall of the fallopian tube

	Infundibulum	Ampulla	Isthmus	Uterine part
Mucosa				
Maze-like pattern on cross section, due to thin longitudinal folds	Well developed ⟶ less developed			
Epithelium	Simple columnar epithelium, with two cell types			
• Ciliated cells	• Columnar cells with pale eosinophilic cytoplasm • Apical nucleus • Cilia are stimulated by estrogen, in the follicular phase, and transport the oocyte towards the uterus			
Abundance	+++	+++	+	+
• Secretory (non-ciliated) cells	• Columnar/cuboidal cells, with acidophilic cytoplasm • Basal nucleus • Apical granules (stains pink with PAS) • Proliferation and secretion are stimulated in the follicular phase			
Abundance	+	+	+++	+++
Lamina propria	Thin layer of loose connective tissue			
Tunica muscularis	• Inner, thicker circular layer of smooth muscle tissue • Outer longitudinally layer of smooth muscle tissue			
• Thickness	Thin ⟶ Thick			
Tunica serosa	• Mesothelium • Thin layer of connective tissue		–	

UTERUS

Structure
- 2 × 5 × 8 cm, 40–50 g (nullipara), 70 g (multipara)
- Wall thickness 1.5 cm
- Hollow, muscular pear-shaped organ

Function
- Site of development of morula to fetus
- Gives rise to the decidual part of placenta
- Contractions during labor, as well as during menstruation

Divided into
- Body, corpus (2/3)
  - With uterine cavity
  - The convex, top part is called fundus
- Isthmus
  - Connecting part between body and cervix
- Cervix (1/3)
  - With the cervical canal
  - Divided into:
    - Supravaginal part
    - Vaginal part/portio

The Wall of the uterine body

Consists of
- Endometrium (mucosa)
  - Epithelium
  - Stroma (lamina propria)
- Myometrium
  - Smooth muscle tissue, continuous with the smooth muscle tissue of the fallopian tube and vagina
  - Works as a syncytium during contractions
- Perimetrium (serosa/adventitia)
  - Visceral peritoneum, continuous with abdominal and pelvic peritoneum.
  - Some of the anterior surface of the uterus is covered with loose connective tissue, adventitia.

Light Microscopy
- Endometrium (mucosa)
  - Single columnar epithelium on a basement membrane
    - Two cell types:
      - Ciliated cells
      - Secretory (non-ciliated) cells
    - Simple, tubular glands run deep into the stroma
  - Stroma (lamina propria)
    - Loose connective tissue, rich in cells and ground substance
- Myometrium
  - Smooth muscle tissue:
    - Internal longitudinal layer
    - Middle, thick, circular/spiral layer
      - Rich in large vessels, called stratum vasculare
    - External longitudinal layer
- Perimetrium (serosa/adventitia)
  - Mesothelium on basement membrane
  - Loose connective tissue

Functional aspect of the endometrial structure

Divided into (Fig. 25.1)

Due to physiological properties, the endometrium is divided into two zones:

- Functional layer (stratum functionale)
  - Luminal zone, which goes through cyclical changes and is expelled during menstruation
    - Spiral arteries (straight → coiled → expelled)
    - Endometrial glands (straight → coiled → filled with glycogen → expelled)
- Basal layer (stratum basale)
  - Basal zone.
  - Stratum functionale regenerates from the stratum basale during each menstrual cycle.
  - Basal part of spiral arteries (straight arteries, basal arteries).
  - Basal part of the endometrial glands.

Endometrial Blood Supply

Consists of

- Uterine artery (a. uterina)
- Arcuate arteries (aa. arcuatae)
- Radial branches (aa. radiales)
- Spiral arteries + straight arteries (basal arteries)
- Well-developed capillary net
- Venous plexus in the endometrium
- Venules
- Venous plexus in the myometrium and lateral to the uterus (plexus venosus uterinus)
- Uterine veins (vv. uterinae)

Menstruation (Endometrial) Cycle

General

- During the fertile period, the endometrium goes through cyclical changes, every month preparing for implantation of an embryo.
- Only the endometrium in the body of the uterus participates in the menstruation.
- The cyclical changes are correlated with follicle development in the ovaries and coordinated by the ovarian sex hormones.

Divided into (Fig. 25.1)
1. Menstrual phase (endometrial thickness: 6 mm → 1 mm)
   - A fall in plasma levels of progesterone (as corpus luteum vanishes) → ischemia in stratum functionale → decomposition.
   - Stratum functionale is discharged during menstruation, together with blood from mucosal blood vessels.
2. Proliferative phase (endometrial thickness, 1 mm → 3 mm)
   - Estrogen from the growing follicles stimulates endometrial proliferation.
   - Epithelial cells from the base of the glands proliferate and migrate to cover the endometrial surface.
   - Stromal glands and blood vessels lengthen.
3. Secretory phase (endometrial thickness, 3 mm → 6 mm)
   - Progesterone from the corpus luteum stimulates secretory changes in the endometrium.
   - Glands grow, become coiled, and their lumina fill up with mucous secretions, rich in glycogen.
   - Spiral arteries elongate and become coiled.
   - The stroma becomes edematous.
   - If pregnancy occurs -
4. Decidual reaction
   - If fertilization occurs the endometrium goes through a "decidual reaction" → stromal cells differentiate into large, pale cells filled with glycogen and lipid (decidual cells).
   - The endometrium is now called decidua and a part of it (decidua basalis) makes up the maternal part of the placenta.

Cervix

Function
- Connects the cavity of uterus with the vagina:
  - Cavity of uterus → internal opening (orificium) → cervical canal → external orificium → vagina
- Carries sperm from the vagina to the uterus.
- Transports menstruation from the cavity of uterus to the vagina.
- Cervical mucus serves as a barrier, protecting the internal reproductive organs as well as the developing fetus against pathogens.

Divided into
- Supravaginal part (2/3)
- Vaginal part (portio) (1/3)

Cervical wall
Consists of
- Mucosa
  - Endocervix
    - Lining of the cervical canal
    - No cyclical changes in the mucosal structure but in the mucus secretions:
      - Mucus is more permeable close to ovulation and less permeable in other times of the cycle.
  - Ectocervix
    - Lining of the vaginal part
- Muscle and connective tissue layer

Light Microscopy
- Mucosa
  - Endocervix
    - Columnar epithelium
    - Large, branched mucous glands
  - Transformation zone
    - Here the columnar epithelium of the endocervix and the squamous epithelium of the ectocervix abruptly meet.
    - Located outside the external os in women of fertile age.
    - Located within the cervical canal in prepubertal and postmenopausal females.
  - Ectocervix
    - Stratified squamous epithelium
- Muscle and connective tissue layer
  - More connective tissue than smooth muscle tissue
  - Abundant elastic fibers

VAGINA

Structure
- Fibro-muscular tube, with an H-shaped lumen, on a cross section
- 7–10 cm long, ⊘ 2–3 cm

Function
Connects the internal reproductive organs to the external environment

Vaginal wall

Consists of

- Mucosa
  - With transverse folds, rugae.
  - In virgins, mucosal folds, *hymen*, protrudes into the distal vaginal lumen (vaginal opening, introitus).
- Muscularis
  - With the bulbospongiosus muscle (m. bulbospongiosus): additional striated skeletal muscle fibers, in the distal part of the vaginal wall
- Adventitia

Light Microscopy

- Mucosa
  - Stratified, squamous, nonkeratinized epithelium on a basement membrane
    - Deep zone: single layer of basophilic basal cells
    - Intermediate zone: several layers of boat-shaped cells, with glycogen granules, stained pink with PAS
    - Outer zone: several layers more flattened acidophilic cells
  - Lamina propria
    - Loose connective tissue directly underneath the epithelial basal membrane
    - Thin-walled veins with erectile function
- Muscularis
  - Smooth muscle tissue
    - Inner circular layer
    - Outer thicker longitudinal layer
- Adventitia
  - Inner layer
    - Dense connective tissue, rich in elastic fibers
  - Outer layer
    - Loose connective tissue, blood vessels, lymphatic vessels, and nerves

The External Reproductive Organs (Vulva)

General

Are formed and developed during the fetal period and further developed during the pubertal period.

Function
- Protection of the internal reproductive organs
- Intercourse

Consist of
- Mons pubis
  - Region superficial to the pubic symphysis
  - Rich in subcutaneous adipose tissue
  - Covered with pubic hair (after puberty)
- Labia majora
  - Two large skin folds on each side of the vestibule
  - Rich in subcutaneous adipose tissue, with connective tissue septa and smooth muscle cells
  - Homologous to the skin of the scrotum
  - With pubic hair and sebaceous and apocrine glands (after puberty)
- Labia minora
  - Two thin, hairless, well-vascularized skin folds
  - Located on each side of the vestibule, medial to the labia majora
  - With large sebaceous glands that produce smegma
  - Surrounds the vestibule
- Erectile bodies
  - Clitoris
    - With two corpora, a glans and a prepuce
    - Rich in sensory nerve endings
    - Located at the anterior of the vulva, where the labia minora meet
    - Homologous to corpora cavernosa of the penis
  - Vestibular bulbs
    - Homologous to corpus spongiosum of the penis
- Vestibule
  - Area between the labia minora
  - Covered in stratified squamous epithelium
  - Contains:
    - Introitus vagina
    - External urethral ostium
- Vestibular glands
  - Major (Bartholin's glands)
    - Paired tubuloalveolar, mucous glands
    - Located in the lateral wall, in the posterior part of the vestibule
  - Minor
    - Numerous mucous glands in the anterior part of the vestibule

Placenta and Umbilical Cord

PLACENTA

General
- Temporary organ, essential during pregnancy
- Unique in being the only organ composed of cells from to genetically different individuals
  - Fetal part: chorion frondosum, derived from the trophoblast
  - Maternal part: decidua basalis, derived from the endometrium

Structure
- Discoid
- $\oslash$ 15–20 cm, 2–3 cm thick, 500 g
- Incompletely divided into 15–25 cotelydons, by septa from decidua basalis

Function
- Exchange
  - Gasses, nutrients, waste products, antibodies (IgG), hormones, electrolytes, etc., between maternal and fetal blood vascular systems
- Synthesis
  - Cholesterol, glycogen, and fatty acids used during early development of the embryo
- Hormone production
  - hCG, human chorionic somatomammotropin (hCS), progesterone, estrogen as well as other hormones and growth factors

Consists of (Fig. 25.2)
- Chorionic plate
  - Fetal part (chorion frondosum), from which villi project
  - Insertion of the umbilical cord
- - - - - Separated by the intervillous space - - - - - - - -
- Basal plate
  - Maternal part (decidua basalis)
  - Facing the myometrium of the uterus

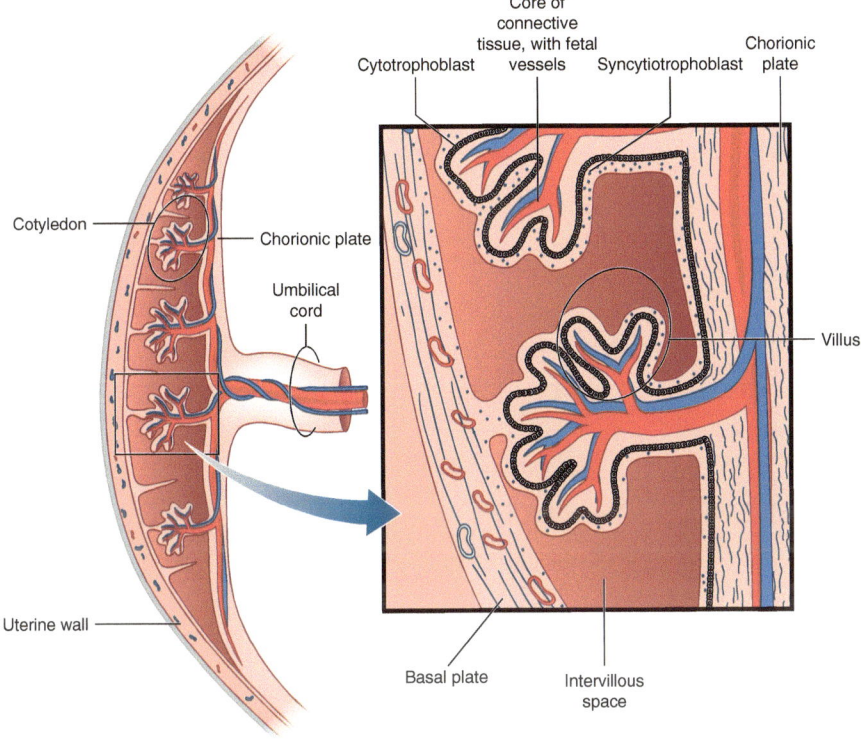

Fig. 25.2 Mature placenta. Villi from the chorionic plate project into the intervillous space, which is filled with maternal blood, and incompletely separated into cotyledons by decidual septa from the basal plate

Formation

See Figs. 25.3 and 25.4

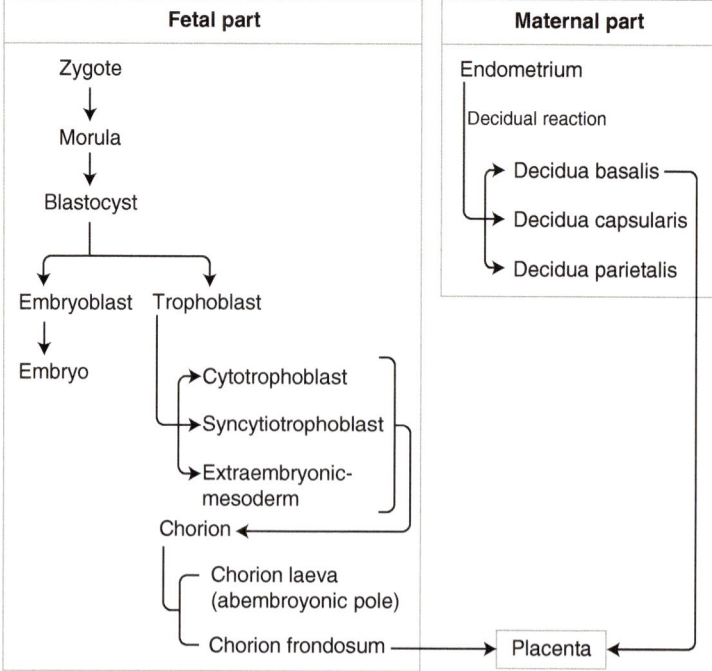

Fig. 25.3   The fetal and maternal parts of placenta

Uteroplacental Circulation

Formation

- Vascular spaces (lacunae) form in the syncytiotrophoblast and fuse to a lacunar network.
- Maternal blood vessels open into the lacunar network, filling it with blood.
  - 80–100 spiral arteries supply the placenta (intervillous space) with maternal blood.
- Cords of cytotrophoblast (primary villi) proliferate into the blood-filled lacunar network of the syncytiotrophoblast:
  1. Primary villi are invaded by chorionic mesenchyme (→ secondary villi).
  2. Capillaries develop in the mesenchymal core (→ tertiary villi).

Villi

General

- Branched extensions of the fetal part of the placental tissue projecting into the blood-filled lacunar network
- Develop and mature during pregnancy:
  - Primary villi → secondary villi → tertiary villi

- The "placental barrier" is the distance between maternal and fetal blood vascular systems.
  - After 20 weeks the placental barrier is optimized, as the layers of cytotrophoblast and chorionic mesenchyme get thinner to facilitate exchange across the barrier.

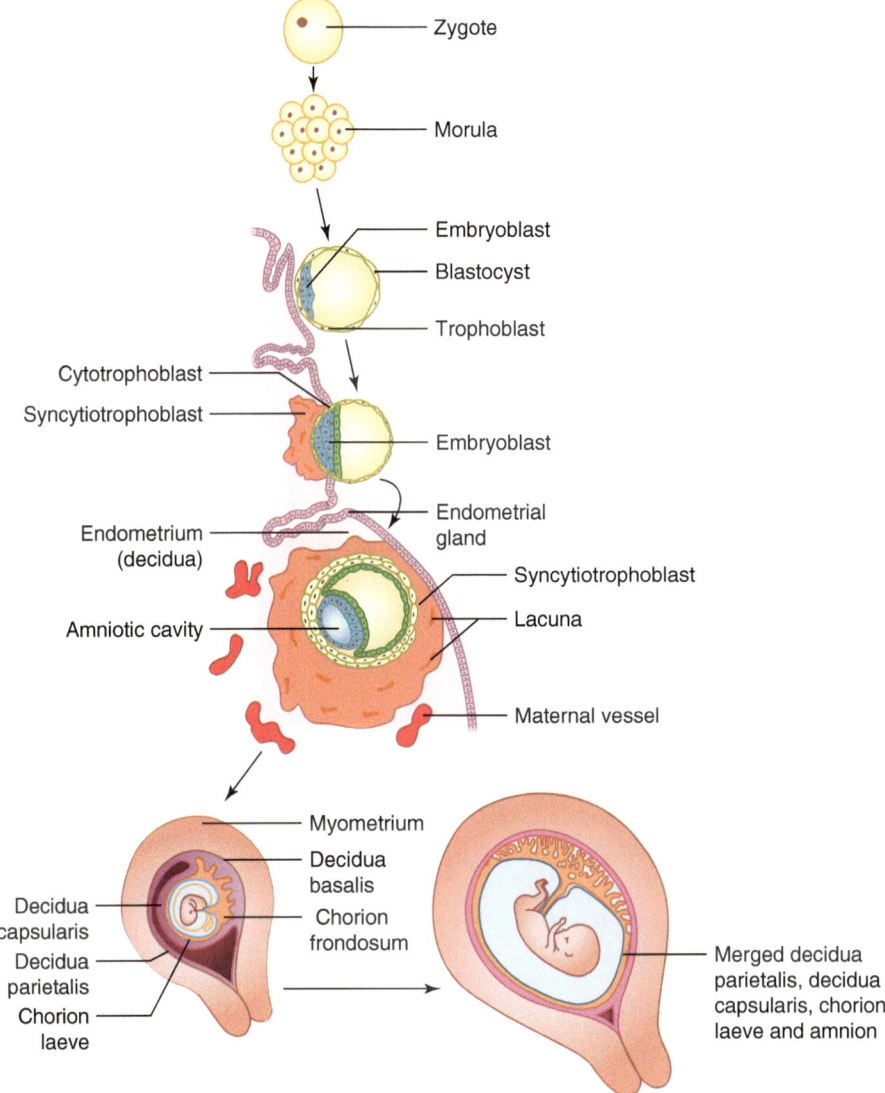

Fig. 25.4 Development of placenta. The zygote develops into a blastocyst with an embryoblastic and a trophoblastic part. The trophoblast invades the decidua (endometrium), and cells from the cytotrophoblast merge into a syncytiotrophoblast. Cords of cytotrophoblast (primary villi) develop into the blood-filled lacunar network of the syncytiotrophoblast. Decidua basalis and chorion frondosum form the placenta, and the decidua parietalis and decidua capsularis merge

Function
Villi increase the surface area from which exchange of substances takes place.

Divided into
- Primary villi
  - Syncytiotrophoblast and cytotrophoblast
- Secondary villi
  - Syncytiotrophoblast, cytotrophoblast, and a core of chorionic mesenchyme
- Tertiary villi
  - Syncytiotrophoblast, cytotrophoblast, a core of chorionic mesenchyme, and capillaries

Light Microscopy
Placental barrier of a tertiary villus consists of (from maternal to fetal blood):
- Syncytiotrophoblast
  - Heavily stained syncytium of cells with several small apical nuclei
  - Ultrastructurally: with microvilli and multiple small vesicles
- Cytotrophoblast
  - Cuboidal, large, pale cells with a central nucleus
  - Discontinuous layer
- Basal lamina of the trophoblast
- Chorionic mesenchyme
  - Loose connective tissue
  - Fibroblasts, smooth muscle cells and phagocytic, antigen-presenting Hofbauer cells
- Basal lamina of the endothelium
- Endothelium of the fetal capillaries

UMBILICAL CORD

General
- Cord connecting the fetus to the placenta.
- The navel (umbilicus) marks the location where the umbilical cord was attached during the fetal life.

Structure
- 50 cm long, ◌ 1–1.5 cm
- Extend from the umbilical region of the fetus to the fetal part of placenta

Function
- Umbilical vein: transports oxygenated blood and nutrients from the placenta to the fetus.
- Umbilical arteries: transports deoxygenated blood and waste products from the fetus to the placenta.

Consists of
- One umbilical vein (v. umbilicalis)
- Two umbilical arteries (aa. umbilicales)
- Wharton's gel:
  - Mucous connective tissue (Chap. 7)
  - Surrounds and cushions the blood vessels

Guide to Practical Histology: The Female Reproductive System

Ovary

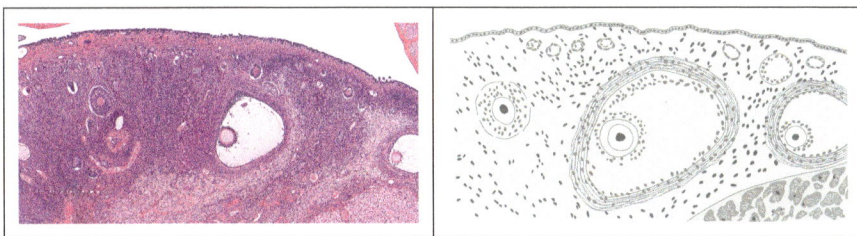

Left: photomicrograph of the ovarian cortex with primordial, primary, and secondary follicles. Magnification: low. Stain: HE (Courtesy of associate professor Steen Seier Poulsen, University of Copenhagen). *Right*: simplified illustration of the ovarian cortex

Characteristics
- Rounded structure
  - The surface is covered with a simple, cuboidal epithelium.
  - A central eosinophilic, well-vascularized medulla.
  - A basophilic cortex, containing numerous follicles in different stages.
- Sometimes a corpus luteum is seen as a large, light mass, spanning the cortex.

Fallopian Tube

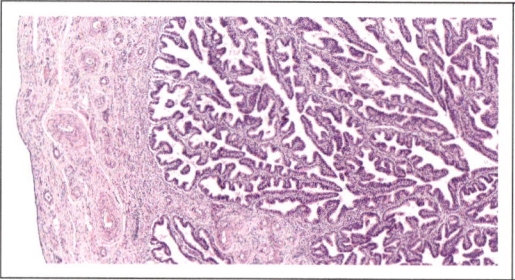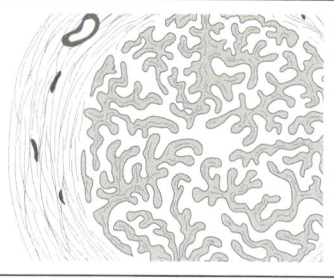

Left: photomicrograph of the fallopian tube with a lumen (to the right), with an extremely folded mucosa. Magnification: low. Stain: HE (Courtesy of associate professor Steen Seier Poulsen, University of Copenhagen). *Right*: simplified illustration of the fallopian tube

Characteristics
Cross section:
- A ring-shaped structure
  - The lumen is lined with columnar epithelium, with ciliated and non-ciliated cells.
  - Mucosa is extremely folded (resembles curly kale).
  - A layer of smooth muscle tissue surrounds the mucosa.

Can be mistaken for
- Ureter
  - A star-shaped lumen
  - Lined with urothelium
- Ductus deferens
  - A star-shaped lumen
  - Lined with pseudostratified epithelium
  - Extremely thick layer of smooth muscle tissue below the mucosa
- Seminal vesicles
  - The tubular gland is extensively coiled → several adjacent cross sections of the lumen of the gland/tube are seen in the same specimen.
  - Lined with low, pseudostratified epithelium.

Uterus

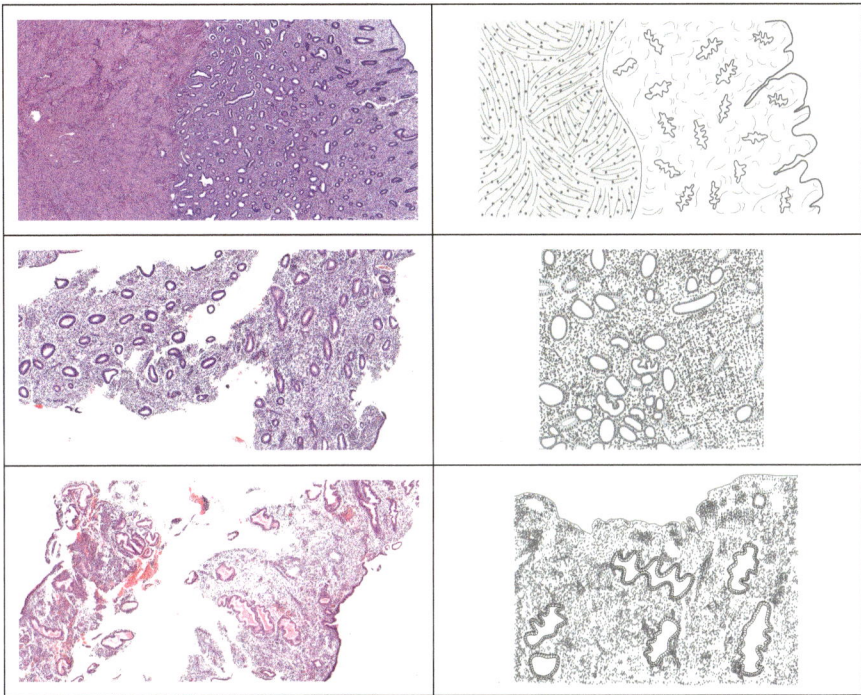

Top panel, *left*: photomicrograph of the uterine wall with endometrium (proliferative phase) to the right and myometrium to the left. Magnification: low. Stain: HE (Courtesy of associate professor Steen Seier Poulsen, University of Copenhagen). *Top panel*, *right*: Simplified illustration of the uterine wall with endometrium in proliferative phase. *Middle panel*, *left*: photomicrograph of an endometrial biopsy (stratum functionale in proliferative phase). Magnification: low. Stain: HE (Courtesy of associate professor Steen Seier Poulsen, University of Copenhagen). *Middle panel*, *right*: simplified illustration of endometrium (stratum functionale) in proliferative phase. *Bottom panel*, *left*: photomicrograph of an endometrial biopsy (stratum functionale in secretory phase). Magnification: low. Stain: HE (Courtesy of associate professor Steen Seier Poulsen, University of Copenhagen). *Bottom panel*, *right*: simplified illustration of endometrium (stratum functionale) in secretory phase

Characteristics
- Simple columnar epithelium on a thick cell-rich stroma (endometrium).
  - The superficial part (stratum functionale) changes during the menstrual cycle:
    - Sloughed off during menstruation
    - Resurfaces and increases in thickness during the proliferative phase:
      - Deep, straight epithelial invaginations into the stroma (endometrial glands)
    - Increases in thickness during the secretory phase:
      - Deep, dilated, sawlike endometrial glands
      - Stroma becomes edematous
- Thick layer of smooth muscle tissue (myometrium) is seen underneath the endometrium:
  - Smooth muscle fibers run in several different directions.

Cervix Uteri

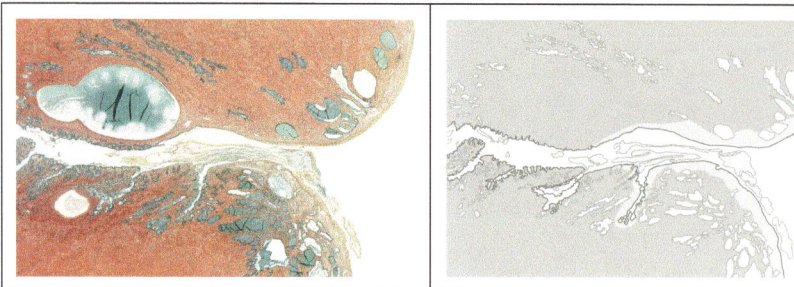

Left: photomicrograph of a longitudinal section of the endocervical canal (portio vaginalis). Transition zone, with columnar epithelium to the left and stratified squamous epithelium of to the right. Magnification: low. Stain: Van Geison and Alcian blue (Courtesy of associate professor Steen Seier Poulsen, University of Copenhagen). *Right*: simplified illustration of the endocervical canal

Characteristics

Longitudinal section

- The transformation zone (junction between two different epithelia) at the vaginal opening of the cervical canal is often visualized in the specimen
  1. Simple columnar epithelium of the cervical canal.
     - Lumen of the cervical canal appears sawlike, because of deep, regular folds of mucosa.
     - Lined with simple columnar epithelium with many mucous-secreting cells.
  2. Nonkeratinized, stratified, squamous epithelium of the vaginal part (portio).
     - Appears smooth.
- Underneath the epithelium is a thick layer of connective tissue and smooth muscle tissue.

Vagina

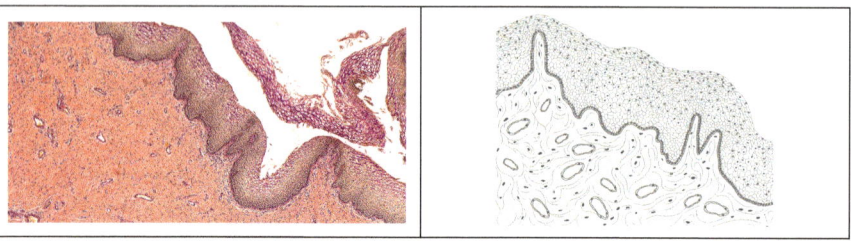

Left: photomicrograph of the vaginal wall (the luminal part of the epithelium is torn off (artifact)). Magnification: low. Stain: PAS (Courtesy of associate professor Steen Seier Poulsen, University of Copenhagen). *Right*: simplified illustration of the luminal part of the vaginal wall

Characteristics
- Lumen is lined with nonkeratinized, stratified, squamous epithelium.
- Cells of epithelium are pale basophilic and boat shaped.
- Below the epithelium:
  - Connective tissue with abundant blood vessels.
  - Irregularly arranged smooth muscle tissue.

Can be mistaken for
- Esophagus:
  - Smooth muscular tissue (muscularis mucosae) is seen between the connective tissue in the lamina propria and the submucosa.
  - With mucous glands in the lamina propria.
- Skin:
  - With keratinized stratified squamous epithelium in epidermis.
    - Cells in the superficial layers have no nuclei.

Special Staining
PAS: stains the epithelium pink, due to the glycogen content

Placenta

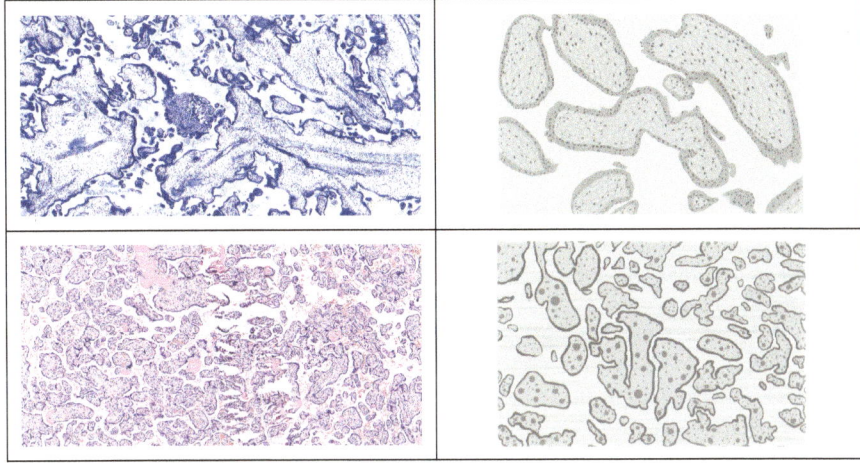

Top panel, *left*: photomicrograph of an early placenta with large villi. Magnification: low. Stain: Toluidine blue (Courtesy of associate professor Steen Seier Poulsen, University of Copenhagen). *Top panel*, *right*: simplified illustration of the early placenta. *Bottom panel*, *left*: photomicrograph of a mature (third trimester) placenta with smaller, more developed villi. Magnification: low. Stain: HE (Courtesy of associate professor Steen Seier Poulsen, University of Copenhagen). *Bottom panel*, *right*: simplified illustration of the mature placenta

Characteristics

- Numerous pale islets (villi)
  - Core of light, loose connective tissue
  - Border of dark, basophilic epithelium
  - Changes during pregnancy
    - Early placenta: few, larger "primary villi"
    - Mature placenta: numerous smaller "tertiary villi," with capillaries in their core
- Blood cells are often seen between the villi (in the intervillous space).

Umbilical Cord

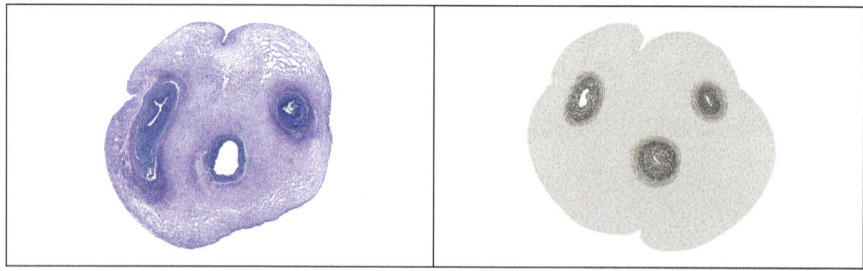

Left: photomicrograph of the umbilical cord. Magnification: low. Stain: Toluidine blue (Courtesy of professor Jørgen Tranum Jensen, University of Copenhagen). *Right*: simplified illustration of the umbilical cord

Characteristics

Macroscopic

- The umbilical cord looks like a face:
  - The two umbilical arteries as eyes.
  - The umbilical vein as a mouth.

References

5, 25, 31, 33, 34, 35, 45.

Chapter 26
The Male Reproductive System

Contents

General

- For a general introduction to both the female and male reproductive systems, see Chap. 25.
- The male reproductive organs form during the fetal period and grow and develop further during puberty.

© Springer International Publishing Switzerland 2017   569
A. Rehfeld et al., *Compendium of Histology*, DOI 10.1007/978-3-319-41873-5_26

Consists of
- Internal reproductive organs
  - Testicles
  - Epididymes   ⎤
  - Ductus deferens   ⎬ Excurrent duct system
  - Ductus ejaculatorius ⎦
  - Prostate gland   ⎤
  - Seminal vesicles   ⎬ Accessory glands
  - Bulbourethral glands (Cowper's glands) ⎦
- External reproductive organs
  - Penis
  - Scrotum

The Internal Reproductive Organs

Consists of
- Testicles (paired)
- Excurrent duct system (paired)
  - Epididymes
  - Ductus deferens
  - Ductus ejaculatorius
- Accessory glands
  - Prostate
  - Seminal vesicles (paired)
  - Bulbourethral glands (paired)

TESTICLE (TESTIS)

General
- Male gonad
- Located in the scrotum (after 26th week of gestation)

Structure
- Paired ovoid organ
- $2 \times 3 \times 4$ cm, 12–20 g

Function
- Spermatogenesis: proliferation and maturation of the male gametes, spermatozoa (sperm cells)
- Production of sex hormones: androgens (primarily testosterone) that are crucial for:
  - Development of a male phenotype during embryonic and fetal life
  - Spermatogenesis
  - Male dimorphism, i.e., behavioral and physical appearance

Consists of (Fig. 26.1)
- Stroma
  - Tunica albuginea: a thick capsule of dense connective tissue
    - External surface covered with mesothelium, tunica vaginalis testis
    - Internal surface covered with well-vascularized loose connective tissue, tunica vasculosa
  - Mediastinum testis: a thickening of the posterior part of the tunica albuginea
  - Septa testis: incomplete septa project from tunica albuginea into the parenchyma and divide it into 200–300 lobules
- Parenchyma (located within the lobules)
  - Interstitial tissue
    - Leydig cells
    - Macrophages
    - Blood vessels and lymphatic vessels
  - Seminiferous tubules
    - 3–4 in each lobule, 50 cm long, $\oslash$ 250 μm
    - Wall consists of:
      - Seminiferous epithelium (spermatozo-producing epithelium)
      - Basal lamina
      - Myoid cells (myofibroblasts): 3–4 layers, flattened contractile cells

Leydig cells

Function
Production of testosterone, under influence of LH

Light Microscopy
- Large, polygonal cell with eosinophilic cytoplasm
- Large, spherical, eccentric nucleus

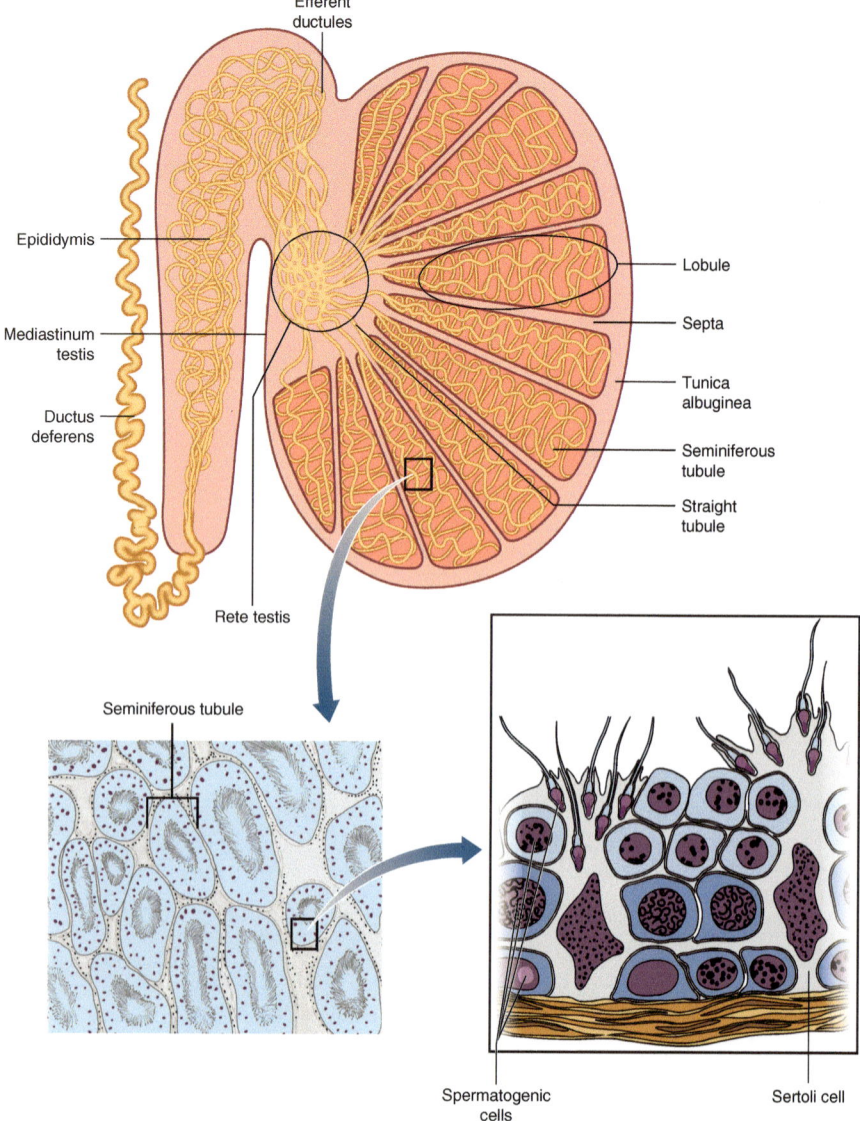

Fig. 26.1 Testicle and seminiferous epithelium. Cross section of a testicle showing seminiferous tubules in lobules, as well as rete testis and the start of the excurrent duct system. Interposed figure shows seminiferous epithelium of the seminiferous tubules

Ultrastructure
- Abundant sER, lipid droplets, and mitochondria with tubulovesicular cristae, characteristic for steroid hormone producing cells
- Lipofuscin pigment (crystals of Reinke)

Seminiferous Epithelium

General

Tall pseudostratified epithelium lining the seminiferous tubules of the testes

Consists of (Fig. 26.1)
- Sertoli cells:
  - Support the spermatogenic cells
  - Tight junctions between the Sertoli cells form the blood–testis barrier
  - Divide the epithelium into a luminal and a basal compartment
- Spermatogenic cells (Table 26.1):
  - Arise from primordial germ cells that migrate from the yolk sac to the gonads in the embryonic life
  - Move from basal lamina to lumen as they develop into spermatozoa

Light Microscopy
- Sertoli cells
  - Tall, columnar cells with abundant sER and rER, mitochondria, and Golgi (seen in electron microscope)
  - Large, indented nucleus
  - Reach all the way from the basal lamina to the lumen, surrounding the spermatogenic cells as they move from the basal lamina to the lumen
- Spermatogenic cells
  - The cells are connected through bridges of cytoplasm, but separate as they reach the lumen as spermatocytes.
  - Developmental stage can be identified in light microscopy by the morphology of the nucleus (Table 26.1)

Spermatogenesis

General (Table 26.1)

- Development of male gametes, spermatozoa (sperm cells)
- Starts shortly before puberty and continues throughout the entire life.
- Meiotic divisions → haploid gametes (spermatids), i.e., containing a single set of chromosomes (1n).
- The cell divisions are initially non-complete → spermatids are connected through thin cytoplasmic bridges.

Table 26.1 Spermatogenesis

		Cell	Chromosomes	Nucleus
Spermatogenesis	Basal compartment	Dark A-spermatogonia (Stem cell, self-renewing) ↓ Mitosis	46×2	Ovoid, dark nucleus
		Pale A-spermatogonia ↓ Mitosis	46×2	Ovoid, pale nucleus
		B-spermatogonia ↓ Mitosis	46×2	Round nucleus with one central nucleolus
		Primary spermatocytes ↓ Meiosis I	46×2	Large, dark nucleus
		- - - - - - - - - - - - - Blood-testis barrier - - - - - - - - - - - - - - -		
	Luminal compartment (Spermiogenesis)	Secondary spermatocytes (Rarely seen since the development to spermatids is fast) ↓ Meiosis II	23×2	Round, dark nucleus
		Spermatids |Differentiation	23×1	• Small nucleus • Most luminal in the epithelium
		Spermatozoa (Fig. 26.2)	23×1	Small nucleus

Spermatozoon (sperm cell)

Consists of (Fig. 26.2)

- Head (1 × 3 × 5 µm)
  - ○ Nucleus: dark, condensed chromatin
  - ○ Acrosome, with
    - ▪ Enzymes for breakdown of the zona pellucida
    - ▪ Stains pink with PAS
  - ○ Basal plate
- Tail (55 µm): flagellum
  - ○ Neck
    - ▪ Centrioles
    - ▪ Connecting piece (origin of outer dense fibers)
  - ○ Middle piece
    - ▪ Axoneme
    - ▪ Outer dense fibers
    - ▪ Mitochondrial sheath
  - ○ Principal piece
    - ▪ Axoneme
    - ▪ Outer dense fibers
    - ▪ Fibrous sheath
  - ○ End piece
    - ▪ Axoneme

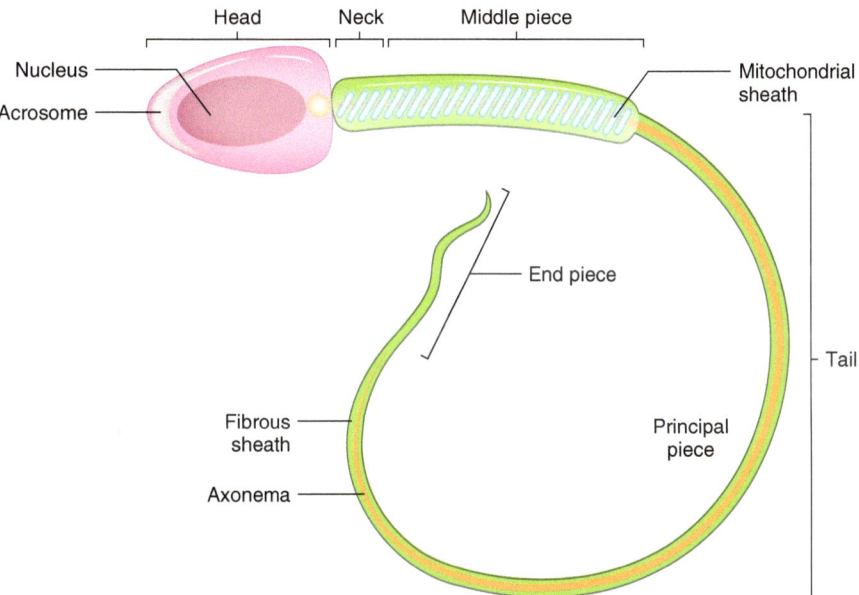

Fig. 26.2 Spermatozoon. Mature sperm cell with head and tail

Spermiogenesis

- Differentiation of spermatids into mature spermatozoa, i.e., the last part of spermatogenesis
- During spermiogenesis, basic organelles form the basis of sperm cell specific structures:
  - ○ Golgi apparatus → acrosome
  - ○ Mitochondria → mitochondrial sheath
  - ○ Centrioles →
    - ▪ Initiates formation of the axoneme (9 + 2 microtubules doublets)
    - ▪ Initiates formation of the connecting piece
  - ○ Remaining organelles and cytoplasm become residual bodies as the spermatids mature into spermatozoa.

Blood–testis barrier

Structure

- A barrier between the blood and the luminal part of the seminiferous epithelium
- Formed by tight junctions between neighboring Sertoli cells
- Divides the epithelium of the seminiferous tubules into a luminal and a basal compartment

Function

- Maintenance of a luminal microenvironment that is ideal for spermatogenesis
- Isolation of the spermatogenic cells from the immune system
- Protection of the spermatogenic cells from potential harmful substances in the blood

Pathway of the sperm

Consists of (Table 26.2)

1. Seminiferous tubules (tubuli seminiferi contorti)
2. Straight seminiferous tubules (tubuli seminiferi recti)
3. Rete testis
4. Efferent ductules
5. Ductus epididymidis
6. Ductus deferens + ductus excretorius (duct of the vesicula seminalis)
7. Ejaculatory duct
8. Urethra

Table 26.2 Pathway of the sperm and the histology of the seminiferous tubules, intratesticular ducts and excurrent duct system

Location	Testis			Epididymidis		Ductus deferens	Prostate
Duct	Seminiferous tubule	Straight seminiferous tubule	Rete testis	Efferent ductules	Ductus epididymidis	Ductus deferens	Ejaculatory duct
Sperm path							
Function	Production	Transportation		• Storage • Maturation		Transportation	• Transportation • Mixing sperm cells with secretions from prostate and seminal vesicles
Transport of spermatozoa	Fluid flow	Fluid flow	Fluid flow	• Fluid flow • Ciliary action	• Fluid flow • Peristaltic waves	Peristaltic waves	Peristaltic waves
Mucosa							
• Epithelium	Tall pseudostratified seminiferous epithelium	Simple, columnar with Sertoli cells	Simple cuboidal	Pseudostratified columnar/cuboidal with clusters of: • Tall ciliated cells • Smaller absorptive cells with microvilli • Cell clusters → festoon-shaped lumen	Pseudostratified: • Principal cells: columnar cells with stereocilia • Basal cells: small round stem cells, lying on the basal lamina • Halo cells: migrating lymphocytes	Pseudostratified: • Columnar cells with stereocilia • Basal cells: small round stem cells lying on the basal lamina • Mucosal folds → star-shaped lumen in cross section	Pseudostratified/simple columnar
• Basal lamina	+	+	+	+	+	+	+
• Lamina propria	Loose connective tissue with: • Myoid cells • Leydig cells			Loose connective tissue	Loose connective tissue	Thin layer of loose connective tissue	Elastic connective tissue
Muscularis							
• Inner layer	–			Thin, circular	Circular	Longitudinal	
• Middle layer				–	–	Particularly thick circular layer	
• Outer layer				–	• Longitudinal • Only in the distal part of the duct	Longitudinal	The surrounding prostate tissue
Adventitia	–			–	–	Dense → loose connective tissue	–

EPIDIDYMIS

Structure (Fig. 26.1)
• Paired crescent-shaped tubular organ
• Coiled into a 7 cm long structure
• Runs on the superior, posterior part of the testicle

Divided into
• Head: efferent ductules (coni vasculosi)
• Body: ductus epididymidis
• Tail: ductus epididymidis

Function
• Maturation of spermatozoa, e.g. making the spermatozoa able to swim once ejaculated
• Storage of spermatozoa
• Transport of spermatozoa (immotile until ejaculation), through:
  ○ Fluid flow
    ▪ Flow is established as fluid is secreted from the seminiferous tubules and absorbed in the efferent ductules.
  ○ Ciliary action, in the efferent ductules.
  ○ Peristaltic waves, only in distal part of ductus epididymidis.

Consists of
• Efferent ductules
  ○ Pass through the superior part of the mediastinum testis and connect the rete testis with ductus epididymidis
  ○ 15–20 cm long tube
  ○ The ductules coil and form approximately 10 conical masses (coni vasculosi)
  ○ Constitute the head of the epididymis
• Ductus epididymidis
  ○ 5–6 m long, coiled tube (ductus epididymidis)
  ○ Constitutes the body and tail of the epididymis
• Connective tissue with blood and lymph vessels
  ○ Surrounds the efferent ductules and the ductus epididymidis

Light Microscopy
See Table 26.2.

DUCTUS DEFERENS

Structure
- Paired organ
- 35–40 cm long, outer $\oslash$ 3–4 mm
- Muscular tube, with star-shaped lumen
  - Proximal end: coiled
  - Distal end (ampulla): enlarged
- Ductus deferens runs:
  1. From the base, on the posterior rim of the testicle
  2. Into the spermatic cord in the inguinal canal
  3. Into the abdomen
  4. Into the prostate where ductus deferens fuses with the duct from the seminal vesicle to form the ejaculatory duct

Function
Transport of spermatozoa during ejaculation

Light Microscopy
See Table 26.2.

Accessory Sex Glands

Function
Production of secretes to assist reproduction

Consist of
- Seminal vesicles
- Prostate
- Bulbourethral glands (Cowper's glands)

SEMINAL VESICLES

Structure
- Paired tubular gland
- 15 cm long, coiled into a 1.5 × 1.5 × 4 cm structure.
- The short duct of the gland, the excretory duct, fuses with the distal end of the ductus deferens (ampulla) → ductus ejaculatorius.
- Developed from an invagination of the early ductus deferens.

Function
- Production of a viscous secrete, containing fructose, amino acids, ascorbic acid, and prostaglandins.
- The secrete is discharged late in the ejaculation.

Seminal Vesicle Wall

Consists of
- Mucosa
  - With numerous folds → increased surface area for secretion
- Muscularis
- Adventitia
  - Loose connective tissue, continuous with the connective tissue that "glues" the coils of the gland together

Light Microscopy
- Tubular gland
  - Highly coiled → several cross sections are seen in a specimen
- The secrete is seen as highly eosinophilic luminal masses.
- Mucosa: with numerous folds.
  - Pseudostratified columnar epithelium
    - Non-ciliated secretory columnar cells with abundant rER and Golgi
    - Small, round stem cells, located basally
  - Lamina propria: thin layer of loose connective tissue
- Muscularis
  - Thin layer of smooth muscle cells
- Adventitia
  - Loose connective tissue

PROSTATE GLAND

Structure
- Chestnut-shaped gland.
- 2 × 3 × 4 cm, 20 g.
- Located just inferiorly to the bladder.
- Urethra and the two ejaculatory ducts pass through the prostate.

Function
- Production of a thin secrete, containing enzymes and citric acid.
- The secrete is discharged early in the ejaculation.

Consists of
- Capsule
  - Dense connective tissue, firmly attached to the stroma
- Stroma
  - Smooth muscle tissue
  - Dense connective tissue
- Parenchyma (glands and ducts)
  - 40 tubuloalveolar glands in three concentric zones:
    1. Periurethral/transitional zone with mucosal glands
    2. Central zone with submucosal glands
    3. Peripheral zone with main glands (main part of the prostate glands)

Prostate parenchyma

Divided into
- Periurethral/transitional zone (5 %)
  - Only in the superior part of the prostate.
  - Mucosal glands.
  - Glands open directly into the urethra.
- Central zone (25 %)
  - Submucosal glands.
  - Ducts open into sinuses in the lateral/posterior wall of urethra.
- Peripheral zone (70 %)
  - Main glands.
  - Alveolar end pieces with varying shape and size.
  - Ducts open into sinuses in the lateral/posterior wall of urethra.

Light Microscopy
- The epithelium is varied, usually pseudostratified, with:
  ○ Luminal columnar/cuboidal cells
  ○ Basal flattened cells
- Corpora amylacea
  ○ Eosinophilic, rounded concretions of secretory material
  ○ Often seen in the lumen of the alveolar end pieces, especially in elder men

BULBOURETHRAL GLANDS

Structure
- Paired gland, located in the urogenital diaphragm.
- 1 × 1 × 1 cm each.
- 3 cm duct, which opens into the penile part of urethra.

Function
Secretion of a mucous fluid during sexual stimulation

Light Microscopy
- Branched tubuloalveolar glands
- End pieces with columnar cells
  ○ Basal nuclei, as the cytoplasm is filled with secretory granules

External Reproductive Organs

PENIS

General
- Size differs with age and erectile state
- Grows and develops during puberty

Function
- Intercourse
- Urination

Consists of

The penis is composed of three erectile bodies:

- Two dorsal corpora cavernosa
- One, ventral corpus spongiosum, containing:
  - Bulb of the penis (bulbus penis)
  - Glans penis

Divided into

- Radix (root), attached to the pubic bone and inferior side of the urogenital diaphragm
  - The crus of the penis: two crura cavernosa
  - The bulb of the penis
- Corpus (body)
  - Two corpora cavernosa
  - Corpus spongiosum
- Glans penis
  - Distal part of the corpus spongiosum

Layers of the Penis

Consist of

Profound → superficial

1. The erectile tissue (with tunica albuginea)
   - Corpora cavernosa and corpus spongiosum
     - Tunica albuginea is a thick capsule, surrounding each corpora cavernosa.
     - Trabeculae divide the erectile tissue into communicating cavernous spaces.
2. The deep fascia of the penis (Buck's fascia)
3. Subcutis
4. The superficial fascia of the penis (tunica Dartos)
   - Continuous with the tunica Dartos of the scrotum
5. Skin
   - Thin, loosely attached (except on the glans).
   - Prepuce (preputium) is a thin skin fold covering the glans (in uncircumcised men).
     - Inner surface of prepuce resembles a mucous membrane.
   - Tyson's glands are seen both on glans and on the inner surface of the prepuce.
     - Modified sebaceous glands
     - Produces smegma

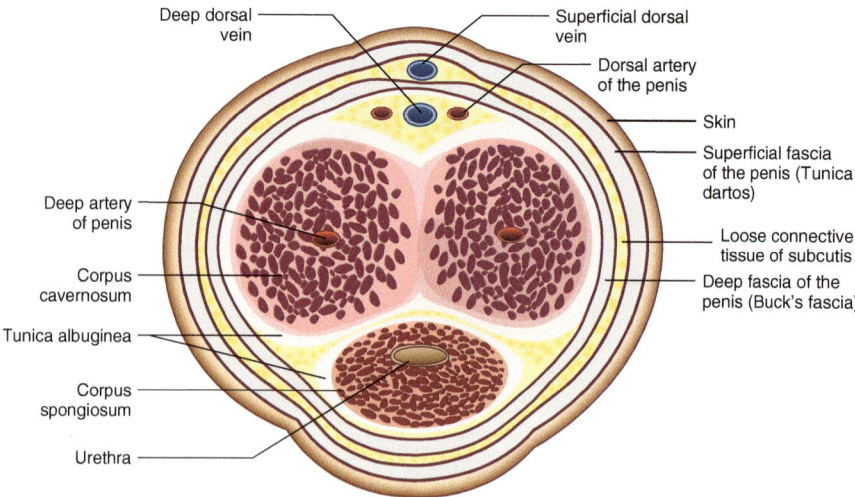

Fig. 26.3 Penis. Cross section, showing the five layers of penis

Light Microscopy
- The erectile tissue (with tunica albuginea)
  - Corpora cavernosa
    - Dense connective tissue, with collagen and elastic fibers
      - Inner circular layer
      - Outer longitudinal layer
    - Trabeculae of connective tissue and smooth muscle tissue extend from the tunica albuginea capsule.
      - Covered with endothelium
      - Divides the erectile tissue into communicating cavernous spaces
  - Corpus spongiosum
    - Structure as corpora cavernosa but with thinner and more elastic tunica albuginea
- The deep fascia of the penis (Buck's fascia)
  - Thin, strong fascia of dense connective tissue and elastic fibers
- Subcutis
  - Thin layer of loose connective tissue
  - Contains no adipose tissue
- The superficial fascia of the penis (tunica Dartos)
  - Smooth muscle tissue
- Skin
  - Thin (see Chap. 20)

Blood Supply of the Penis

General

The blood supply of the penis can be divided into:
- Nutritive
- Functional (erection mechanism) (Table 26.3)

Consists of
- Arterial supply
  - The pained internal pudendal artery (a. pudenda interna) contributes with four branches, to each side of the penis.
    - The artery of bulb of penis (a. bulbi penis) to corpus spongiosum
    - The urethral artery (a. urethralis) to corpus spongiosum
    - The dorsal artery of the penis (a. dorsalis penis) to corpus cavernosum
    - The deep artery of the penis (a. profunda penis) to corpus cavernosum (primarily functional)
- Venous drainage
  - Two sets of veins:
    - The superficial dorsal vein of the penis (v. dorsalis superficialis penis)
    - The profound dorsal vein of the penis (v. dorsalis profunda penis)

Table 26.3 Functional blood supply of the corpora cavernosa

Vessel(s)	Run(s)	Feature(s)
The deep artery of the penis ↓	Axially in the two corpora cavernosa	
Helicine arteries of the penis ↓	In the trabeculae of the corpora cavernosa	Empty into the cavernae
Cavernous spaces ↓		Spaces between the trabeculae of the corpora cavernosa
Post-caverneal venules ↓	Just underneath the tunica albuginea	Form a venous plexus
Deep veins of the penis ↓	Diagonal through the tunica albuginea	Thick wall
The profound dorsal vein of the penis		

The Erection Mechanism

Consists of

- Initiation:
  1. Sexual arousal → increased parasympathetic activity → nitric oxide (NO) is secreted from endothelial cells in the penis.
  2. NO induces relaxation of smooth muscle cells in the trabeculae and the helicine arteries → increased blood flow into the cavernous spaces of the erectile tissue.
  3. Blood accumulates in the cavernous spaces → compression of post-caverneal venules against tunica albuginea as well as of the veins running through the tunica albuginea → more blood accumulates in the erectile tissue and the pressure raises → erection.
- Termination:
  1. Sympathetic activity → contraction of smooth muscle cells in the trabeculae and the helicine arteries → decreased blood flow into the cavernous spaces → decreased pressure.
  2. Lower pressure permits venous drainage → erection terminates.

SCROTUM

Structure

Skin bag holding the testicles and epididymes

Function

Regulation of the temperature of the testicles (2–3 °C below body temperature), which is essential for the spermatogenesis

The wall of the scrotum

Consists of

Seven layers, profound → superficial:
1. Tunica vaginalis testis
   - Visceral layer: derived from peritoneum
   - - Potential space, containing a minimal amount of serous fluid - - -
   - Parietal layer: derived from peritoneum
2. Fascia spermatica interna
   - Derived from the transverse fascia (fascia transversalis) of the abdominal wall
3. Fascia cremasterica
   - Derived from internal abdominal oblique muscle

4. Fascia spermatica externa
   - Derived from the aponeurosis of the external abdominal oblique muscle
5. Subcutis
   - Without adipose tissue
6. Tunica Dartos
   - Thin layer of smooth muscle tissue
   - Derived from fascia abdominalis superficialis
7. Skin
   - With pubic hair, apocrine sweat glands, and sebaceous glands
   - Highly pigmented, especially in the midline called raphe scroti

Guide to Practical Histology: The Male Reproductive System

Testicle

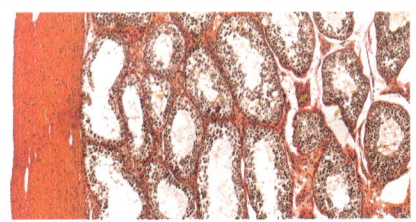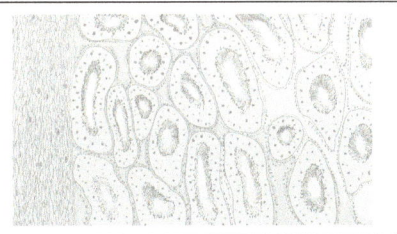

Left: photomicrograph of the testicle (a thick connective capsule (tunica albuginea) is seen to the left and seminiferous tubules to the right). Magnification: low. Stain: Van Gieson (Courtesy of associate professor Steen Seier Poulsen, University of Copenhagen). *Right*: simplified illustration of the capsule (tunica albuginea) and seminiferous tubules

Characteristics
- Macroscopic:
  - Round structure with a thick capsule of dense connective tissue (tunica albuginea).
  - Septa of dense connective tissue divide the organ into lobules.
- Microscopic:
  - The lobules contain multiple cross sections of tubules (seminiferous tubules) with irregular lumina.
    - High, pseudostratified epithelium.
    - Nuclei of different appearance in the different levels of the epithelium.

Efferent Ductules

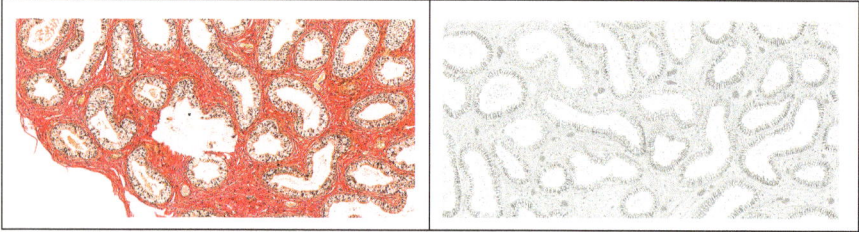

Left: photomicrograph of several cross sections of efferent ductules. Magnification: low. Stain: Van Gieson (Courtesy of associate professor Steen Seier Poulsen, University of Copenhagen). *Right*: simplified illustration of the efferent ductules

Characteristics
- Usually seen in the same specimen as ductus epididymidis
- Several cross sections with irregular lumina
  - Festoon-shaped luminal border, as groups of tall columnar cells, are seen alternating with groups of smaller cuboidal cells.
  - The basal surface of the ductules has a smooth border.

Can be mistaken for
Ductus epididymidis in the body and tail of the epididymis:
- More "rough" structure
- Larger ⊘
- Thicker epithelium
- No festoon-shaped luminal border

Ductus Epididymidis

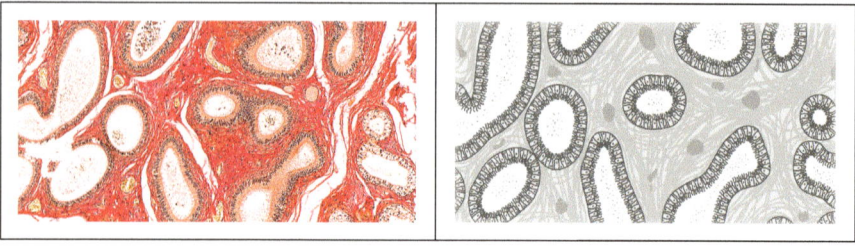

Left: photomicrograph of several cross sections of ductus epididymidis. Magnification: low. Stain: Van Gieson (Courtesy of associate professor Steen Seier Poulsen, University of Copenhagen). *Right*: simplified illustration of cross sections of ductus epididymidis

Characteristics

- Usually seen in the same specimen as efferent ductules
- Several cross sections of irregular lumina
  - Pseudostratified columnar epithelium
    - Particularly high columnar cells with basal nuclei
    - Long stereocilia project into the lumen

Can be mistaken for

Efferent ductules:

- More "delicate" structures
- Smaller ⊘
- Thinner epithelium
- Festoon-shaped luminal border

Ductus Deferens

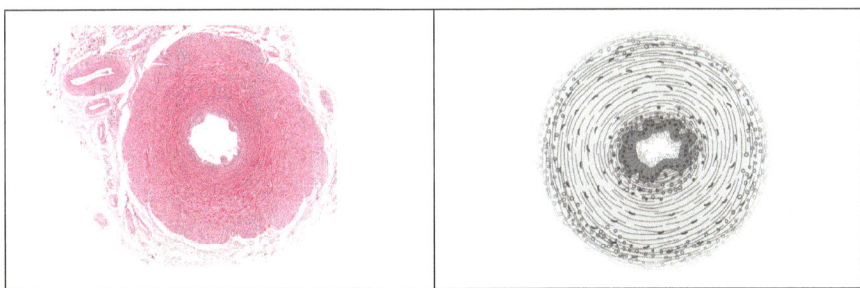

Left: photomicrograph of the ductus deferens. Magnification: low. Stain: HE (Courtesy of associate professor Steen Seier Poulsen, University of Copenhagen). *Right*: simplified illustration of a cross section of ductus deferens

Characteristics

Cross section:

- A ring-shaped structure with a small star-shaped lumen
- Lined with pseudostratified columnar epithelium
- The lumen is surrounded by an extremely thick layer of smooth muscle tissue

Can be mistaken for

- Ureter
  - Lined with urothelium
- Fallopian tube
  - Lined with simple columnar epithelium
  - Extremely folded mucosa (looks like curly kale)

Prostate Gland

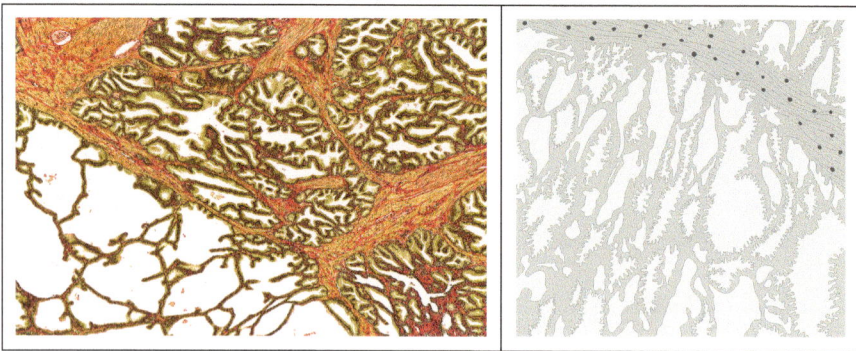

Left: photomicrograph of the prostate gland with secretory alveoli of different size and shape. Magnification: low. Stain: Van Gieson (Courtesy of associate professor Steen Seier Poulsen, University of Copenhagen). *Right*: simplified illustration of the prostate gland

Characteristics
- Eosinophilic capsule of dense connective tissue
- Eosinophilic stroma of connective tissue and smooth muscle tissue
- Basophilic cross sections of alveolar secretory end pieces:
  - Great variation in size and shape of the secretory end pieces.
    - Often with large visible lumina.
  - Concentric, eosinophilic bodies (corpora amylacea) are often seen in the lumina.

Can be mistaken for
Mammary gland (lactating)
- More organized structure.
- Smaller lumina of alveolar end pieces.
- Larger interlobar ducts, sometimes with eosinophilic secretions (milk).
- No corpora amylacea are seen.

Special Staining
Van Gieson
- Stains connective tissue red
- Stains cytoplasm of the epithelial and smooth muscle cells yellowish

Seminal Vesicle

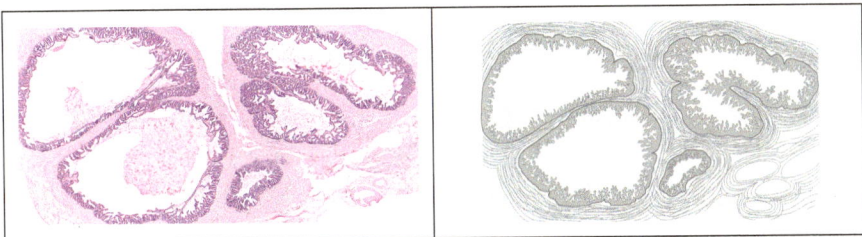

Left: photomicrograph of the seminal vesicle with several cross sections of the coiled tubular gland. The mucosa is extensively folded. Magnification: low. Stain: HE (Courtesy of associate professor Steen Seier Poulsen, University of Copenhagen). *Right*: simplified illustration of the seminal vesicle

Characteristics

Cross section:

- The tubular gland is extensively coiled → several cross sections of the lumen are seen in the specimen.
- Extremely folded mucosa.
  - Folds appear to branch with each other.
  - Lined with low, pseudostratified columnar epithelium.
- Surrounded by loose connective tissue and smooth muscular tissue.

Can be mistaken for

Fallopian tube

- Lined with simple columnar epithelium
- Extremely folded mucosa (looks like curly kale)

Penis

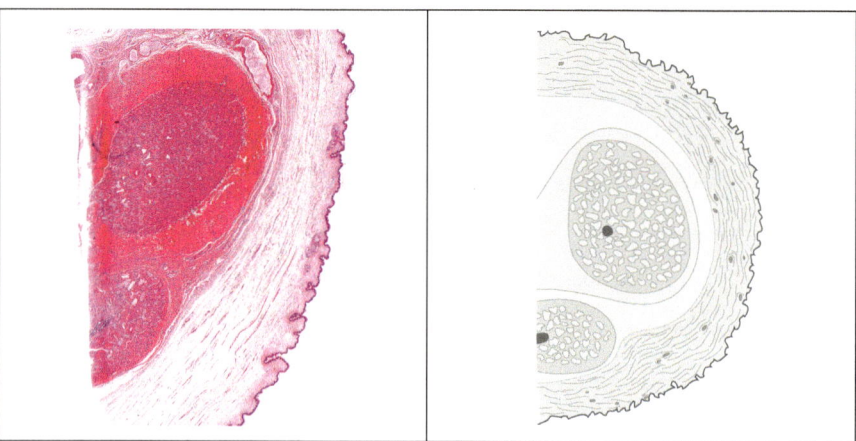

Left: photomicrograph of a cross sectioned penis (showing a part of the "monkey face," corpus cavernosum to the top right (one eye) and half the circumference of corpus spongiosum in the bottom (the mouth)). Magnification: low. Stain HE (Courtesy of associate professor Steen Seier Poulsen, University of Copenhagen). *Right*: simplified illustration of a cross section of the penis

Characteristics

Cross section:

- Macroscopic
  - ○ Resembles of the face of a monkey
    - ▪ The two deep arteries of the penis (centrally in the two corpora cavernosa) represent the eyes.
    - ▪ The urethra (centrally in the corpus spongiosum) represents the mouth.
- Microscopic:
  - ○ The cavernous bodies have a thick wall of dense connective tissue (tunica albuginea).
  - ○ Trabeculae of dense connective tissue extend from the wall into the cavernous tissue.
  - ○ The cavernous spaces between the trabeculae are filled with blood.

References

5, 25, 31, 33, 34, 35, 45.

Chapter 27
The Breast

Contents

General

- The breast (mamma) is a paired exocrine gland embedded in adipose and connective tissue.
- The appearance varies with sex, age, reproductive status, and menstrual cycle.
- The glands develop during the fetal period from the mammary ridges (milk lines), two ectodermal thickenings, which run from the axilla to the inguinal.
- Matures under influence of sex hormones.
  - Equal development in male and female until puberty, hereafter
    - Estrogens and progesterone → further growth and development in females
    - Testosterone → inhibition of further growth and development in males

Structure

Paired glandular organ:
- Exocrine tubuloalveolar gland: 15–20 separate glands, each with their own duct system
- Embedded in the subcutaneous adipose tissue and connective tissue

© Springer International Publishing Switzerland 2017
A. Rehfeld et al., *Compendium of Histology*, DOI 10.1007/978-3-319-41873-5_27

Function
Production and secretion of breast milk

Consists of
- Parenchyma
  - Exocrine tubuloalveolar glands (gll. mammaria)
  - Duct system
- Stroma
  - Connective tissue
  - Adipose tissue

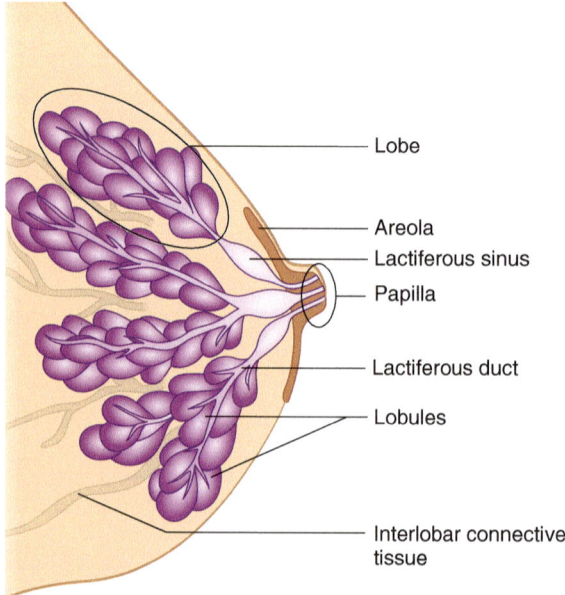

Fig. 27.1 Breast. Cross section through the breast and papilla showing the duct system and the connective tissue of the breast

Divided into (Fig. 27.1)
- Lobes
  - 15–20 per breast
  - Radiating from the papilla
  - Separated by interlobar connective tissue
  - Further divided into lobules, by interlobular connective tissue
- Lobules
  - Also called terminal duct lobular units (TDLUs)
  - Separated by interlobular connective tissue
  - A lobule is a cluster of:
    - Intralobular ducts (collecting ducts): from the terminal ductules

- Terminal ductules
  - Terminal duct endings (rudimentary alveoli): Develop into mature alveoli (alveolar secretory end pieces) in the active, lactating gland
- Intralobular loose connective tissue

PARENCHYMA OF THE BREAST

General

The epithelial and myoepithelial cells constitute the parenchymal part of the mammary glands:
- Epithelial cells line the ducts and alveoli.
- The myoepithelial cells are located between the epithelial cells and their basement membrane.

Light Microscopy

Differs with the level of activity:
- Active, lactating gland
  - Glandular and ductal components are described in Table 27.1
  - Lumina are filled with granular, eosinophilic material with lipid droplets
- Inactive gland
  - More connective tissue than ductal components
  - No alveoli

Table 27.1 Lactating mammary gland

Part	Epithelium	Surrounded by	
Lactiferous ducts	Stratified squamous keratinized (near opening at papilla) → two-layered cuboidal/columnar (deeper)	Myoepithelial cells	Basement membrane
Interlobular ducts	Single columnar	Myoepithelial cells	Basement membrane
Intralobular ducts	Single columnar/cuboidal	Myoepithelial cells	Basement membrane
Alveoli (alveolar end pieces)	Single cuboidal: • Basal nucleus • Basophilic cytoplasm, due to abundant rER • Supranuclear pale area is often seen, corresponding to the Golgi apparatus • Apical secretory vesicles and lipid droplets • Irregular convex apical border	Myoepithelial cells	Basement membrane

Myoepithelial cells

Function

Contractions in the myoepithelial cells → the secretory product (breast milk) produced in the alveoli is expelled.

Light Microscopy

- Stellate, flattened cells
- Organized in a network, surrounding and epithelial cells
- Located between the epithelial cells and the basement membrane

Changes during pregnancy

General

- Volume of the secretory parenchyma and duct system increases gradually:
    1. Lengthening and branching of terminal ducts
    2. Differentiation of alveoli from terminal duct endings
    3. Maturation of alveoli
- Volume of the adipose and connective tissue decreases gradually.
    ○ Lymphocytes and plasma cells infiltrate the stroma from the second trimester.

DUCT SYSTEM

Consists of (Fig. 27.1)

- Lactiferous ducts (ducti lactiferi)
    ○ 2–4.5 cm
    ○ Open through a narrow opening in the papilla
    ○ Lactiferous sinus: Dilated part located close to the papilla
    ○ Branch into interlobular ducts
- Interlobular ducts
    ○ Branch into intralobular ducts
- Intralobular ducts (collecting ducts)
    ○ Last branches are called terminal ductules, which develop into alveoli in the active gland.

CONNECTIVE TISSUE OF THE BREAST

General

Bands of connective tissue separate the lobes and lobules of the mammary gland and suspend the gland by attaching to the dermis.

Consists of (Fig. 27.1)
- Interlobar connective tissue
  - Dense connective tissue
  - Divides the breast into lobes, i.e., separates the 15–20 glands
- Interlobular connective tissue
  - Dense connective tissue
  - Divides the lobes into lobules
- Intralobular connective tissue
  - Loose connective tissue
  - Surrounds the alveoli in the lobules
  - Houses plasma cells and lymphocytes after the second trimester of pregnancy
- Suspensory ligaments (Cooper's ligaments, ligamentum suspensorium mammae)
  - Attached to the dermis, to support the gland

PAPILLA AND AREOLA

General
- Papilla, nipple
  - Contains the outlets of the lactiferous ducts (one from each lobe).
  - At the apex of the breast.
  - The nipple has abundant sensory nerve endings.
- Areola
  - Pigmented area, surrounding the papilla

Consists of
- Skin of the papilla and areola:
  - Epidermis
    - Highly pigmented
    - Melanocytes are stimulated by estrogen in puberty and further in pregnancy
  - Dermis
    - High dermal papillae
    - Glands of the areola:
      - Areolar glands (glands of Montgomery), modified mammary glands
      - Sebaceous glands
      - Sweat glands:
        - Eccrine
        - Apocrine
    - Smooth muscle tissue is found deeper in the areola and nipple:
      - Radially ⎤
      - Circumferentially ⎦ → papilla erection, in response to different stimuli
  - Subcutis
- Outlets of the lactiferous ducts

HORMONAL CONTROL OF THE MAMMARY GLAND

During puberty

Estrogen and progesterone from the ovaries →
- Initial enlargement and development of:
  - The mammary gland
  - The connective and adipose tissue
- Formation of terminal duct lobular units

During menstrual cycle

Estrogen and progesterone from the ovaries → minor changes in the gland tissue:
- Estrogen → proliferation of duct components
- Progesterone →
  - Accumulation of a small amount of secretion in the lumen of the ducts
  - Swelling of intralobular loose connective tissue

During pregnancy

- Estrogen and progesterone from the corpus luteum and placenta
- Prolactin from the adenohypophysis   } → 1. and 2.
- Human chorionic somatomammotropin (hCS) from the placenta
    1. Changes in parenchyma:
       - Volume of the secretory parenchyma and duct system increases
       - As the pregnancy proceed
         1. Lengthening and branching of terminal ducts
         2. Differentiation of alveoli from terminal duct endings
         3. Maturation of alveoli
    2. Changes in stroma:
       - Volume of the adipose and connective tissue decreases

During lactation

- Initiation of lactation:
  - Estrogen and progesterone inhibit the lactogenic effect of prolactin, during pregnancy.
  - After delivery the abrupt fall in plasma levels of estrogen and progesterone, due to loss of placenta, allows prolactin to undertake it's lactogenic effect.
- Maintenance of lactation:
  - Stimulation of the papilla (suckling) → nerve impulses to the hypothalamus → two reflexes:
    1. Secretion of prolactin (PRL) from the adenohypophysis → stimulation of production of breast milk in the mammary gland

   2. Secretion of oxytocin (OX) from the neurohypophysis → contraction in
      myoepithelial cells in the duct system and alveoli → ejection of milk
   ○ If suckling does not occur, the absence of PRL will cause the production of
     milk to cease
• Cessation of lactation:
   ○ When breastfeeding stops, the main part of the alveoli developed during
     pregnancy and lactation degenerates:
      ▪ Epithelial cells undergo apoptosis and are removed by macrophages.
      ▪ Duct system returns to inactive state.

After menopause

Decreased levels of sex hormones cause regression of glandular tissue and
connective tissue.

BREAST MILK

Consists of
• Lipids
• Proteins
• Antibodies:
   ○ Provide passive immunity to the newborn
   ○ Produced by the plasma cells of the stroma
• Carbohydrates: primarily lactose

Divided into
• Colostrum:
   ○ The first portions of breast milk
   ○ Rich in protein, vitamin A, Cl^- and Na^+ and antibodies (primarily secretory
     IgA)
   ○ Less lipid, carbohydrate, and K^+ content than ordinary breast milk
• Regular breast milk:
   ○ Replaces colostrum after a few days of lactation

Types of secretion

Divided into
• Merocrine secretion:
   ○ Secretion of protein component by exocytosis
• Apocrine secretion:
   ○ Secretion of lipid component
   ○ Small lipid droplets in the cytoplasm fuse into larger droplets
   ○ The large droplets are located apically in the cell and are discharged with a
     surrounding brim of plasmalemma.
   ○ This type of secretion is only seen in the lactating mammary gland.

Guide to Practical Histology:
The Breast

Mammary Gland (Inactive)

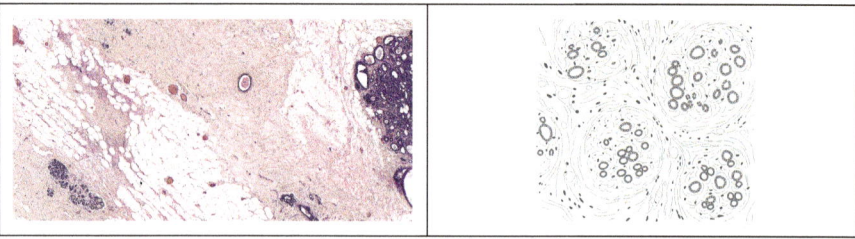

Left: photomicrograph of an inactive mammary gland with abundant connective tissue and adipose tissue with small, basophilic islets of glandular components. Magnification: low. Stain: HE (Courtesy of associate professor Steen Seier Poulsen, University of Copenhagen). *Right*: simplified illustration of inactive mammary glands

Characteristics
- Irregular eosinophilic connective tissue with many adipocytes and few basophilic cells
- Small islets with groups of cross sections of ducts and non-developed alveoli with basophilic epithelial cells

Mammary Gland (Lactating)

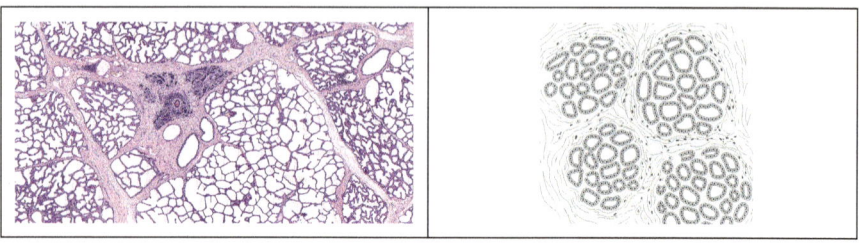

Left: photomicrograph of a lactating mammary gland with abundant glandular tissue and sparse connective tissue. Magnification: low. Stain: HE (Courtesy of associate professor Steen Seier Poulsen, University of Copenhagen). *Right*: simplified illustration of lactating mammary gland

Characteristics
- Abundant cross sections of basophilic alveolar secretory end pieces and ductal components separated by eosinophilic connective tissue septa.
- Cells of alveolar end pieces are basophilic and vacuolated.
- Larger interlobar ducts, sometimes with eosinophilic secretions (milk) are seen.

Can be mistaken for
Prostate gland:
- Less organized structure.
- The lumina of the alveolar end pieces are wider than those of the lactating mammary gland.
- Concentric, eosinophilic bodies (corpora amylacea) often seen in the lumina.

References
5, 25, 31, 33, 34, 35, 45.

Chapter 28
The Eye

Contents

Consists of
- Eyeball (paired)
- Optic nerve (paired)
- Accessory structures of the eye (paired):
  - Eyebrow
  - Eyelid
  - Extrinsic muscles
  - Conjunctiva
  - Lacrimal apparatus

© Springer International Publishing Switzerland 2017
A. Rehfeld et al., *Compendium of Histology*, DOI 10.1007/978-3-319-41873-5_28

Eyeball (Bulbus Oculi)

General
- Spherical structure, located in the orbital cavity
- Surrounded by fat tissue

Structure (Fig. 28.1)
- The wall of the eyeball consists of three layers:
  - The outer layer (fibrous tunic, fibrous layer, corneoscleral coat)
    - Cornea
    - Limbus
    - Sclera
  - The middle layer (vascular coat, uvea)
    - Iris
    - Ciliary body
    - Choroid
  - The inner layer (retina)
    - Retinal pigment epithelium
    - Neural retina
- Intraocular structures
  - The lens
  - The vitreous body

THE OUTER LAYER OF THE EYEBALL (FIBROUS TUNIC)

Function
- Forms a protective capsule around the two inner layers of the eyeball
- Attachment site of the extrinsic eye muscles

Consists of (Fig. 28.1)
- Cornea, anterior $\frac{1}{6}$
- Limbus
  - The transition zone between cornea and sclera.
- Sclera, posterior $\frac{5}{6}$

Divided into
The three parts are subdivided into several layers. (Table 28.1)

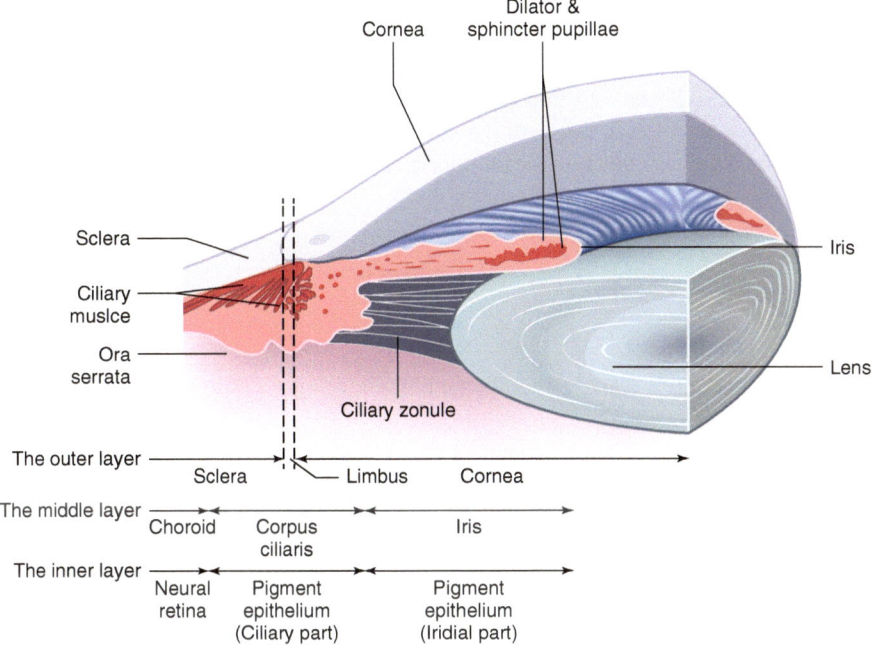

Fig. 28.1 The layers of the eyeball

Table 28.1 Subdivision of the outer layer of the eyeball

	Cornea	Limbus	Sclera
Superficial → profound	1. Corneal epithelium →	1. Conjunctival epithelium (→ the bulbar conjunctiva)	–
	2. Anterior basement membrane (Bowman's membrane)	2. Tenon's capsule	–
	–	3. Episcleral layer →	1. Episcleral layer
	3. Substantia propria (corneal stroma) →	4. Limbal stroma →	2. Substantia propria (scleral stroma, sclera proper)
	4. Posterior basement membrane (Descemet's membrane)	–	3. Lamina fusca
	5. Corneal endothelium	–	–

Cornea

General (Fig. 28.1 and Table 28.1)
- Forms the anterior ⅙ of the outer layer of the eyeball
- Recieves nutrition through diffusion from:
  - The aqueous humor in the anterior chamber (primary source)
  - The interstitial fluid supplied by the peri-corneal blood vessels

Structure
- Convex and avascular
- ⊘ 11.5 mm
- 0.5–1 mm thick
- Consists of 80 % water and collagen fibrils
- Transparent:
  - Uniform organization of the collagen fibrils within the lamellae of the substantia propria → transparency.
  - Cells of the corneal endothelium regulate the transport of fluid and solutes between the aqueous humor and corneal stroma → regulate transparency.

Function
The main refractive element of the eye

Light Microscopy
See Table 28.2.

Limbus

General (Fig. 28.1, Table 28.1)
- The transition zone between cornea and sclera
- 2 mm wide and 2 mm thick

Function
Maintenance of the intraocular pressure by drainage of the aqueous humor through the canal of Schlemm

Light Microscopy
See Table 28.3.

Table 28.2 The layers of the cornea

	Layer	General	Light microscopy	Continuous with
Superficial → profound	1. Corneal epithelium	Contains numerous free nerve endings → high sensibility	Nonkeratinized stratified squamous epithelium • Cells are connected through desmosomes and tight junctions • Five to six cell layers	The outermost layer of limbus
	2. Anterior basement membrane	Consists of randomly organized collagen fibrils	Thin homogeneous layer	Exists only in cornea
	3. Substantia propria	Constitutes the majority of cornea	Composed approximately of 60 lamellae, organized parallel with the surface and consisting of: • Parallel collagen fibrils • Fibroblasts (keratocytes) • Ground substance	The fourth layer of limbus
	4. Posterior basement membrane	Basal lamina of the corneal endothelium.	Thin homogenous layer	The trabecular meshwork of fibrils in the iridocorneal angle.
	5. Corneal endothelium	• Cells are connected by tight junctions • The cells transport fluid and solutes between the aqueous humor and corneal stroma → regulate transparency	A single layer of squamous cells	An endothelial layer, covering the trabecular meshwork in the iridocorneal angle

Table 28.3 The layers of limbus

	Layer	General	Light microscopy	Continuous with
Superficial ↓ profound	1. Conjunctival epithelium	Contains blood vessels that nourish the peripheral cornea	Nonkeratinized stratified squamous epithelium	• The outermost layer of cornea • The bulbar conjunctiva (mucous membrane), which lines the sclera
	2. Tenon's capsule		Dense, collagenous, connective tissue	Exists only in limbus
	3. Episcleral layer		Thin layer of loose connective tissue	The outermost layer of sclera

	4. Limbal stroma	• Most abundant layer
		 • Transition zone between:
		   ○ The corneal stroma with parallel collagen fibrils
		   ○ The scleral stroma with collagen fibrils organized in different directions
			Composed of:
			 • Collagen fibrils
			 • Fibroblasts (keratocytes)
			 • Ground substance
				• The third layer of cornea
				 • The second layer of sclera

Sclera

Structure (Fig. 28.1, Table 28.1)
- White, opaque, membrane that forms the posterior ⅚ of the outer layer of the eyeball.
- Continuous with the dura mater that covers the optic nerve.
  - The nerve fibers from the neural retina pierce the sclera at the lamina cribrosa and form the optic nerve.

Function
- Forms a protective capsule around the two inner layers of the eyeball
- Attachment site of the extrinsic eye muscles

Light Microscopy
See Table 28.4.

Table 28.4 The layers of sclera

	Layer	General	Light microscopy	Continuous with
Superficial → profound	1. Episcleral layer	Contains blood vessels	Loose, vascularized connective tissue	The third layer of limbus
	2. Substantia propria	Almost avascular	• A dense network of bundles of thick collagen fibers ○ Parallel to the surface, but in different directions • Sparse ground substance	The fourth layer of limbus
	3. Lamina fusca	Dark color due to melanin granules in the: • Melanocytes • Macrophages	• Fibers ○ Thin bundles of collagen fibers ○ Elastic fibers • Cells ○ Fibroblasts ○ Melanocytes ○ Macrophages	• Exists only in limbus • Profound part is connected to the suprachoroid layer in the choroid

THE MIDDLE LAYER OF THE EYEBALL (UVEA)

General
- A well-pigmented and well-vascularized layer between the innermost and outermost layers of the eyeball.
- Contains the muscles that control:
  - The pupil ⊘
  - The shape of the lens

Structure
- Well pigmented
- Well vascularized

Function
- Absorption of light → minimizing glare within the eye.
- Provide nutrients to retina.
- Production of the humor aquosus.

Consists of
- Iris
- Ciliary body
- Choroid

Divided into
The three parts that are subdivided into several layers (Table 28.5)

Iris

General (Table 28.5, Fig. 28.1)
- The iris extends posteriorly to the cornea and anteriorly to the lens.
- Separates the anterior chamber and the posterior chamber.
- The color of the iris, the "eye color", depends on the number of melanocytes in the iris.
- Surface runs from the ciliary (peripheral) margin to the pupillary (central) margin.
- The pupil is the central circular aperture.

Structure
- 0.5 mm thick diaphragm
- ⊘ 12 mm
- Contains two muscles:
  - The sphincter pupillae muscle
  - The dilator pupillae muscle

Table 28.5 Subdivision of the middle layer of the eyeball

	Iris	Ciliary body	Choroid
Superficial → profound	1. Anterior limiting layer ⟶	1. Supraciliary layer ⟶	1. Suprachoroid layer
		2. Ciliary muscle	
	2. Stroma of the iris ⟶	3. Stroma of the ciliary body ⟶	2. Stroma of the choroid
			3. Choriocapillary layer
		4. Basal lamina (Bruch's membrane) ⟶	4. Basal lamina (Bruch's membrane)
	3. Anterior pigment myoepithelium ⟶	5. Pigmented epithelium (→ retina)	
	4. Posterior pigment epithelium ⟶	6. Nonpigmented epithelium (→ retina)	

Function

Controls the amount of light that passes through the pupil to the retina by changing the diameter of the pupil:

- The sphincter pupillae muscle: constricts the pupil
- The dilator pupillae muscle: dilates the pupil

Light Microscopy

See Table 28.6.

Table 28.6 The layers of iris

	Layer	General	Light microscopy	Continuous with
Superficial → profound	1. Anterior limiting layer	An inconsistent layer: • The aqueous humor in the anterior camera is in contact with the stroma of the iris	Abundant fibroblasts and melanocytes	The first layer of the ciliary body
	2. Stroma of iris	• Contains the sphincter pupillae muscle • Blood vessels here are branches from the major arterial circle of the iris • Tight junctions of the endothelium and in the ciliary epithelium form the blood–aqueous barrier	• Loose connective tissue • Highly vascularized • Smooth muscle cells of the sphincter pupillae muscle	The third layer of the ciliary body

	3. Anterior pigment myoepithelium	• Contains the dilator pupillae muscle
		• Forms the iridial part of the nonphotosensitive region of retina, together with the fourth layer of iris
			• Basal (anterior):
			  ○ Smooth muscle cells of the dilator pupillae muscle
			• Apical (posterior):
			  ○ Pigmented single cuboidal epithelium
			  ○ Cannot be distinguished from the posterior pigment epithelium
				The fifth layer of the ciliary body

	4. Posterior pigment epithelium	Forms the iridial part of the nonphotosensitive region of retinae, together with the third layer of iris	• Simple columnar epithelium that cannot be visualized due to extensive pigmentation • The pigmentation decreases towards the ciliary body, where it disappears	The sixth layer of the ciliary body

The sphincter pupillae muscle

General
- Located centrally in the second layer of iris
- Muscle fibers arranged circumferentially near the pupillary (central) margin
- Innervation:
  - Parasympathetic nerve fibers: preganglionic nerve fibers (oculomotor nerve, cranial nerve III) → ciliary ganglion → postganglionic fibers (short ciliary nerves) → contraction of the pupil (miosis)
  - Similar as for the ciliary muscle

Function
Constriction of the pupil upon:
- Accommodation
- Bright light
  - Pupillary light reflex: increased intensity of light → constriction of the pupil (miosis)

Consists of
Smooth muscle cells

The dilator pupillae muscle

General
- Located peripherally in the third layer of the iris
- Innervation:
  - Sympathetic: postganglionic nerve fibers (superior cervical ganglion) → short and long ciliary nerves → dilating pupil (mydriasis)

Function
Dilation of the pupil upon:
- Dim light.
- High sympathetic activity, e.g., during the "fight-or-flight reflex"

Consists of
Smooth muscle cells (multiunit type) (Chap. 13)
- Sometimes referred to as myoepithelial cells

Ciliary Body

General (Fig. 28.1)
- Extends from the root of the iris, posterior to the ora serrata
  - Ora serrata: The transitional zone between the ciliary body and the photosensitive part of the retina
- Houses the ciliary muscle

Structure
- A "ring-shaped" structure surrounding the lens.
- On a cross section of the "ring", the ciliary body has the shape of a triangle.
  - Approximately 6 mm in length
  - The apex is continuous with the choroid (the posterior part of the middle layer of the eyeball).

Function
- Production of the aqueous humor, in the sixth layer of the ciliary body
- Suspension of the lens via the ciliary zonula fibers
- Accommodation of the lens via the ciliary muscle

Divided into
- Anterior part:
  - Approximately 2 mm long
  - Contains:
    - 70–80 radial ridges (ciliary processes)
    - Grooves separating the ridges
      - The ciliary zonula fibers arise from the grooves and constitute the suspensory ligament of the lens.
- Posterior part:
  - Approximately 4 mm long
  - Flat and highly pigmented
  - Continuous with the choroid at the ora serrata

Consists of
Six layers (Table 28.7)

Table 28.7 The layers of the ciliary body

	Layer	General	Light microscopy	Continuous with
Superficial → profound	1. Supraciliary lamina	Contains branches from: • The long posterior ciliary arteries • The anterior ciliary arteries	• Loose connective tissue • Well vascularized	• The first layer of iris • The first layer of the choroid
	2. Ciliary muscle	Constitute the bulk of the ciliary body	Smooth muscle tissue	Exists only in the ciliary body
	3. Ciliary stroma	Blood vessels here form the major arterial circle of the iris	• Highly vascularized loose connective tissue • Extend up into the ciliary processess	• The second layer of the iris • The second layer of the choroid
	4. Basal lamina (Bruch's membrane)	Basement membrane of the fifth layer of the ciliary body	Dense network of elastic fibers	The fourth layer of the choroid
	5. Pigmented epithelium	Forms the ciliary part of the nonphotosensitive region of retina, together with the sixth layer of the ciliary body	One layer of cuboidal cells, with abundant melanin granules	• The third layer of iris • Retina (retinal pigment epithelium)
	6. Nonpigmented epithelium	• Forms the ciliary part of the nonphotosensitive region of retina, together with the fifth layer of the ciliary body. • Produces the aqueous humor • Tight junctions here and in the vascular endothelium of the iris form the blood–aqueous barrier	Columnar cells	• The fourth layer of the iris • Retina (neural retina)

Ciliary muscle

General

Circular smooth muscle tissue located in the ciliary body

Divided into
- Outer meridional portion:
  - The most external part
  - Embedded in the stroma of the choroid
- Middle radial portion:
  - Muscle cells attach to the connective tissue of the ciliary processes.
- Inner circular portion:
  - Circumferentially arranged muscle cells, which act as a sphincter.

Consists of
Smooth muscle cells

Structure
Innervation
- Parasympathetic:
  - Preganglionic nerve fibers (oculomotor nerve, cranial nerve III) → ciliary ganglion → postganglionic fibers (short ciliary nerves) → contraction of the ciliary muscle → accommodation.
  - Similar as for the sphincter pupillae muscle
- Sympathetic:
  - Postganglionic nerve fibers from the superior cervical ganglion innervate the muscle through the short ciliary nerves.
  - Function is unclear.

Function
Accommodation:
- Contraction → ciliary zonula fibers relax → reduces the tension on the lens → increase the convexity of the lens → increased refraction (accommodation).

Blood supply of the ciliary body
Divided into
- Arterial:
  - Abundant vessels in the ciliary stroma creates the major arterial circle of iris
  - Consists of vessels from:
    - The long ciliary arteries
    - The anterior ciliary arteries
  - Located in the anterior part of the ciliary body, close to the basis of the iris
- Venous:
  - The four vorticose (vortex) veins

The aqueous humor

General

- A transparent fluid, produced in the sixth layer (nonpigmented epithelium) of the ciliary body
- Similar to the composition of blood plasma, but with less protein
- Route:
  - From the ciliary body → posterior chamber → through the pupil → the anterior chamber → the trabecular network of the iridocorneal angle → canal of Schlemm → veins

Function

- Maintenance of the intraocular pressure
- Nourishment of avascular structures, e.g.:
  - Cornea
  - Lens

Drainage of the aqueous humor

General

The drainage of aqueous humor is important for the normal function of the eye.

Consists of

Two draining pathways (both passive processes):
1. Drainage through the iridocorneal angle, 80–90 %:
   - The trabecular meshwork:
     - Located in the iridocorneal angle
     - Connective tissue covered by an endothelial layer, continuous with the corneal endothelium
     - Provides resistance to the outflow of aqueous humor
     - After crossing the trabecular meshwork, the aqueous humor exits into the scleral venous sinus, which drains directly to the aqueous veins
   - Scleral venous sinus (canal of Schlemm, Schlemm's canal):
     - Located at the limbus
     - Formed from the gaps in the trabecular meshwork
     - Endothelium-lined
     - The aqueous humor exits the canal of Schlemm through 25–35 collecting vessels that end in the ophthalmic vein
2. Uveoscleral drainage, 10–20 %:
   - A nondistinctive pathway where the aqueous humor leaches out through surrounding tissues and into the veins

Choroid

General
- 0.25–0.1 mm thick, macroscopically brown membrane.
- Extends posteriorly from the ciliary body.
- The choroid is continuous with the meninges, pia mater, and arachnoid that ensheath the optic nerve.

Structure
- An uneven, well-pigmented layer with abundant blood vessels
- Composed mainly of blood vessels surrounded by:
  - Connective tissue
  - Melanocytes
  - Nerves

Function
- Nourishes the outer layers of the retina (primary function).
- Reduces glare by absorbing scattered and reflected light.

Light Microscopy (Table 28.8)
The four layers of the choroid are difficult to distinguish from each other the light microscope.

Table 28.8 The layers of the choroid

	Layer	General	Light microscopy	Continuous with
Superficial → profound	1. Suprachoroid layer	Dark color due to melanin granules in the melanocytes	Pigmented loose connective tissue with: • A network of thin collagen and elastic fibers • Fibroblasts • Melanocytes	The first layer of the ciliary body

	2. Choroidal stroma	• Forms the bulk of the choroid
		• Contains a dense network of blood vessels:
		  ○ Arteries: branches from the ciliary arteries
		  ○ Veins: small veins → larger veins → the four vorticose (vortex) veins
			Pigmented loose connective tissue with:
			• Melanocytes
			• Macrophages
			• A dense network of blood vessels
				The third layer of the ciliary body

	3. Choriocapillary layer	• Contains branches from the blood vessels in the choroidal stroma • Nourish the outer part of retina (layers 1–5)	• A network of fenestrated capillaries • A few thin collagen and elastic fibers	Exists only in the choroid
	4. Basal lamina (Bruch's membrane)	• The innermost layer of the choroid • Thickest near the optic disc, thinner towards the periphery	Dense network of elastic fibers	The fourth layer of the ciliary body

THE INNER LAYER OF THE EYEBALL (RETINA)

General (Figs. 28.1 and 28.2)
- The innermost layer of the eyeball
- Divided into two continuous regions, separated by the ora serrata:
  ○ The anterior nonphotosensitive region
    ▪ Described under the middle layer of the eyeball
  ○ The posterior photosensitive region
    ▪ The part usually referred to as "retina"

Structure
- The nonphotosensitive region
  - ○ Located anterior to ora serrata
  - ○ Composed of:
    - ▪ The anterior continuation of the retinal pigment epithelium
    - ▪ The anterior continuation of the neural retina
  - ○ Forms the two innermost layers of:
    - ▪ The ciliary body
    - ▪ The iris
  - ○ Described under the middle layer of the eyeball
- The photosensitive region
  - ○ Located posterior to the ora serrata
  - ○ Lines ⅔, of the inner surface of the eye
  - ○ Forms the neural retina

The Photosensitive Region of Retina (Neural Retina)

Divided into (Figs. 28.1 and 28.2, Table 28.9)
- The retinal pigment epithelium
  - ○ The outermost layer (layer 1)
- The neural retina (retina proper)
  - ○ A multilayered structure (layers 2–10)

Consists of (Fig. 28.2)
- Retinal pigment epithelium
- Neurons:
  - ○ Photoreceptor neurons (Table 28.11)
    - ▪ Rod cells
    - ▪ Cone cells
  - ○ Conducting neurons
    - ▪ Bipolar cells
    - ▪ Ganglion cells
  - ○ Associating neurons
    - ▪ Horizontal cells
    - ▪ Amacrine cells
- Glial cells
  - ○ Müller cells
  - ○ Astroglia
  - ○ Microglia

Divided into (Fig. 28.2)

Ten recognizable layers (superficial → profound):

1. Retinal pigment epithelium
2. Layer of rods and cones
3. Outer limiting membrane
4. Outer nuclear layer
5. Outer plexiform layer
6. Inner nuclear layer
7. Inner plexiform layer
8. Ganglion cell layer
9. Nerve fiber layer
10. Inner limiting membrane

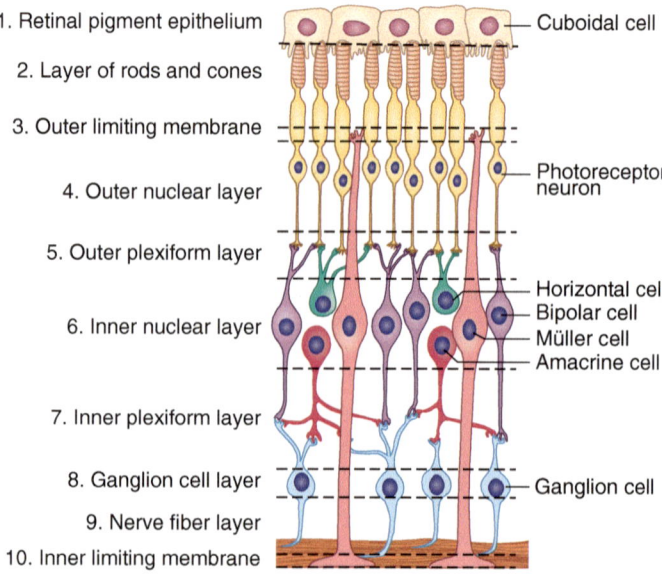

Fig. 28.2 The ten layers of retina

Function

Phototransduction

Light Microscopy

See Tables 28.9 and 28.10.

Table 28.9 The layers of retina

	Layer	General	Light microscopy
Superficial → profound	1. Retinal pigment epithelium	• Attached to the choroid • Prevents reflection of light by absorbing light • Regulates the exchange of materials from the blood vessels in the choroid to the retina: ○ Tight junctions here and in the vascular endothelium form the blood–retinal barrier • Phagocytosis of shedded discs from the rod and cone cells	• Single layer of cuboidal cells • Ovoid nuclei • Multiple melanin granules • Rest on the basal lamina Bruch's membrane, the fourth layer of the choroid
	2. Layer of rod and cone cells	Contains parts of the rod and cone cells (photoreceptor neurons): • The outer segment • The connecting stalk • Parts of the inner segment	The outer and inner segments of the photoreceptor cells are arranged in palisades → vertical striations
	3. Outer limiting membrane	A dense line formed by zonula adherents between: • Part of the inner segment of the rod and cone cells • The apical end of the Müller cells	A continuous line
	4. Outer nuclear layer	Consists of the nuclei of photoreceptor neurons: • Nuclei of the cone cells are located in several levels • Nuclei of the rod cells form a line at one level	• The cell bodies of the rod and cone cells • Difficult to distinguish between the cells
	5. Outer plexiform layer	Composed of the synapses between: • The terminal processes of the rod cells, called spherules • The terminal processes of the cone cells, called pedicles • Horizontal cell processes • Bipolar cell dendritic processes	Lack nuclei

	6. Inner nuclear layer	• Capillaries from the retinal vessels
		• The cell bodies of:
		  ○ Müller cells
		  ○ Bipolar cells
		  ○ Horizontal cells
		  ○ Amacrine cells
			• A thick layer of nuclei
			• Impossible to distinguish cells from each other.

	7. Inner plexiform layer	Contains synapses between:
		• Axons of:
		  ○ Bipolar cells
		  ○ Amacrine cells
		• Dendrites of:
		  ○ Ganglion cells
			Lack nuclei

(continued)

Table 28.9 (continued)

Layer	General	Light microscopy
8. Ganglion cell layer	Cell bodies of the ganglion cells • Multipolar nerve cells • One ganglion cell forms synapses with more than a hundred bipolar cells	A thick layer of large nuclei of the ganglion cells.
9. Nerve fiber layer	Consists of: • Unmyelinated axons of the ganglion cells • Blood vessels from both the central retinal vein and artery	Lack nuclei
10. Inner limiting membrane	A thin membrane consisting of the expanded terminal portions of Müller cells	A thin membrane

Table 28.10 Location of the cell parts of the most important cells of retina

Layer	Photoreceptor cells		Conducting neurons		Associating neurons		Glial cells
	Rod cells	Cone cells	Bipolar cells	Ganglion cells	Horizontal cells	Amacrine cells	Müller cells
1. Retinal pigment epithelium	–	–	–	–	–	–	–
2. Layer of rods and cones	The outer and inner segment	The outer and inner segment	–	–	–	–	–
3. Outer limiting membrane	Part of the inner segment	Part of the inner segment	–	–	–	–	Apical end
4. Outer nuclear layer	Cell body	Cell body	–	–	–	–	Cell extension
5. Outer plexiform layer	The terminal process (spherule)	The terminal process (pedicle)	Dendrite	–	Axon and dendrite-like process	–	Cell extension
6. Inner nuclear layer	–	–	Cell body	–	Cell body	Cell body	Cell body
7. Inner plexiform layer	–	–	Axon	Dendrite	–	Axon and dendrite-like process	Cell extension
8. Ganglion cell layer	–	–	–	Cell body	–	–	Cell extension
9. Nerve fiber layer	–	–	–	Axon	–	–	Cell extension
10. Inner limiting membrane	–	–	–	–	–	–	Basal end

Superficial → profound

Neurons of the Retina

Function
Transduce light (photons) into electrical signals

Divided into
- Photoreceptor neurons
  - Rod
  - Cone
- Conducting neurons
  - Bipolar cells
  - Ganglion cells
- Association neurons
  - Horizontal cells
  - Amacrine cells

Photoreceptor cells of the retina
General
See Tables 28.10 and 28.11.

Conducting neurons of the retina
General
See Tables 28.9 and 28.10.

Function
Conduct the signals from the photoreceptor neurons to the brain.

Divided into
- Bipolar cells
  - Cone bipolar cells
  - Rod bipolar cells
- Ganglion cells
  - Contain a large round nucleus.
  - The axons form the nerve fiber layer of retina.
  - Divided into several types, named after the size of the cell.

Associating neurons of the retina
General
Interneurons

Function
Modulation of the signals from the rod and cone cells

Divided into
- Horizontal cells
- Amacrine cells

Table 28.11 The photoreceptor cells of retina

	Rod cell	Cone cell
Abundance	120 million	6–7 million
Light sensitivity	• Sensitive • Responds to single photons	• Less sensitive • Specialized for color vision in bright light
Size	⊘ 1.5 µm, 120 µm long	⊘ 5 µm, 70 µm long
Composed of		
• Outer segment	• Cylindrical (rod) shaped • Photosensitive • Contains 600–1000 horizontal flattened membranous discs with visual pigments	• Conical (cone) shaped
• Connecting stalk	• A narrow area that joins the inner and outer segment • Structure similar to that of a cilium (Chap. 5)	
• Inner segment	• Divided into: ○ Outer ellipsoid part ○ Inner myoid part • Contain the nucleus and the organelles	
• Nucleus	Align in the same level in adjacent cells	Located in several levels in adjacent cells
• Inner terminal expanded portion	Called a spherule	Called a pedicle
• Discs	• Formed by invaginations of the plasma membrane • Loose contact with the plasma membrane shortly after they are formed • Shed apically every 10 days → engulfed by retinal pigment epithelium	• Formed by invaginations of the plasma membrane • Retain the contact with the plasma membrane • Shed apically less frequently than in rod cells → engulfed by retinal pigment epithelium
Function	Black and white vision	Divided into three functional cell types, which are sensitive to different wavelengths, with a maximum in either the red, blue, or green spectrum of light
Visual pigment	Rhodopsin	Iodopsin

Phototransduction

1. Light (photons) reach the visual pigments of the rod and cone cells
2. Photochemical reaction in the discs of the outer segment
3. Change of membrane potential → membrane hyperpolarization
4. Less glutamate is released to the bipolar cells
5. Further processing and modulation of the signal by the other neurons in retina
6. Signal is transmitted to the visual centers of the brain

Glial Cells of the Retina

Divided into
- Müller cells
- Astroglia (astrocytes)
- Microglia

Müller cells

Structure
- Large cells
- Flattened nuclei

Function
Mechanical support of retina

Astroglia (astrocytes)

General
- Fattened cell with several radiating processes (Chap. 14)
- Almost only present in the 9th layer (nerve fiber layer) of the retina

Function
Unclear

Microglia

General
- Small cell with short, thin cell extensions (Chap. 14)
- Found in every layer of the retina

Function
Can be activated to reactive microglia with phagocytic and antigen presenting functions.

Blood Ocular Barrier

General
Essential for visual function

Consists of
- Blood–aqueous barrier
  - A barrier formed by tight junctions in:
    - The nonpigmented ciliary epithelium of the ciliary body
    - The vascular endothelium of the vessels in iris

- Blood–retinal barrier
  - ◦ A barrier that regulates ion, protein, and water transport into and out of the retina.
  - ◦ Formed by tight junctions in:
    - ▪ The vascular endothelium of the retinal capillary network
    - ▪ The retinal pigment epithelium

Function

Regulate the exchange of solutes to keep the intraocular fluid composition constant.

Specialized Areas of the Retina

Consists of
- Macula lutea
- Fovea centralis
- Optic disc

Macula lutea

Structure
- ⊘ 5.5 mm.
- Area surrounding the fovea centralis.
- All layers of the retina are present.
- Contains abundant carotenoids (part of the visual pigment) → yellow (lutea) color.

Fovea centralis

General (Fig. 28.3)
- ⊘ 1.5 mm.
- A shallow depression, located in the center of the macula lutea

Structure
- Only cone cells are represented centrally → precise visual acuity.
- Bipolar and ganglion cells are located at the periphery.
- Blood vessels and nerve fibers diverge away from the center to not cover this area.

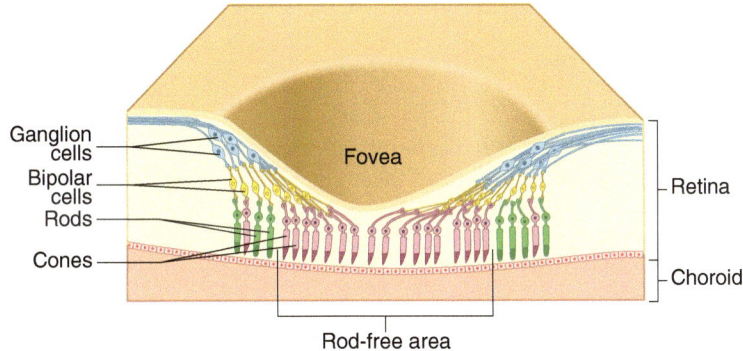

Fig. 28.3 The organization of the layers in the fovea centralis

Optic disc (Blind spot, Optic papilla)

General
- Area where the optic nerve leaves the retina and the central retinal artery enters the eyeball.
- Located posteriorly in the eyeball.
- A blind spot in the visual field due to lack of photoreceptor cells.

Blood Vessels of the Retina

General (Table 28.12)
- Two arterial circulations:
  - External circulation: Supplied by the ophthalmic artery
  - Internal circulation: Supplied by the central retinal artery
- One central retinal vein, which follows the central retinal artery

Table 28.12 The retinal blood supply

	Nutrition of layers in retina	Location of the blood vessels	Source
External circulation	Layers 1–5	In the third layer of the choroid	The ophthalmic artery
Internal circulation	Layers 6–10	In the ninth layer of the retina, giving off small branches that reach the sixth layer of the retina	The central retinal artery, an end artery from the ophthalmic artery

Optic Nerve

General
- The optic nerve, also referred to as cranial nerve II, is a paired nerve.
- The optic nerve is an extension of the brain and surrounded by the three meninges.

Structure
Divided into two parts:
- Intraocular part:
  - ○ Unmyelinated nerve fibers (ganglions cell axons)
  - ○ Astrocytes
- Extraocular part:
  - ○ Nerve fibers penetrate the sclera at the lamina cribrosa.
  - ○ The nerve fibers become myelinated by oligodendrocytes, at the lamina cribrosa.

Refractive Media of the Eye

General
The refractive media of the eye that bend and refract the incoming light → focus light on the fovea centralis of the retina.

Consists of
- Cornea (page 606)
- Aqueous humor (page 616)
- Lens
- Vitreous body

LENS

General
- The lens continues to grow throughout life → gradual loss of elasticity and the ability to accommodate.
- Attached to the ciliary body by the suspensory ligament of the lens (ciliary zonula fibers).

Structure
- Biconvex, transparent structure.
- Avascular, nourished by diffusion from:
  - Aqueous humor
  - The vitreous body
- Thickness changes during accommodation.

Function
- Refraction of light
- Accommodation:
  - Contraction of the ciliary muscle → ciliary zonula fibers relax → reduces the tension on the lens → increases the convexity of the lens → increased refraction of the light (accommodation)

Consists of (Fig. 28.4)
- Lens capsule:
  - A thick basal lamina.
  - Mainly composed of collagen type IV.
  - Synthesized by the lens epithelium.
- Lens epithelium:
  - The subcapsular lens epithelial cells located on the internal anterior surface of the lens.
  - The lens epithelial cells serve as progenitors for new lens fiber cells:
    1. The cells located near the equator of the lens increase in size.
    2. Differentiate into lens fiber cells.
    3. The lens fiber cells are pushed towards the core of the lens as they elongate.
- Lens fiber cells:
  - Form the bulk of the lens.
  - Derived from the subcapsular epithelial cells.
  - Formed continuously → the size of the lens continues to increase throughout life.

Light Microscopy
- Lens capsule:
  - Acellular, homogeneous layer
- Subcapsular epithelium:
  - A simple cuboidal epithelium
- Lens fiber cells:
  - Elongated cells.
  - Lose the nucleus as they mature and move towards the core of the lens.

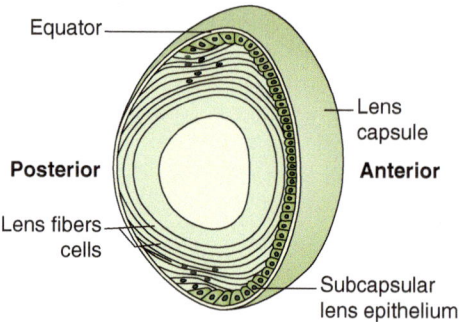

Fig. 28.4 The lens. The subcapsular lens epithelial cells are only located on anterior surface and are progenitors for the lens fiber cells

VITREOUS BODY

Structure
- Transparent structure that occupies the main part of the eyeball
- Loosely attached to surrounding structures
- Gel-like in the periphery, liquefied in the core
- Avascular, nourished through diffusion from the surroundings

Function
- Refraction of light
- Mechanical support of the eyeball structures by exerting pressure

Consists of
- Water (99 %)
- Hyaluronan
- Collagen fibers
- Hyalocytes:
  - Few
  - Responsible for the production of hyaluronan and collagen fibers

Accessory Structures of the Eye

Consists of
- Eyelid
- Conjunctiva
- Lacrimal apparatus
- Extrinsic skeletal muscles (not described)

EYELID (PALPEBRA)

General
Paired, moveable skinfolds covering the eyeball

Function
- Protection of the eyeball
- Regulation of the amount of light reaching the eye
- Distribution of the tear film across the surface of the eye
  - Achieved during blinking
  - Important for protection of the eyeball

Divided into
- Superior eyelid
  - The largest
- Inferior eyelid
  - The smallest

Consists of
- Skin with eyelashes
- Subcutaneous tissue
- Orbicularis oculi muscle (palpebral portion):
  - Skeletal (voluntary) muscle that closes the eyelid
- Fibrous layer:
  - Tarsal plate
  - Orbital septum
- Conjunctiva (palpebral portion)

The Eyelashes

Structure
- Short, terminal hairs that emerge from the anterior edge of the eyelid margin
- Organized in double or triple rows.
- Hair follicles of the eyelashes are associated with:
  - Glands of Zeis: sebaceous glands
  - Glands of Moll: modified apocrine sweat glands

Tarsal Plate and the Orbital Septum

General
- The tarsal plate and the orbital septum are continuous.
- Constitute the fibrous core in the eyelid.

Structure
- The superior and inferior tarsal plates continue in the orbital septum that inserts on the orbital rim.
- The orbital septum separates the orbital tissue from the eyelid tissue.
- The superior tarsal plate blends with the tendon of the levator palpebrae superioris muscle.

Light Microscopy
- Dense irregular and elastic connective tissue
- Tarsal muscle (superior and inferior):
  - Smooth muscle cells.
  - The superior muscle blends with the superior levator palpebrae muscle (skeletal muscle).
- The tarsal glands (Meibomian glands):
  - Sebaceous glands, embedded in the tarsal plates

The tarsal glands (Meibomian glands)

General
- Modified sebaceous glands
- Embedded in the tarsal plates

Structure
- Run vertically in separate, parallel strands.
- Approximately 30 in each eyelid.

Function
Secretion of an oily substance that:
- Prevents evaporation of the tear film as the oily layer covers the tear film
- Prevents tear leakage to the skin
- Forms a thin oily layer on the rims of the eyelids that enables the eyelids to close tightly

CONJUNCTIVA

Structure
- A thin, transparent mucous membrane that lines:
  - The inside of the eyelids:
    - Palpebral conjunctiva
  - The sclera:
    - Bulbar conjunctiva

- The junctions between the palpebral and bulbar parts are called:
  - Fornix conjunctiva superior
  - Fornix conjunctiva inferior

Function

Lubrication of the surface of the eyeball:
- Goblet cells of conjunctiva produce mucus, a component of the tear film

Light Microscopy
- Epithelium:
  - Nonkeratinized, stratified squamous to columnar epithelium
  - Numerous goblet cells
- Lamina propria:
  - Loose connective tissue

LACRIMAL APPARATUS

Consists of (Fig. 28.5)
- Lacrimal gland (paired)
- Lacrimal ducts (paired)
- Lacrimal canaliculi (paired)
- Lacrimal sac (paired)
- Nasolacrimal duct (paired)

Pathway of the tears

1. Lacrimal gland
   - Production of tears
   - Secretion through approximately 12 lacrimal ducts
2. Surface of the eyeball
3. Lacrimal canaliculi
4. Lacrimal sac
5. Nasolacrimal duct
6. Nasal cavity

Lacrimal Gland

General

- A tubuloacinar serous gland
  - ○ Divided into several separate lobules.
  - ○ Approximately 12 secretory ducts secrete into the fornix conjunctiva superior.
- Located in the upper lateral side of the orbital cavity

Function

Production of tears

Light Microscopy

- Serous end pieces with large lumina, lined with columnar glandular epithelial cells
- Myoepithelial cells located between columnar cells and basal lamina
- Basal lamina

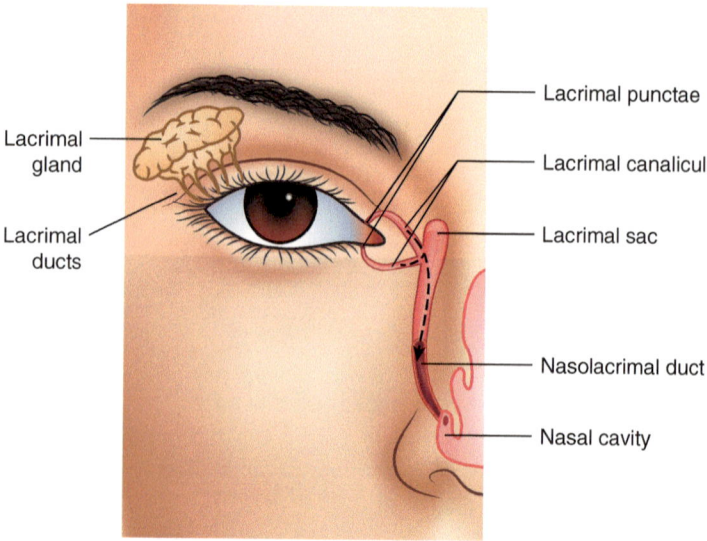

Fig. 28.5 The lacrimal apparatus

Lacrimal Canaliculi

General

- Form a duct from the eye to the lacrimal sac
- A superior and an inferior canaliculus

Structure
Lined with nonkeratinized stratified squamous epithelium

Function
Transportation of tears

Lacrimal Sac and Nasolacrimal Duct

General
Constitute the connection between the lacrimal canaliculi and the nasal cavity

Structure
- Lined with pseudostratified ciliated epithelium (respiratory epithelium)
- The nasolacrimal duct drains to the inferior nasal meatus under the inferior nasal conchae

Function
Transportation of tears

Guide to Practical Histology: The Eye

Anterior Part of the Eye

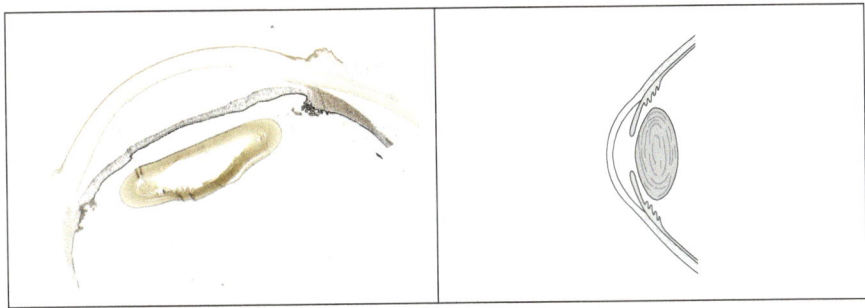

Left: photomicrograph of the anterior part of the eye. Magnification: macroscopic. Stain: osmium (Courtesy of professor Jørgen Tranum-Jensen, University of Copenhagen). *Right*: simplified illustration of the anterior part of the eye

Characteristics

Macroscopic:

- A convex part (cornea) on each side connected to a thinner and less convex part (sclera).
- Posterior to the cornea is a large biconvex homogenous structure (lens).
- Between the cornea and the lens are one or two thin highly pigmented stands (iris).

Posterior Part of the Eye

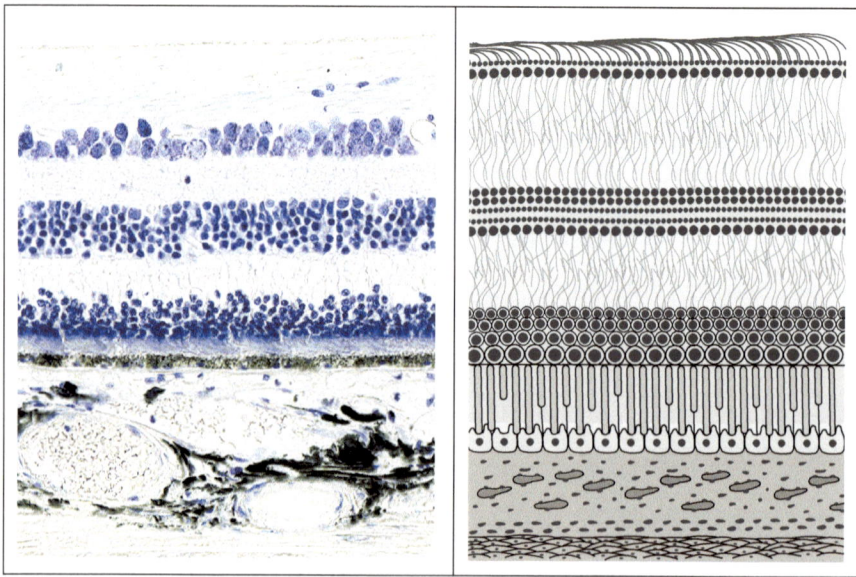

Left: photomicrograph of the posterior part of the eye. Magnification: low. Stain: HE (Courtesy of professor Jørgen Tranum-Jensen, University of Copenhagen). *Right*: simplified illustration of posterior part of the eye

Characteristics

Concave surface lined with retina:

- A thick, multilayered, highly ordered structure
- Three densely basophilic layers are seen:
    1. Outer nuclear layer (fourth layer of the retina)
    2. Inner nuclear layer (sixth layer of the retina)
    3. Ganglion cell layer (eighth layer of the retina)

Eyelid (Palpebra)

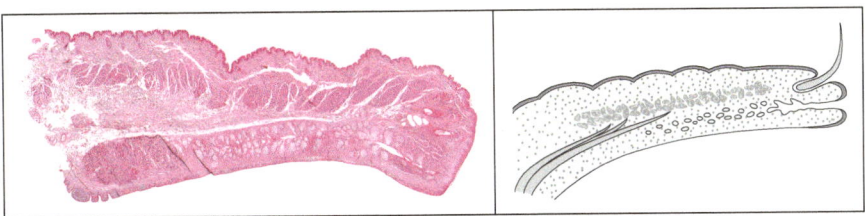

Left: photomicrograph of the palpebra. Magnification: low. Stain: HE (Courtesy of professor Jørgen Tranum-Jensen, University of Copenhagen). *Right*: simplified illustration of the palpebra

Characteristics

- Macroscopic:
  - Shape like a little finger
  - A pale central core
- Microscopic:
  - Two surfaces that meet at the apex:
    - Outer surface:
      - Keratinized stratified squamous epithelium
    - Inner surface:
      - Nonkeratinized stratified squamous to columnar epithelium, with multiple goblet cells.
      - Abundant sebaceous glands (Meibomian glands) are seen under the inner surface near the apex.

Can be mistaken for

Lips:
- Nonkeratinized stratified epithelium without goblet cells
- No sebaceous glands below surface with nonkeratinized epithelium

Lacrimal Gland

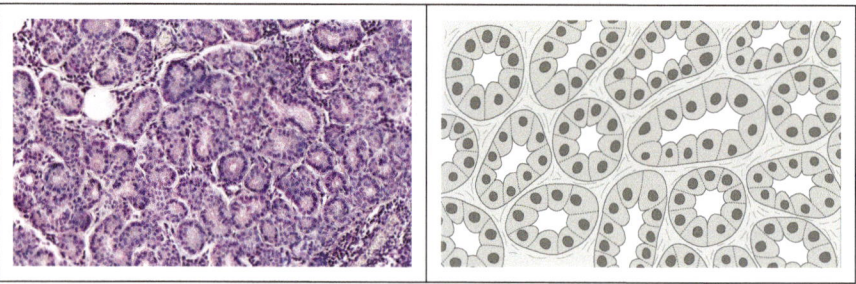

Left: photomicrograph of the lacrimal gland. Magnification: low. Stain: HE (Courtesy of professor Jørgen Tranum-Jensen, University of Copenhagen). *Right*: simplified illustration of the lacrimal gland

Characteristics
- Tubular and acinar serous end pieces (Chap. 6).
- The lumen of the end pieces is large and easily recognizable.

Can be mistaken for
- The parotid gland:
  - Have abundant fat infiltrations.
  - The lumen of the serous end pieces is smaller and not easily recognizable.
- Kidney:
  - Have renal corpuscles (with capillary coils)

References

3, 5, 8, 25, 26, 33, 34.

Chapter 29
The Ear

Contents

General

A paired auditive and balance organ located in the temporal bone of the cranium.

Consists of (Fig. 29.1)

- External ear
  - Auricle
  - External acoustic meatus
- Middle ear
  - Tympanic membrane
  - Tympanic cavity
  - Mastoid antrum and mastoid air cells
  - Auditory tube
- Internal ear
  - Bony labyrinth
  - Membranous labyrinth

© Springer International Publishing Switzerland 2017
A. Rehfeld et al., *Compendium of Histology*, DOI 10.1007/978-3-319-41873-5_29

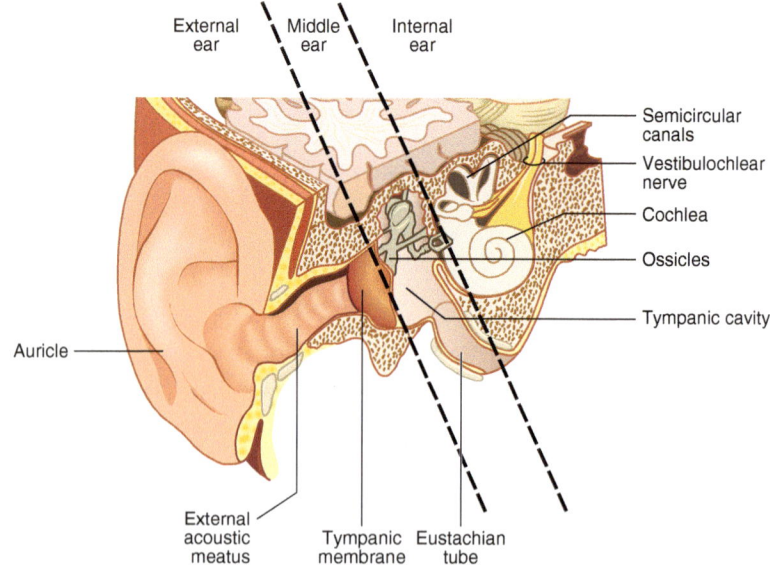

Fig. 29.1 The division of the ear

External Ear

General
The external portion of the ear

Divided into (Fig. 29.1)
- Auricle (pinna)
- External acoustic meatus (ear canal)

Function
- Collection of sound waves
- Direction of the sound waves towards the tympanic membrane
- Localization of the source of the sound
- Protection of the middle and internal ear from incoming particles

AURICLE

General
- Oval-shaped structure with complex folds.
- A core of elastic cartilage covered with skin.
- The skin and elastic cartilage continue in the external auditory meatus.

Light Microscopy
- Skin:
  - Keratinized stratified squamous epithelium
  - Thin layer of dermis with:
    - Hair follicles
    - Sebaceous glands
- Elastic cartilage
  - Constitute the core
  - Not present in the earlobe, where connective tissue forms the core

Function
- Collection of sound waves
- Direction of the sound waves towards the tympanic membrane
- Localization of the source of the sound

EXTERNAL ACOUSTIC MEATUS

General
- 3.5 cm long canal
- Limits:
  - External limit: the tragus, a part of the auricle
  - Internal limit: the tympanic membrane

Function
- Transportation of sound waves from the auricle to the tympanic membrane
- Protection and cleaning of the external acoustic meatus and the tympanic membrane by:
  - Terminal hairs
  - Cerumen (earwax)
    - Produced by the ceruminous glands and sebaceous glands

Divided into
- Cartilaginous part, $\frac{2}{5}$:
  - The lateral part, a continuation of the auricle
  - Covered with skin containing:
    - Terminal hairs

- Glands:
  - Ceruminous glands
  - Sebaceous glands
- Core of elastic cartilage
- Bony part, $\frac{2}{5}$:
  - The medial part
  - Located in the temporal bone
  - Covered with skin containing:
    - A few hairs and glands

Middle Ear

General (Fig. 29.1)
- An air-filled space in the temporal bone containing various structures.
- Lined primarily with a mucosal membrane.
- The auditory tube is lined with respiratory epithelium.

Function
Houses several structures that are important for the transduction of sound waves:
- Tympanic membrane
- Ossicles

Consists of
- Tympanic membrane
- Tympanic cavity
- Mastoid antrum and mastoid air cells
- Auditory tube (Eustachian tube)

Transduction of sound waves in the middle ear
1. Sound waves from the external ear reach the tympanic membrane.
2. Vibrations in the tympanic membrane.
3. Vibrations in ossicles.
4. Waves in the fluid within the internal ear.

TYMPANIC MEMBRANE

Structure
- ⊘10 mm, 0.1 mm thick
- Pellucid, conical-shaped membrane
- Separates the external acoustic meatus from the tympanic cavity
- The medial surface is connected to the malleus

Function
- Conversion of sound waves into mechanical vibrations
- Works together with the ossicles

Light Microscopy
See Table 29.1.

Table 29.1 The layers of the tympanic membrane

	Epidermal layer	Fibrous layer	Mucous membrane layer
Location	Forms the lateral surface	Forms the main, central part	Form the medial surface
Light microscopy	Stratified squamous epithelium	Loose connective tissue with collagen fibers arranged in two layers	• Simple squamous epithelium • Thin lamina propria
Other	Continuous with the epithelium of the acoustic meatus	Inconsistent in the flaccida area of the tympanic membrane	A continuation of the mucosal membrane that lines the tympanic cavity

TYMPANIC CAVITY

Structure
- An air-filled space in the petrous part of the temporal bone
- $15 \times 15 \times 4$ mm
- Communicates with:
  - Anteriorly: the nasal cavity
    - Through the Eustachian tube
  - Posteriorly: the mastoid air cells
    - Through the mastoid antrum
  - Laterally: the external ear
    - Through the tympanic membrane
  - Medially: the internal ear
    - Through:
      - The oval (vestibular) window
      - The round (cochlear) window

Consists of

The tympanic cavity houses several structures:

- Ossicles
- Ligaments
  - Associated with the ossicles
- Chorda tympani
  - A nerve branch from the facial nerve (cranial nerve VII)
  - Carries the parasympatic innervation to the submandibular and sublingual gland, and taste from the anterior 2/3 of the tongue
- Skeletal muscles:
  - Tensor tympani muscle
  - Stapedius muscle

Light Microscopy

Lined primarily by simple squamous or cuboidal epithelium (mucosal membrane).

- Near the opening of the auditory tube, the epithelium changes to ciliated, pseudostratified columnar epithelium (respiratory epithelium).

Ossicles

General (Fig. 29.1)

- A chain of bones that connect the tympanic membrane with the oval window.
- Synovial joints connect the bones.

Structure

Composed of compact bone, except from stapes that is partly composed of hyaline cartilage

Function

- Conversion of sound waves into mechanical vibrations
- Works together with the tympanic membrane
- Amplification of the sound signal:
  - Increases the amplitude of the vibration from the tympanic membrane to the fluid within the internal ear
  - Works analogous to a lever system

Consists of

Three small bones:

- Malleus (hammer):
  - Connected to:
    - The tympanic membrane
    - The incus

- Incus (anvil)
  - Connected to:
    - The malleus
    - The stapes
- Stapes (stirrup):
  - Connected to:
    - The incus
    - The oval window

The skeletal muscles of the middle ear

General
Two small skeletal muscles located in the middle ear, associated with the ossicles

Function
Protection of the inner ear through the attenuation reflex:
- Loud sound → contraction of the muscles → the tympanic membrane and the ossicle chain get rigid → reduced transmission of the vibrations to the fluid within the internal ear

Divided into
- Tensor tympani muscle
  - Arises in relation to the Eustachian tube.
  - Inserts at the neck of malleus.
  - Contraction of the muscle increases tension of the tympanic membrane.
  - Innervation: a branch of the mandibular nerve from the trigeminal nerve (cranial nerve V).
- Stapedius muscle
  - Arises from the posterior wall in the tympanic cavity.
  - Inserts at the neck of stapes.
  - Contraction of the muscle dampens the movements of the stapes at the oval window.
  - Innervation: the stapedius nerve from the facial nerve (cranial nerve VII).

MASTOID ANTRUM AND MASTOID AIR CELLS

General
- Cavities that extend into the osseous mastoid process of the temporal bone.
- The mastoid antrum connects the mastoid air cells to the tympanic cavity.

Structure
- Various cavities of different sizes.
- Both the mastoid antrum and the mastoid air cells are covered with a mucosal membrane, continuous with the mucosal membrane of the tympanic cavity.

AUDITORY TUBE

General (Fig. 29.1)
- A 3.5 cm long tube.
- The lumen is normally collapsed, but opens during, e.g., swallowing.
- Connects the tympanic cavity with the nasopharynx.

Structure
- Posterolateral part:
  - $\frac{1}{3}$, closest to the tympanic cavity
  - Outer "skeleton" of bone
- Anteromedial part
  - $\frac{2}{3}$, closest to the nasopharynx
  - Outer "skeleton" of elastic cartilage

Function
Facilitates communication between the tympanic cavity and the nasopharynx
- Equalization of the air pressure between the tympanic cavity and the external environment
- Drainage of the middle ear, e.g., of fluid

Consists of
- Mucosal membrane, ciliated pseudostratified columnar epithelium
- Connective tissue
- Outer skeleton of either bone or elastic cartilage

Light Microscopy
- Ciliated pseudostratified columnar epithelium (respiratory epithelium).
- Goblet cells appear near the nasopharynx.
- Connective tissue containing:
  - Seromucous glands
  - Diffuse lymphoid tissue
- Outer border of either bone or elastic cartilage

Internal Ear

General (Table 29.2, Figs. 29.1 and 29.2)
- Located in the petrous part of the temporal bone
- Formed from two compartments:
  ○ The bony outer part (bony labyrinth)
  - - - - - - separated by perilymph - - - - - - -
  ○ The membranous central part (membranous labyrinth)

Consists of (Table 29.2)
Two functionally different systems
- Vestibular system (balance)
- Auditory system (hearing)

Divided into
Structurally different parts:
- The bony labyrinth
- The membranous labyrinth
  ○ Located inside the bony labyrinth
- Fluid-filled spaces
  ○ The perilymphatic space
    ▪ Located between the bony labyrinth and the membranous labyrinth
    ▪ Filled with perilymph
  ○ The endolymphatic space
    ▪ Located inside the membranous labyrinth
    ▪ Filled with endolymph
  ○ The corticolymphatic space
    ▪ Located within the tunnels of the organ of Corti
    ▪ Filled with corticolymph

Table 29.2 Nomenclature and relations of the bony and membranous labyrinth

	Vestibular system		Auditory system
Bony labyrinth	Semicircular canals	Vestibule	The cochlea
Membranous labyrinth	Semicircular ducts	Saccule Utricle	The cochlear duct (scala media)
Function	Balance sensory organ		Hearing sensory organ

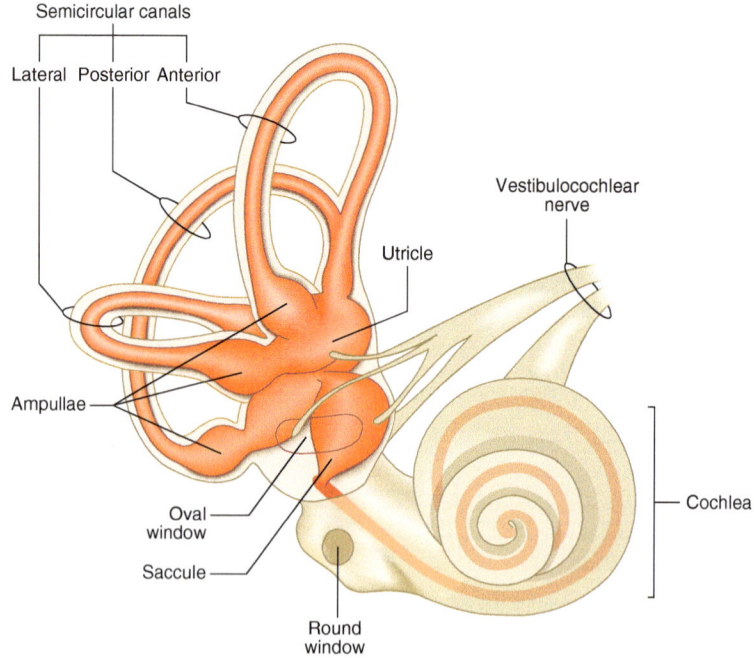

Fig. 29.2 The internal ear, showing the outer bony part and the central membranous part

BONY LABYRINTH

General (Fig. 29.2)
- Interconnected canals and cavities within the temporal bone.
- The membranous labyrinth lies within the bony labyrinth, surrounded by perilymph.

Consists of
- Semicircular canals
- Vestibule
- The cochlea

Semicircular Canals

General
- Three communicating bony canals, each forming three quarters of a circle
- Attached to the vestibule at both ends
  - One end of the anterior and posterior semicircular canal join in a common leg, so only five openings attach to the vestibule
- Oriented in three planes, at right angles to one another

Structure
At one of the ends of each semicircular canal is a dilatation, the ampulla.

Divided into
- Anterior semicircular canal
  - In the sagittal plane
- Lateral semicircular canal
  - In the horizontal plane
- Posterior semicircular canal
  - In the frontal plane

Vestibule

General
- Oval bony cavity
- Forms the center of the bony labyrinth
- The saccule and utricle of the membranous labyrinth are located within the vestibule
- Communicates:
  - Anteriorly with the cochlea
  - Posteriorly with the three semicircular canals

The Cochlea

General (Fig. 29.3)
- Bony tunnel that coils 2.5 turns → appearance of a snail shell
- Two openings, the oval and the round window:
  - Located at the basal end of the coil
  - Closed by membranes
  - Communicates with the tympanic cavity
- The apical end of the coil is called helicotrema

Structure
- Modiolus:
  - Central pillar in the cochlea
  - Spongy bone tissue
  - Contains the spiral ganglia
- Spiral lamina
  - Partial shelf of bone projecting form the modiolus.
  - The basilar membrane attaches to the spiral lamina, forming the floor in the cochlear duct (scala media).

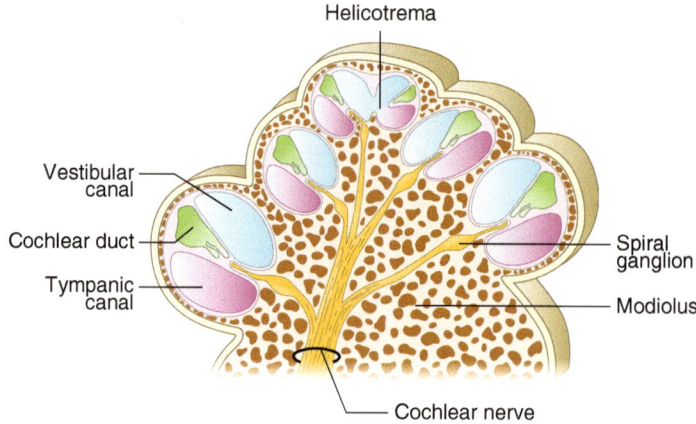

Fig. 29.3 Cochlear. The cochlear canal is divided into the vestibular canal, cochlear duct, and tympanic canal

Divided into (Fig. 29.3)

The membranous cochlear duct (scala media) runs within the bony cochlea and divides it into three parallel compartments:

- Vestibular canal (scala vestibuli)
  - Contains perilymph
  - Fuses with the tympanic canal at the helicotrema
- Cochlear duct (scala media)
  - Contains endolymph
- Tympanic canal (scala tympani)
  - Contains perilymph
  - Fuses with the vestibular canal at the helicotrema

MEMBRANOUS LABYRINTH

General

- Several communicating membranous sacs and ducts
- Suspended in perilymph within the bony labyrinth
- Contains endolymph

Consists of

- Epithelium
- Connective tissue

Divided into
- The vestibular system
  - Semicircular ducts
  - Utricle
  - Saccule
- The cochlear system
  - Cochlear duct (scala media)

Semicircular Ducts

General
- Located within their respective bony semicircular canals.
- Connect to the utricle through five holes, since one end of the anterior and posterior canal joins in a common leg.
- The ampulla is a dilatation in one end of each duct.
  - Contains the receptor epithelium, in the crista ampullaris

Function
Role in the vestibular (balance) system

Crista ampullaris
General
- Contains the sensory receptors for angular accelerations of the head
- Projects into the lumen of the semicircular canals

Function
Registration of angular acceleration:
1. During rotational movement of the head, the bony semicircular canals move.
2. The endolymph does not move instantly due to inertia.
3. The difference in movement between the endolymph and the crista ampullaris of the semicircular canals leads to movement of the cupula.
4. The movement of the cupula leads to deflection of the stereocilia, which generate nerve impulses (mechanoelectric transduction).

Consists of (Tables 29.4 and 29.8)
- An epithelial ridge
  - Located in the wall of the ampulla of the membranous semicircular canals
  - Consists of cells with the same histology as in the macule of the utricle and saccule:
    - Hair cells
      - Two types:
        - Type I
        - Type II
      - With stereocilia
    - Supporting cells
- The cupula
  - Attached to the luminal surface of the epithelium
  - A gelatinous mass that projects into the lumen of the semicircular canals
  - Surrounded by endolymph

Light Microscopy
See Table 29.4.

Saccule and Utricle

General
- Also referred to as the otolith organs due to the otolithic membrane
- Part of the vestibular (balance) system
- Communicate with the rest of the membranous labyrinth

Function
See Table 29.3.

Macula of the saccule and utricle

General
- Contain the sensory receptors for linear accelerations.
- A macula projects into the lumen of the utricle and the saccule.

Function
Reception of linear acceleration:
- During linear accelerations, the stereocilia of the hair cells are deflected due to displacement of the otolithic membrane.
- The deflection of the stereocilia generates nerve impulses (mechanoelectric transduction).

Table 29.3 Characteristics of the two otolith organs, saccule and utricle

	Shape	Location	Communicate	Sensory organ	Stimulus	Function
Saccule	• The smallest of the two otolith organs • Round	The vestibule of the bony labyrinth	• Caudally with the ductus cochlearis through the canalis reunions • Posteriorly with the utricle through the ductus utriculosaccularis	Macula of the sacculi: • Horizontally orientated • In the medial wall of the saccule	Sensitive to vertical acceleration of endolymph	Translation of movement of endolymph into nerve impulses
Utricle	• The biggest of the two otolith organ • Irregular elongated shape	The vestibule of the bony labyrinth	• Posteriorly with the semicircular ducts • Anteriorly with the saccule through ductus utriculosaccularis	Macula of the utricle: • Vertically oriented • In the lateral wall of the utricle	Sensitive to horizontal acceleration of endolymph	Translation of movement in endolymph into nerve impulses

Consists of (Tables 29.4 and 29.8)
- An epithelium ridge
  - Located in the wall of the saccule and utricle
  - Consists of cells with the same histology as in the crista ampullaris
    - Hair cells
      - Two types
        - Type I
        - Type II
      - With stereocilia
    - Supporting cells
- Otolithic membrane
  - Attached to the luminal surface of epithelium.
  - A gelatinous mass that projects into the lumen of the utricle and the saccule
  - Surrounded by endolymph.
  - The outer surface contains otoliths, structures made of calcium carbonate and protein.

Light Microscopy
See Table 29.4.

Table 29.4 The hair cells and supporting cells of the vestibular system

	Hair cell, type I	Hair cell, type II	Supporting cells
Location	• Crista ampullaris • Macula of the saccule and utricle	• Crista ampullaris • Macula of the saccule and utricle	• Crista ampullaris • Macula of the saccule and utricle
Shape	Flask shape	Cylindrical	Cylindrical
Nucleus	• Round • Basal	• Round • Central	• Round • Basal
Apical specialization	• Few stereocilia • One kinocilium	• Many stereocilia • One kinocilium	None
Initiation of action potential	Mechanically gated ion canals: • Bending of stereocilia → action potential	Mechanically gated ion canals: • Bending of stereocilia → action potential	None

Innervation	• Afferent:
	  ○ A single nerve fiber surrounds most of the hair cell
	• Efferent:
	  ○ A few nerve fibers form synapses with the afferent nerve fiber
	  ○ No synapses are formed directly with the hair cell
		• Afferent:
		  ○ Hair cell forms synapses with several nerve fibers
		• Efferent:
		  ○ Several nerve fibers form synapses directly with the hair cell
			None

Function	Mechanoelectric transduction	Mechanoelectric transduction	Mechanical support of the hair cells

The Cochlear Duct (Scala Media)

General
- Membranous canal that follows the coils of the bony cochlea
- Runs between the vestibular canal (superiorly) and the tympanic canal (inferiorly)
- Seen as a triangular space in a transverse section
- Houses:
  - The receptor organ of hearing, the organ of Corti
  - The production site of endolymph, stria vascularis

Consists of (Fig. 29.4)
- Upper wall
  - Separates the cochlear duct from the vestibular canal
  - Called Reissner's membrane (Vestibular membrane)

- Floor
  - ○ Separates the cochlear duct from the tympanic canal
  - ○ Consist of:
    - ▪ The basilar membrane
      - ○ The organ of Corti rests on the membrane.
      - ○ Extend from the bony spiral lamina of the cochlea to the lateral wall.
      - ○ Contains collagen fibers that change shape from the basis to the apex of cochlea (Table 29.5).
- Lateral wall
  - ○ Consist of the spiral ligament
    - ▪ Not a "true" ligament but a part of the periost of the cochlea
    - ▪ Contains a luminal specialization, the stria vascularis
      - • A vascularized epithelium

Light Microscopy (Fig. 29.4)
- Reissner's membrane
  - ○ Two layers of simple squamous epithelium. The cells are arranged basis to basis.
  - ○ Separated by a shared basal lamina.
- Basilar membrane
  - ○ Collagen fibers
  - ○ Ground substance
- Lateral wall
  - ○ Periphery: connective tissue of the periost
  - ○ Luminal surface: vascularized epithelium

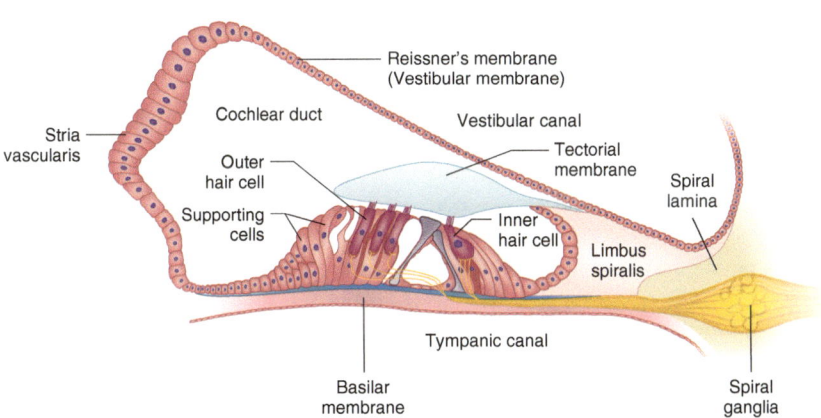

Fig. 29.4 The cochlear duct with the organ of Corti

Table 29.5 The basilar membrane: fibril characteristics in the basis and apex of the cochlear duct

	Basis	Apex
Length of collagen fibrils	40 μm	⟶►500 μm
⃠ of collagen fibrils	1.5 μm	⟶►0.5 μm
Stiffness of collagen fibrils	High stiffness ⟶►Low stiffness	
The optimal frequency (resonance) that induces oscillations of the basilar membrane	High frequency⟶►Low frequency 20.000 Hz	20 Hz

Stria vascularis

General
- A specialized epithelium on the luminal part of the spiral ligament
- Encloses a capillary network

Function
Production of the endolymph:
- Flows from the organ of Corti to the other parts of the membranous labyrinth

Consists of
- Stratified epithelium:
  - Marginal cells
  - Intermediate pigment-containing cells
  - Basal cells
- Capillary network
  - Enclosed within the epithelium

The Organ of Corti

General (Fig. 29.4, Table 29.8)
- The receptor organ for hearing
- Located within the cochlear duct
- Rests on the basilar membrane, the floor of the cochlear duct

Consists of (Tables 29.6 and 29.7)
- Sensory cells:
  - Inner hair cells
  - Outer hair cells
- Supporting cells:
  - Inner border cells
  - Inner phalangeal cell

- ○ Inner pillar cells
- ○ Outer pillar cells
- ○ Outer phalangeal cells
- ○ Outer border cells
- Tunnels with corticolymph:
  - ○ Outer tunnel
  - ○ Inner tunnel
  - ○ Tunnel of Corti
- Tectorial membrane

Sensory cells (hair cells) of the organ of corti

General (Table 29.6)
- Sensory cells of the auditive system
- Two types of cells, similar to the hair cells in the vestibular system:
  - ○ Inner hair cells
  - ○ Outer hair cells

Function (Table 29.8)
- Inner hair cells transduce vibrations (originating from sound waves) into nerve impulses (auditory signal).
- Outer hair cells modulate the auditory signal.

Light Microscopy
See Table 29.6.

Table 29.6 Overview of the hair cells of the organ of Corti

	Row(s)	Numbers of cells	Shape	Relation to supporting phalangeal cells	Nucleus	Apical specialization	Initiation of action potential	Function
Inner hair cells	1	3.000–3.500	Pear shaped	Completely surrounded by the inner phalangeal cell, except the apical part	• Round • Central	• Approximately 50 stereocilia • Not in direct contact with the tectorial membrane	Mechanically gated ion canals: • Bending of stereocilia → action potential	Transduction of sound waves into auditory signals
Outer hair cells	3–5	10.000–12.000	Cylindrical	Only the most basal part is surrounded of the outer phalangeal cells	• Round • Basal	• Approximately 100 stereocilia • Embedded within the tectorial membrane	Mechanically gated ion canals: • Bending of stereocilia → action potential	Modulation of the auditory signals

Table 29.7 Overview of the inner supporting cells of the organ of Corti

	Shape	Nucleus	Arranged in	Other
Inner border cells	Columnar	Central	Several rows	Increases in height towards the periphery
Inner phalangeal cell	Columnar	Basal	One row	• Form junctions with the inner hair cells • Inner hair cell is located in an invagination of the inner phalangeal cell
Inner pillar cells (rod)	Irregular	Basal	One row	• Broad apical and basal surface • Located on the bony spiral lamina
Outer pillar cells (rod)	Irregular	Basal	One row	• Broad apical and basal surface • Located on the basilar membrane
Outer phalangeal cells (Deiter's cells)	Columnar	Central	Several rows	• Form junctions with the outer hair cells and neighboring phalangeal cells • The basal part of the outer hair cell is located in an invagination of the outer phalangeal cell
Outer border cells (Hensen's cells)	Columnar	Central	Several rows	• 1–2 layers • Apical surface with numerous microvilli

Table 29.8 Sensory epithelium of the membranous labyrinth

	Location	Function	Hair cells nomenclature	Kinocilium	Gelatinous mass
Crista ampullaris	Semicircular ducts	Reception of angular acceleration	• Type I • Type II	+	The cupula
Macula of: • Utricle • Saccule	Utricle Saccule	Reception of linear acceleration	• Type I • Type II	+	The otolithic membrane
Organ of Corti	Cochlear duct (scala media)	Sense vibrations (originating from sound waves)	• Inner • Outer	–	The tectorial membrane

Supporting cells of the organ of corti

General (Table 29.7)

Mechanical and biochemical support of the hair cells

Structure

- Inner supporting cells:
  1. Inner border cells
  2. Inner phalangeal cell
  3. Inner pillar cells
  4. Outer pillar cells
  5. Outer phalangeal cells
  6. Outer border cells

- Outer supporting cells:
  - Not a part of the organ of Corti
  - Line a part of the luminal surface of the cochlear duct, the external spiral sulcus
  - 1–2 layers of cuboidal cells
    - Claudius cells: located luminally, in relation to the endolymph
    - Boettcher cells: located profound to the Claudius cells

Function
- Mechanical support of the hair cells
  - For example, regulation of the environment that surrounds the hair cells
- Recycling of K^+ from the organ of Corti to the stria vascularis
  - As endolymph has a high K^+ concentration

Light Microscopy
See Table 29.7.

Tunnels of the organ of corti

General
Intercellular spaces
- Filled with corticolymph which is similar to extracellular fluid
- Communicate with each other, but not with the endolymphatic or perilymphatic spaces

Function
The corticolymph is assumed to facilitate the function of the hair cells.

Divided into
- Outer tunnel
  - Between the outer border cells and the outer phalangeal cells
- Inner tunnel
  - Between the outer pillar cells and the complex of the outer hair cells and outer phalangeal cells
- Tunnel of Corti
  - Between the inner and outer pillar cells

Tectorial membrane

General
- A gelatinous acellular structure.
- Attached to the spiral limbus (Fig. 29.4)
- Extends over the cells of the organ of Corti.
- The stereocilia of the outer hair cells are embedded within the membrane.

Consists of
- Ground substance
- Collagen fibers

Function
Stimulation of the outer hair cells of the organ of Corti

Auditory transduction

General
1. Sound waves (vibrations) reach the inner ear from the surroundings:
    I. From the external ear
    II. The tympanic membrane
    III. The ossicles
    IV. The oval window membrane
2. Vibrations travel in the perilymph of the vestibular and tympanic canals
3. Vibrations of the basilar membrane → vibrations in the endolymph
4. Stereocilia of the hair cells bend:
    - Outer hair cells: stereocilia are bent due to their embedding in the tectorial membrane
    - Inner hair cells: stereocilia are bent due to vibrations in the endolymph
5. Mechanically gated ion canals open
6. Depolarization of the hair cells initiates nerve impulses in afferent nerve fibers to the brain

Innervation of the internal ear

General
- The vestibulocochlear nerve (cranial nerve VII)
- Runs in the internal acoustic meatus, a bony canal in the petrous part of the temporal bone

Function
Leads impulses from the internal ear to the temporal lobe

Divided into
- The vestibular nerve
    ○ Associated with the vestibular (balance) system.
    ○ The vestibular ganglion is located in the internal acoustic meatus.
    ○ Transports impulses from the sensory receptors in the vestibular system:
        ▪ The crista ampullaris of semicircular canals
        ▪ The macula of utricle and saccule
    ○ The nerve terminates in the vestibular nuclei located in the brain stem.

- The cochlear nerve
  - ○ Associated with the auditory (hearing) system.
  - ○ The spiral ganglion is located in the modiolus of the cochlea.
  - ○ The nerve fibers form synapses with the hair cells:
    - ▪ 90% with inner hair cells
    - ▪ 10% with outer hair cells
  - ○ The nerve terminates in:
    - ▪ The cochlear nuclei located in the brain stem
    - ▪ The auditory cortex located in the cerebral temporal lope

Guide to Practical Histology: The Ear

Auricle

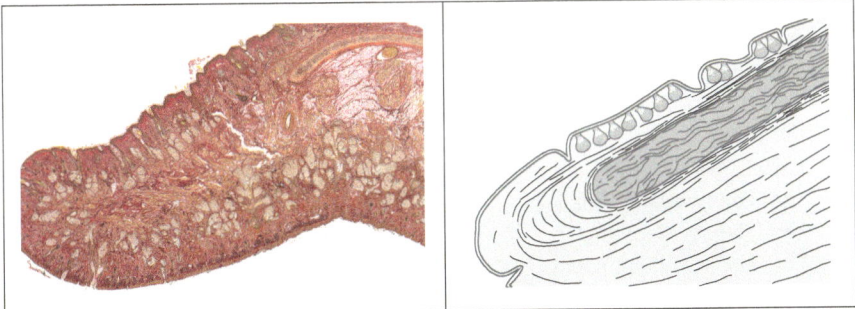

Left: photomicrograph of the auricle. Magnification: low. Stain: orcein. Courtesy of professor Jørgen Tranum-Jensen, University of Copenhagen. *Right*: simplified illustration of the auricle

Characteristics
- A core of elastic cartilage and dense connective tissue
- Covered with keratinized stratified squamous epithelium
- Contains multiple sebaceous glands below the epithelium

Can be mistaken for
Epiglottis:
- Covered with nonkeratinized stratified squamous epithelium on one surface and pseudostratified epithelium with cilia and scattered goblet cells on the other surface
- Contains exocrine seromucous glands surrounding the elastic cartilage, but no sebaceous glands

Cochlea

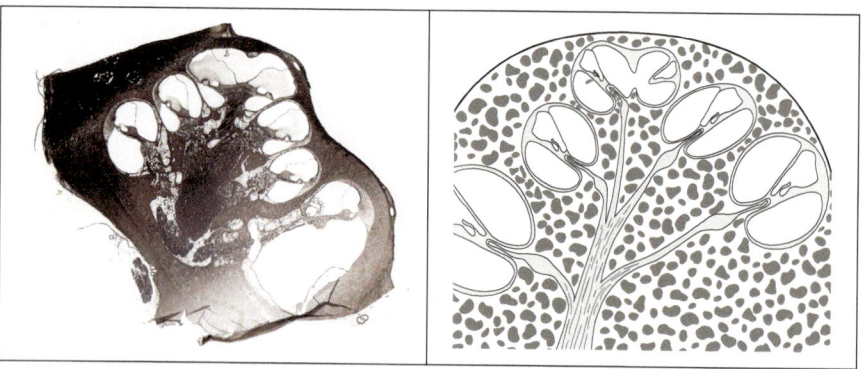

Left: photomicrograph of the cochlea. Magnification: macroscopic. Stain: osmium tetroxide. Courtesy of Professor Jørgen Tranum-Jensen, University of Copenhagen. *Right*: simplified illustration of the cochlea

Characteristics
- Macroscopic:
  - Resembles a snail shell cut in half
- Microscopic:
  - Each "turn" of the snail shell houses three compartments:
    - The tympanic canal
    - The cochlear duct
    - The vestibular canal

References

5, 25, 33, 34, 35.

References

1. Alberts B, Bray D, Hopkin K, Johnson AD, Lewis J, Raff M, Roberts K, Walter P. Essential cell biology. 4th ed. New York: Garland Science; 2013.
2. Baumann N, Pham-Dinh D. Biology of oligodendrocyte and myelin in the mammalian central nervous system. Physiol Rev. 2001;81:871–927.
3. Borges-Giampani AS, Giampani Jr J. Anatomy of ciliary body, ciliary processes, anterior chamber angle and collector vessels. In: Rumelt S, editor. Glaucoma – basic and clinical aspects. Rijeka: InTech; 2013.
4. Borlotti A, Park C, Parker KH, Khir AW. Reservoir and reservoir-less pressure effects on arterial waves in the canine aorta. J Hypertens. 2015;33:564–74.
5. Brüel A, Christensen EI, Geneser F, Tranum-Jensen J, Qvortrup K. Genesers Histologi. 1st ed. Copenhagen: Munksgaard; 2012.
6. Carlsen F, Behse F. Three dimensional analysis of Schwann cells associated with unmyelinated nerve fibres in human sural nerve. J Anat. 1980;130:545–57.
7. Clarke B. Normal bone anatomy and physiology. Clin J Am Soc Nephrol. 2008;3(Suppl 3): S131–9.
8. Cunha-Vaz JG. The blood-ocular barriers: past, present, and future. Doc Ophthalmol. 1997;93:149–57.
9. Fazan VPS, Borges CT, Da Silva JH, Caetano AG, Filho OAR. Superficial palmar arch: an arterial diameter study. J Anat. 2004;204:307–11.
10. Fix JD. BRS Neuroanatomy. 4th ed. Philadelphia: Lippincott Williams & Wilkins; 2008.
11. Földi M, Földi E, editors. Földi's textbook of lymphology. 3rd ed. München: Urban & Fischer; 2012.
12. Friesema ECH, Jansen J, Jachtenberg J-W, Visser WE, Kester MHA, Visser TJ. Effective cellular uptake and efflux of thyroid hormone by human monocarboxylate transporter 10. Mol Endocrinol. 2008;22:1357–69.
13. Hai CM, Murphy RA. Cross-bridge phosphorylation and regulation of latch state in smooth muscle. Am J Physiol. 1988;254:C99–106.
14. Hall CN, Reynell C, Gesslein B, Hamilton NB, Mishra A, Sutherland BA, et al. Capillary pericytes regulate cerebral blood flow in health and disease. Nature. 2014;508:55–60.
15. Hansen NE, Haunsø S, Schaffalitzky De Muckadell OB (editors). Medicinsk Kompendium, Bind 2. 16th ed. Copenhagen: Nyt Nordisk Forlag Arnold Busck; 2004.
16. Helander HF, Fändriks L. Surface area of the digestive tract – revisited. Scand J Gastroenterol. 2014;49:681–9.
17. Jelkmann W. Regulation of erythropoietin production. J Physiol. 2011;589:1251–8.

© Springer International Publishing Switzerland 2017

A. Rehfeld et al., *Compendium of Histology*, DOI 10.1007/978-3-319-41873-5

18. Johanson CE, Duncan JA, Klinge PM, Brinker T, Stopa EG, Silverberg GD. Multiplicity of cerebrospinal fluid functions: new challenges in health and disease. Cerebrospinal Fluid Res. 2008;5:10.

19. Kumar R, Ghyselinck N, Ishiguro K, Watanabe Y, Kouznetsova A, Höög C, et al. MEI4 – a central player in the regulation of meiotic DNA double-strand break formation in the mouse. J Cell Sci. 2015;128:1800–11.

20. Lee MG, Ohana E, Park HW, Yang D, Muallem S. Molecular mechanism of pancreatic and salivary gland fluid and HCO3 secretion. Physiol Rev. 2012;92:39–74.

21. Linke WA, Krüger M. The giant protein titin as an integrator of myocyte signaling pathways. Physiology (Bethesda). 2010;25:186–98.

22. Louveau A, Smirnov I, Keyes TJ, Eccles JD, Rouhani SJ, Peske JD, et al. Structural and functional features of central nervous system lymphatic vessels. Nature. 2015;523:337–41.

23. Lozupone E, Favia A. The structure of the trabeculae of cancellous bone. 2. Long bones and mastoid. Calcif. Tissue Int. 1990;46:367–72.

24. McMahill MS, Sham CW, Bishop DK. Synthesis-dependent strand annealing in meiosis. PLoS Biol. 2007;5:e299.

25. Mescher AL. Junqueira's basic histology, text and atlas. 13th ed. New York: McGraw-Hill/Medical; 2013.

26. Van Buskirk EM. The anatomy of the limbus. Eye (Lond). 1989;3(Pt 2):101–8.

27. Miller JD, Pegelow DF, Jacques AJ, Dempsey JA. Skeletal muscle pump versus respiratory muscle pump: modulation of venous return from the locomotor limb in humans. J Physiol. 2005;563:925–43.

28. Ochei J, Kolhatkar A. Medical laboratory science. Theory and practice. 1st ed. New Delhi: Tata Mcgraw-Hill; 2000.

29. de Almeida PDV, Grégio AMT, Machado MAN, de Lima AAS, Azevedo LR. Saliva composition and functions: a comprehensive review. J Contemp Dent Pract. 2008;9:72–80.

30. Phillips MN, Jones GT, van Rij AM, Zhang M. Micro-venous valves in the superficial veins of the human lower limb. Clin Anat. 2004;17:55–60.

31. Putz R, Pabst R. Sobotta – Atlas of human anatomy. 13th ed. Philadelphia: Lippincott Williams & Wilkins; 2001.

32. Ralphs JR, Benjamin M. The joint capsule: structure, composition, ageing and disease. J Anat. 1994;184(Pt 3):503–9.

33. Rehfeld A, Nylander M, Karnov KKS. Histologikompendium. 2nd ed. Copenhagen: Munksgaard; 2013.

34. Ross MH, Pawlina W. Histology: a text and atlas: with correlated cell and molecular biology. 7th ed. Philadelphia: Wolter Kluwer; 2015.

35. Rostgaard J, Tranum-Jensen J, Qvortrup K, Holm-Nielsen P. Hovedets, halsens og de indre organers anatomi. 10th ed. Copenhagen: Munksgaard; 2006.

36. Rozenberg G. Microscopic haematology: a practical guide for the laboratory. 3rd ed. London: Churchill Livingstone; 2011.

37. Sasaki H, Matsui Y. Epigenetic events in mammalian germ-cell development: reprogramming and beyond. Nat Rev Genet. 2008;9:129–40.

38. Shima H, Ohno K, Michi K, Egawa K, Takiguchi R. An anatomical study on the forearm vascular system. J Craniomaxillofac Surg. 1996;24:293–9.

39. Snider J, Lin F, Zahedi N, Rodionov V, Yu CC, Gross SP. Intracellular actin-based transport: how far you go depends on how often you switch. Proc Natl Acad Sci U S A. 2004;101:13204–9.

40. Sofroniew MV. Astrocyte barriers to neurotoxic inflammation. Nat Rev Neurosci. 2015;16:249–63.

41. Tabibian JH, Masyuk AI, Masyuk TV, O'Hara SP, LaRusso NF. Physiology of cholangiocytes. Compr Physiol. 2013;3:541–65.

42. Valecchi D, Bacci D, Gulisano M, Sgambati E, Sibilio M, Lipomas M, et al. Assessment of internal diameters of abdominal and femoral blood vessels in 250 living subjects using color Doppler ultrasonography. Ital J Anat Embryol. 2010;115:180–4.
43. Voeltz GK, Rolls MM, Rapoport TA. Structural organization of the endoplasmic reticulum. EMBO Rep. 2002;3:944–50.
44. Witherspoon JW, Smirnova IV, McIff TE. Neuroanatomical distribution of mechanoreceptors in the human cadaveric shoulder capsule and labrum. J Anat. 2014;225:337–45.
45. Young B, O'Dowd G, Woodford P. Wheater's functional histology: a text and colour atlas. 6th ed. London: Churchill Livingstone; 2014.

Index